Saurav Mallik, Zubair Rahaman, Soumita Seth, Anjan Bandyopadhyay, Sujata Swain, Somenath Chakraborty (Eds.)
Drug Discovery and Telemedicine

Also of Interest

Machine Learning in Healthcare
Data-Driven Decisions, Predictive Modelling, Personalized Medicine
Edited by Saurav Mallik, Sandeep Kumar Mathivanan, S. K. B. Sangeetha,
Ben Othman Soufiene, Saravanan Srinivasan, Aimin Li, 2025
ISBN 978-3-11-154107-5, e-ISBN (PDF) 978-3-11-154123-5

The Mathematics of Machine Learning
Maria Han Veiga, François Gaston Ged, 2024
ISBN 978-3-11-128847-5, e-ISBN (PDF) 978-3-11-128899-4

Artificial Intelligence for Medicine
People, Society, Pharmaceuticals, and Medical Materials
Yoshiki Oshida, 2021
ISBN 978-3-11-071779-2, e-ISBN (PDF) 978-3-11-071785-3

Smart Computing Applications
Edited by Prasenjit Chatterjee, Dilbagh Panchal, Dragan Pamucar,
Sharfaraz Ashemkhani Zolfani
ISSN 2700-6239, e-ISSN 2700-6247

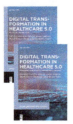
Digital Transformation in Healthcare 5.0
Edited by Rishabha Malviya, Sonali Sundram, Rajesh Kumar Dhanaraj,
Seifedine Kadry, 2024
Volume 1: IoT, AI and Digital Twin
ISBN 978-3-11-132646-7, e-ISBN (PDF) 978-3-11-132785-3
Volume 2: Metaverse, Nanorobots and Machine Learning
ISBN 978-3-11-139738-2, e-ISBN (PDF) 978-3-11-139854-9

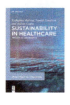
Sustainability in Healthcare
mHealth, AI, and Robotics
Rishabha Malviya, Sonali Sundram, Babita Gupta, 2024
ISBN 978-3-11-143635-7, e-ISBN (PDF) 978-3-11-143643-2

Drug Discovery and Telemedicine

—

Through Artificial Intelligence, Computer Vision, and IoT

Edited by
Saurav Mallik, Zubair Rahaman, Soumita Seth,
Anjan Bandyopadhyay, Sujata Swain, Somenath Chakraborty

DE GRUYTER

Editors

Dr. Saurav Mallik
University of Arizona
Deptartment of Pharmacology and Toxicology
USA
smallik@arizona.edu

Dr. Zubair Rahaman
VITAS Healthcare
USA
Zubair.Rahaman@vitas.com

Dr. Soumita Seth
Future Institute of Engineering and Management
Department of Computer Science & Engineering
India
soumita.seth@teamfuture.in

Dr. Anjan Bandyopadhyay
Kalinga Institute of Industrial Technolology
Department of Computer Science and Engineering
India
anjan.bandyopadhyayfcs@kiit.ac.in

Dr. Sujata Swain
Kalinga Institute of Industrial Technolology
Department of Computer Science and Engineering
India
sujata.swainfcs@kiit.ac.in

Dr. Somenath Chakraborty
West Virginia Institute of Technology
Department of Computer Science and Information Systems
USA
somenath.chakraborty@mail.wvu.edu

ISBN 978-3-11-150398-1
e-ISBN (PDF) 978-3-11-150466-7
e-ISBN (EPUB) 978-3-11-150476-6

Library of Congress Control Number: 2025935629

Bibliographic information published by the Deutsche Nationalbibliothek
The Deutsche Nationalbibliothek lists this publication in the Deutsche Nationalbibliografie; detailed bibliographic data are available on the Internet at http://dnb.dnb.de.

© 2025 Walter de Gruyter GmbH, Berlin/Boston, Genthiner Straße 13, 10785 Berlin
Cover image: Just_Super / iStock / Getty Images Plus
Typesetting: VTeX UAB, Lithuania

www.degruyter.com
Questions about General Product Safety Regulation:
productsafety@degruyterbrill.com

Contents

List of Contributing Authors —— VII

Songita Sett, Soumita Seth, and Saurav Mallik
1   Introduction: fundamentals of drug discovery, telemedicine, artificial intelligence, computer vision, and IoT —— 1

Siddhartha Roy
2   Machine learning transformations in drug discovery: a paradigm shift in development strategies —— 11

Debmitra Ghosh, Dharmpal Singh, and Biswarup Neogi
3   Explainable AI approaches in drug classification from biomarkers of epileptic seizure —— 27

Prateek Kumar, Vishal Pradhan, Vivek Panwar, and Anjan Bandyopadhyay
4   Harnessing predictive analytics and machine learning in personalized medicine: patient outcomes and public health strategies —— 41

Edeh Michael Onyema, Sharanya S, Karthikeyan S, Prabukavin B, and Deepak Arun Annamalai
5   A data-driven framework for future healthcare diagnosis through predictive analytics —— 59

Songita Sett, Soumita Seth, and Saurav Mallik
6   Revolutionizing home healthcare: telemedicine, predictive analytics, and AI-driven drug discovery —— 71

Saboor Uddin Ahmed, Preetam Suman, Akshara Makrariya, and Rabia Musheer Aziz
7   AI-driven insights: a machine learning approach to lung cancer diagnosis —— 91

Abrar Yaqoob, Navneet Kumar Verma, G. V. V. Jagannadha Rao, and Rabia Musheer Aziz
8   Efficient gene selection for breast cancer classification using Brownian Motion Search Algorithm and Support Vector Machine —— 109

Abrar Yaqoob, Navneet Kumar Verma, G. V. V. Jagannadha Rao, and Rabia Musheer Aziz
9   A hybrid feature gene selection approach by integrating variance filter, extremely randomized tree, and Cuckoo Search algorithm for cancer classification —— 127

Kingshuk Kirtania, Anogh Dalal, and Pawan Kumar Singh
10 HySleep_Net: a hybrid deep learning model for automatic sleep stage detection from polysomnographic signals —— 151

Debangshu Ghosh, Arundhuti Mukhopadhyay, and Radha Krishna Jana
11 Ambulance booking and tracking website —— 183

Amalendu Si
12 Entropy based emergency rescue location selection with uncertain travel time —— 207

Anomitro Das, Shayambhu Chaudhuri, Ashfaq Murshed, Rohini Basak, and Pawan Kumar Singh
13 Performance comparison of different deep learning ensemble models for sentiment classification of movie reviews —— 225

Aarya Vilas Karanjawane, Suresh Jagtap, Anupam Mukherjee, and Varsha Umesh Ghate
14 Elevating standards in homoeopathic medicine: chemometric standardization of medicinal plant for quality assurance —— 253

Varsha Umesh Ghate, Ajay G. Namdeo, Abhay Harsulkar, Anupam Mukherjee, Yashwant Chavan, Suresh Jagtap, Devasis Pradhan, and Mehdi Gheisari
15 Evaluation of genetic diversity in *Rauvolfia* species using Random Amplification of Polymorphic DNA (RAPD) technique —— 259

Index —— 269

List of Contributing Authors

Saboor Uddin Ahmed
School of Computing Science and Engineering
VIT Bhopal University
Kothrikalan
Sehore
Madhya Pradesh – 466114
India
E-mail: saboor.ahmed2021@vitbhopal.ac.in

Deepak Arun Annamalai
Saveetha School of Engineering
Saveetha Institute of Medical and Technical Sciences
Chennai
India
E-mail: deepakarun@saveetha.com

Rabia Musheer Aziz
Researcher Officer (Technical)
State Planning Institute (New Division)
Planning Department
Lucknow
Utter Pradesh 226001
India
E-mail: rabia.aziz2010@gmail.com

Anjan Bandyopadhyay
School of Computer Engineering
Kalinga Institute of Industrial Technology (KIIT-DU)
Bhubaneswar
Odisha
India, 751024
E-mail: anjan.bandyopadhyayfcs@kiit.ac.in

Rohini Basak
Department of Information Technology
Jadavpur University
Jadavpur University Salt Lake Campus, Plot No. 8,
Salt Lake Bypass, LB Block, Sector III, Salt Lake City
Kolkata 700106
West Bengal
India
E-mail: visitrohinihere@gmail.com

Shayambhu Chaudhuri
Department of Information Technology
Jadavpur University
Jadavpur University Salt Lake Campus, Plot No. 8,
Salt Lake Bypass, LB Block, Sector III, Salt Lake City
Kolkata 700106
West Bengal
India
E-mail: shayambhuchaudhuri7@gmail.com

Yashwant Chavan
R & D Department
geneOmbio Technologies Pvt Ltd
Vedant, Sr. No. 39/3, Yogi Park, Baner
Pune 411045
India
E-mail: yashvant.chavan@geneombiotechnologies.com

Anogh Dalal
Department of Information Technology
Jadavpur University
Jadavpur University Second Campus, Plot No. 8,
Salt Lake Bypass, LB Block, Sector III, Salt Lake City
Kolkata 700106
West Bengal
India
E-mail: anogh25@gmail.com

Anomitro Das
Department of Information Technology
Jadavpur University
Jadavpur University Salt Lake Campus, Plot No. 8,
Salt Lake Bypass, LB Block, Sector III, Salt Lake City
Kolkata 700106
West Bengal
India
E-mail: anomitro02@gmail.com

Varsha Umesh Ghate
Department of Homoeopathic Pharmacy
Bharati Vidyapeeth (Deemed to be University)
Homoeopathic Medical College & Post Graduate
Research Centre, Hospital
Pune 411043
India
E-mail: varshaghate29@gmail.com

Mehdi Gheisari
Department of Cognitive Computing
Institute of Computer Science and Engineering
Saveetha School of Engineering
Saveetha Institute of Medical and Technical Sciences
Chennai 602105
India
E-mail: mehdi.ghesari61@gmail.com

Debangshu Ghosh
Department of Computer Science and Engineering
JIS University
48, Shibtala Ghoshpara
Kolkata 700122
West Bengal
India
E-mail: shadebangshu155@gamil.com

Debmitra Ghosh
CSE/JIS University
36, B.M. Banerjee Road, Belghoria
Kolkata 700056
India
E-mail: debmitraghosh@jisuniversity.ac.in

Abhay Harsulkar
Department of Pharmaceutical Biotechnology
Bharati Vidyapeeth (Deemed to be University)
Poona College of Pharmacy
Pune 411038
India
E-mail: abhay.harsulkar@bharatividyapeeth.edu

Suresh Jagtap
Department of Herbal Medicine
Interactive Research School for Health
Affairs (IRSHA)
Bharati Vidyapeeth (Deemed to be University)
Pune 411043
India
E-mail: suresh.jagtap@bharatividyapeeth.edu

Radha Krishna Jana
Department of Computer Science and Engineering
JIS University
Kolkata
India
E-mail: radhakrishnajana@gmail.com

Aarya Vilas Karanjawane
Department of Homoeopathic Pharmacy
Bharati Vidyapeeth (Deemed to be University)
Homoeopathic Medical College & Post Graduate
Research Centre, Hospital
Pune 411043
India
E-mail: aarya.karanjawane@bharatividyapeeth.edu

Karthikeyan S
Department of Aerospace Engineering
BS Abdur Rahman Crescent Institute of Science and
Technology
Vandalur
India

Kingshuk Kirtania
Department of Information Technology
Jadavpur University
Jadavpur University Second Campus, Plot No. 8,
Salt Lake Bypass, LB Block, Sector III, Salt Lake City
Kolkata 700106
West Bengal
India
E-mail: bttb.kingshukk@gmail.com

Prateek Kumar
School of Applied Science
Kalinga Institute of Industrial Technology (KIIT-DU)
Bhubaneswar
Odisha
India, 751024

Akshara Makrariya
School of Advanced Sciences and Language
VIT Bhopal University
Kothrikalan
Sehore
Madhya Pradesh – 466114
India
E-mail: akshara.makrariya@vitbhopal.ac.in

Saurav Mallik
Department of Pharmacology and Toxicology
University of Arizona
Tucson, AZ 85721
USA
Department of Environmental Health
Harvard T. H. Chan School of Public Health

Boston, MA 02115
USA
E-mail: smallik@arizona.edu

Anupam Mukherjee
Department of Health and Family Welfare
West Bengal Homoeopathic Health Service
Government of West Bengal
Kolkata 700091
India
E-mail: anupam.dr.98@gmail.com

Arundhuti Mukhopadhyay
Department of Computer Science and Engineering
JIS University
Kolkata
India
E-mail: arnamukherjee4@gmail.com

Ashfaq Murshed
Department of Information Technology
Jadavpur University
Jadavpur University Salt Lake Campus, Plot No. 8, Salt Lake Bypass, LB Block, Sector III, Salt Lake City
Kolkata 700106
West Bengal
India
E-mail: ashfaqmurshed.2024@gmail.com

Ajay G. Namdeo
Department of Pharmaceutical Sciences
HNB Garhwal Central University
Srinagar 246174
Uttarakhand
India
E-mail: ajay.namdeo@bharatividyapeeth.edu

Biswarup Neogi
ECE
JISCE
36, B.M. Banerjee Road, Belghoria
Kolkata 700056
India

Edeh Michael Onyema
Department of Mathematics and Computer Science
Coal City University
Enugu

Nigeria
Adjunct Faculty, Saveetha School of Engineering
Saveetha Institute of Medical and Technical Sciences
Chennai 602105
India
E-mail: mikedreamcometrue@gmail.com

Vivek Panwar
School of Advanced Engineering
UPES
Dehradun
Uttarakhand
India, 248007

Prabukavin B
Department of Data Science and Business Systems
SRM Institute of Science and Technology
Kattankulathur
India
E-mail: ceaserkavin@gmail.com

Devasis Pradhan
Department of Electronics & Communication Engineering
Acharya Institute of Technology
Bangalore 560107
Karnataka
India
E-mail: devasispradhan@acharya.ac.in

Vishal Pradhan
School of Applied Science
Kalinga Institute of Industrial Technology (KIIT-DU)
Bhubaneswar
Odisha
India, 751024
E-mail: vishal.pradhanfma@kiit.ac.in

G. V. V. Jagannadha Rao
Associate Professor & Head
Department of Mathematics
Kalinga University
Naya Raipur 492001
India

Siddhartha Roy
Dept. of Computer Science and Engineering
(IoT, CS, BT)

UEM
5/10, Sevak Baidya Street
Kolkata 700029
West Bengal
India
E-mail: siddhartha_r24@yahoo.com

Soumita Seth
Department of Computer Science and Engineering
Future Institute of Engineering and Management
Narendrapur
Kolkata 700150
West Bengal
India
Department of Computer Science and Engineering
Aliah University
Kolkata 700160
West Bengal
India
E-mail: soumita.seth@teamfuture.in

Songita Sett
Department of Management and Business Administration in Business Analytics
Maulana Abul Kalam Azad University of Technology
Haringhata
Nadia 741249
West Bengal
India
E-mail: songita.sett@gmail.com

Sharanya S
Department of Data Science and Business Systems
SRM Institute of Science and Technology
Kattankulathur
India
E-mail: sharanys1@srmist.edu.in

Amalendu Si
Department of Computer Applications
Maulana Abul Kalam Azad University of Technology
NH-12, Simhat
Nadia 741249
West Bengal
India
E-mail: siamalendu@gmail.com

Dharmpal Singh
CSE/JIS University
81, Nilgunj Rd, Jagarata Pally,
Deshpriya Nagar, Agarpara
Kolkata 700109
India

Pawan Kumar Singh
Department of Information Technology
Jadavpur University
Jadavpur University Second Campus, Plot No. 8,
Salt Lake Bypass, LB Block, Sector III, Salt Lake City
Kolkata 700106
West Bengal
India
Shinawatra University
99, Moo 10, Bang Toei
Sam Khok
Pathum Thani
Thailand, 12160
E-mail: pawansingh.ju@gmail.com

Preetam Suman
School of Computing Science and Engineering
VIT Bhopal University
Kothrikalan
Sehore
Madhya Pradesh – 466114
India
E-mail: preetam.suman@vitbhopal.ac.in

Navneet Kumar Verma
VIT Bhopal University's School of Advanced Science and Language located at Kothrikalan
Sehore
Bhopal 466114
India

Abrar Yaqoob
VIT Bhopal University's School of Advanced Science and Language located at Kothrikalan
Sehore
Bhopal 466114
India
E-mail: abraryaqoob77@gmail.com

Songita Sett, Soumita Seth, and Saurav Mallik

1 Introduction: fundamentals of drug discovery, telemedicine, artificial intelligence, computer vision, and IoT

Abstract: Rapid technological convergence is changing businesses and transforming conventional procedures in fields like research and healthcare. This chapter highlights the revolutionary functions and interrelated applications of the core concepts of drug discovery, telemedicine, artificial intelligence (AI), computer vision (CV), and the Internet of Things (IoT). Artificial intelligence (AI)-driven predictive models and computational tools have transformed drug discovery, which was once a time-consuming and costly process. This has accelerated the development of new therapies. Particularly in remote areas, telemedicine has helped close the healthcare access gap, thanks to wearable technology and digital communication tools. In domains such as autonomous systems and diagnostics, AI and CV are improving decision-making, automating difficult processes, and increasing precision. In order to provide real-time monitoring and predictive analytics across multiple industries, the IoT ecosystem includes smart devices. These technologies work together to create a data-driven future that is innovative, efficient, and accessible. This chapter provides a thorough overview of their core ideas and applications, along with thoughts on how they could revolutionize today's society.

Keywords: Drug discovery, telemedicine, artificial intelligence, computer vision, Internet of Things

1.1 Introduction

In today's constantly evolving technological age, the combination of science, engineering, and technology is changing conventional methods for industrial applications, research, and healthcare. The disciplines of drug discovery, telemedicine, and artificial intelligence (AI), computer vision (CV), and the Internet of Things (IoT) are combining

---

Songita Sett, Department of Management and Business Administration in Business Analytics, Maulana Abul Kalam Azad University of Technology, Haringhata, Nadia 741249, West Bengal, India, e-mail: songita.sett@gmail.com
Soumita Seth, Department of Computer Science and Engineering, Future Institute of Engineering and Management, Narendrapur, Kolkata 700150, West Bengal, India; and Department of Computer Science and Engineering, Aliah University, Kolkata 700160, West Bengal, India, e-mail: soumita.seth@teamfuture.in
Saurav Mallik, Department of Pharmacology and Toxicology, University of Arizona, Tucson, AZ 85721, USA; and Department of Environmental Health, Harvard T. H. Chan School of Public Health, Boston, MA 02115, USA, e-mail: smallik@arizona.edu

https://doi.org/10.1515/9783111504667-001

to provide groundbreaking answers to some of the most important global issues. This chapter explores the foundations of the various fields, emphasizing their applications, intersections, and transformative power.

Here, we analyze these transformative domains in detail. The modern healthcare and pharmaceutical industries are undergoing unprecedented advancements, from revolutionizing the way drugs are discovered and tested to delivering healthcare services remotely via telemedicine, demonstrating the synergy between data-driven methodologies and cutting-edge technologies. At the same time, areas such as AI and CV are improving decision-making processes, automating complex tasks, and creating pathways for innovation across multiple sectors. IoT further amplifies these capabilities by seamlessly connecting devices, enabling real-time monitoring, and facilitating predictive analytics.

1.2 Fundamental terms

1.2.1 Drug discovery

A key component of modern medicine is drug discovery, which focuses on developing safe and effective treatments. In the past, this method depended on trial and error, sometimes taking decades to produce effective medication. Today, target selection, lead optimization, and clinical trial simulation rely heavily on computational technologies and artificial intelligence, which significantly reduces development timelines [1, 2].

Emerging techniques such as structure-based drug design and machine learning models allow researchers to predict biological activity and toxicity with greater accuracy. Moreover, omics technologies and big data analytics facilitate personalized medicine by tailoring treatments to individual genetic and molecular profiles, marking a shift toward precision medicine [3].

1.2.2 Telemedicine

The digital revolution in healthcare delivery is exemplified by telemedicine. Healthcare professionals can diagnose, treat, and monitor patients remotely using communication technologies. This strategy is particularly effective in addressing healthcare inequalities in underserved or rural areas. Some of the most popular applications include teleradiology, remote patient monitoring, and virtual consultations [2].

The integration of AI-driven diagnostic tools and wearable devices increases the effectiveness of telemedicine. For example, AI chatbots assist with initial patient triage, while connected health devices monitor vital signs and send real-time alerts to healthcare providers. However, challenges such as data security and regulatory compliance remain critical barriers that must be addressed [3].

1.2.3 Artificial intelligence (AI)

AI is at the core of the current technology revolution because it can solve complicated issues by simulating human cognition. AI has revolutionized treatment planning, predictive analytics, and diagnostics in the healthcare industry. For example, medical imaging data is analyzed by deep learning algorithms that provide remarkably accurate abnormality detection [3, 5].

AI models are used in drug discovery to predict molecular interactions, accelerating the development of new treatments. AI is driving developments in sectors beyond healthcare, including manufacturing, shipping, and finance. For AI to be used responsibly, ethical factors such as transparency and bias removal are essential [3].

1.2.4 Computer vision (CV)

A branch of artificial intelligence called computer vision is concerned with giving machines the ability to understand and analyze visual data. Diagnostic accuracy has increased as a result of its use in healthcare, including image-based cancer detection and microscopic slide analysis. CV is extensively used in industry for autonomous navigation systems, facial identification, and automated quality control [4]. Recent breakthroughs in neural networks, especially convolutional neural networks (CNNs), have expanded the capabilities of CV, enabling real-time image and video analysis for applications in security, entertainment, and augmented reality.

1.2.5 Internet of Things (IoT)

Devices in the IoT ecosystem are connected to easily collect and share data. Wearables and implanted sensors are examples of IoT-enabled smart devices that provide real-time health monitoring and predictive healthcare solutions in the healthcare industry. Industrial IoT technologies are improving energy management, supply chain optimization, and predictive maintenance [6].

The transformative potential of IOT is driven by advancements in edge computing, 5G networks, and robust cyber security protocols. Despite challenges such as interoperability and data privacy concerns, IoT continues to redefine how people interact with technology.

1.3 Summary of developed works

The pharmaceutical industry is undergoing a massive transformative revolution through the integration of machine learning (ML) into drug discovery and development processes. A comprehensive overview of the paradigm shift brought about by ML techniques, including predictive modeling, virtual screening, and de novo drug design is presented in Chapter 2. The applications of ML in target identification, compound screening, and lead optimization disclose their potential to significantly accelerate the drug development pipeline. Innovative ML-driven approaches are reshaping preclinical and clinical trials, leading to more efficient trial designs, patient stratification, and treatment response prediction. Moreover, advancements in explicable AI are addressing the interpretability concerns associated with complex ML models and building trust between researchers and clinicians. This chapter investigates into successful case studies, including Atomwise's Ebola drug discovery and DeepMind's AlphaFold for protein folding, which highlight the tangible impact of ML in identifying new drug candidates. However, challenges such as limited data availability, interpretability, ethical considerations, and integration with traditional processes require collaborative efforts and strategic solutions to realize the full potential of ML. ML promises accelerated drug development timelines, precision medicine personalized to individual patient profiles, cost reduction through resource optimization, and the emergence of a collaborative ecosystem involving pharmaceutical companies, research institutions, and regulatory bodies. As ethical guidelines and regulatory frameworks evolve, the role of ML role in drug discovery will be guided to revolutionize healthcare by addressing current challenges and advancing the frontiers of medical science.

In Chapter 3, machine learning is used for drug classification which is a key task in drug discovery. The machine learning algorithms that are used for drug classification are Logistic Regression, Support Vector Machine (SVM), Decision Tree, Random Forest, XGBoost, and Stacking Logistics Regression Random Forest Decision Tree model (SLRD). This study primarily focuses on drug prediction. From some user-given data such as age, gender, blood pressure, cholesterol level, and sodium level, the model can classify the person to a certain disease, and then the model itself predicts which drug is the most suitable for the person or user. Finally, we discuss the challenges and opportunities of using ML for drug classification.

Chapter 4 discusses the use of predictive analytics and machine learning in personalized medicine. Predictive analytics is crucial for comparing risk by reading genetic predispositions, lifestyle choices, and scientific history to create personalized risk scores. It makes it easier to prioritize high-risk sufferers and optimize proactive strategies. Machine learning knowledge complements customized medicine by inspecting genomic and proteomic records, figuring out the markers related to vulnerability, and predicting remedy responses. This results in customized remedy plans that enhance affected person outcomes. In public fitness, ML allows stay evaluation of fitness records for early detection of disease outbreaks, enabling organizations to respond proactively and allocate assets effectively. In pharmaceutical co-vigilance, it prioritizes poor activities within the FDA Adverse Event Reporting System (FAERS), supporting targeted protection measures. In drug discovery, knowledge-based algorithms examine organic and chemical datasets to predict drug efficacy and discover new healing targets, significantly reducing drug improvement time and costs. They automate drug improvement pipelines, accelerate the charge of discovery and optimize medical trial designs. Regardless of these advantages, issues like data quality, algorithmic bias, and adherence ought to be addressed for a broader reputation in healthcare. This take a look at makes a specialty of sequential knowledge acquisition and recommender systems, that are crucial methodologies within the swiftly evolving biomedical landscape.

Advancements in AI-based predictive analytics are revolutionizing healthcare by enhancing patient care and reducing costs. Chapter 5 introduces a healthcare predictive analytics framework capable of handling diverse medical data to provide actionable insights. The framework employs deep learning and machine learning models for knowledge discovery and disease prediction, and includes a recommendation system for personalized suggestions to aid patients and hospital management in operational planning. Key areas of focus include treatment cost-effectiveness and adverse event prediction. Future extensions may incorporate privacy-preserving protocols and the use of new AI models to further improve healthcare efficiency.

A revolutionary home healthcare system that integrates telemedicine, predictive analytics, and AI-driven drug discovery is presented in Chapter 6. The adoption of modern technologies like telemedicine, predictive analytics, and artificial intelligence (AI) has significantly altered the home healthcare (HHC) landscape. This chapter examines how new technologies can revolutionize patient care, increase accessibility, and improve healthcare results. The importance of telemedicine in facilitating prompt treatments and lowering the need for hospital visits is highlighted, especially in the context of remote consultations and ongoing patient monitoring for patients with chronic conditions. With the help of artificial intelligence (AI) and machine learning, predictive analytics analyzes enormous volumes of patient data to forecast disease progression, improve treatment regimens, and avert consequences. Additionally, by customizing therapies based on genetic composition, sophisticated genomics opens up new possibilities for individualized care by increasing medication efficacy and reducing risks. The significance of blockchain technology in protecting private telemedicine contacts and safeguarding sensitive health data is also covered in this chapter. Furthermore, by lowering the carbon footprint of healthcare delivery systems, green logistics—which includes the use of electric vehicles (EVs) and optimized routing algorithms—contribute to the sustainability of HHC. Through case studies in emergency response, diabetes control, and cancer treatment, this chapter demonstrates how these technologies are currently being used in practical contexts to improve patient outcomes, lower healthcare costs, and increase the overall effectiveness of home healthcare. As the need for home healthcare keeps increasing, these developments will be crucial in determining how healthcare systems evolve in the future to become more sustainable, patient-centered, and efficient.

Chapter 7 represents a novel contribution toward enhancing early lung cancer detection by introducing an advanced computational framework to support radiological diagnosis. Lung discomfort frequently arises as an early symptom during cancer treatment, yet timely diagnosis remains a challenge due to delays in radiologist assessments.

To address this issue, the chapter presents a multi-tiered prognostic model grounded in cutting-edge machine learning (ML) methodologies.The segmentation stage integrates a threshold-based approach with a marker-controlled watershed algorithm, supported by a dual-classifier system that enhances data refinement and diagnostic precision. The model is trained on a carefully curated dataset to ensure high sensitivity, which is essential in accurately identifying cancerous conditions. Various ML algorithms are employed, including Support Vector Machine (SVM), K-Nearest Neighbors (KNN), Decision Tree (DT), Logistic Regression (LR), Naive Bayes (NB), and Random Forest (RF). Among these, the Random Forest classifier demonstrates superior performance, achieving an accuracy of 88.5 %. This chapter underscores the transformative potential of combining advanced machine learning techniques with expert radiological analysis, thereby offering a promising approach to revolutionize early-stage lung cancer diagnosis and ultimately improving patient outcomes.

Gene expression datasets provide extensive information about various biological processes, but identifying important genes in high-dimensional data is challenging due to redundancy and irrelevant genes. To overcome this challenge, numerous feature selection (FS) techniques have been developed to identify significant genes amidst complex biological data. Chapter 8 introduces a novel approach that combines the Brownian Motion Search Algorithm (BMSA) with Support Vector Machine (SVM) for gene selection in breast cancer classification. Using the breast cancer dataset, our method efficiently identifies relevant gene subsets using BMSA and uses SVM for accurate classification. The BMSA navigates the high-dimensional feature space to select relevant genes by simulating random movements, reducing redundancy and irrelevant genes. SVM evaluates these gene subsets for accurate classification. We assess the performance of the algorithm using various metrics, including the confusion matrix for accuracy and error distribution, the precision-recall curve for precision and recall balance, and the ROC curve for diagnostic ability. The findings demonstrate the effectiveness of our proposed approach in achieving high classification accuracy. Specifically, the method achieves a best classification accuracy of 99.14 % on 16 genes, along with notable mean and worst-case performances. These results highlight the potential of the BMSA-SVM approach to provide accurate classifications and valuable insights into breast cancer-associated gene biomarkers, representing a significant advancement in bioinformatics and cancer research.

Chapter 9 discusses the challenge of handling high-dimensional gene expression data in biomedical data mining, where the number of genes often exceeds the number of samples, posing a significant hurdle for accurate classification and analysis. To address this issue, this paper introduces a novel three-step hybrid gene selection approach that combines a variance filter, an extremely randomized tree, and the Cuckoo Search Algorithm. Initially, the variance filter reduces the dimensionality of the gene space by eliminating genes with low variability. Subsequently, the extremely randomized tree method further refines this subset, prioritizing those with strong associations to the target phenotype. Finally, the Cuckoo Search Algorithm identifies the optimal feature gene subset from this refined pool. The proposed methodology was evaluated on a breast cancer gene expression dataset using four classifiers: Random Forest, Linear Regression, K-Nearest Neighbors (KNN), and Support Vector Machine (SVM). Experimental results showed that the proposed method consistently outperformed the Extremely Randomized Tree and Variance Filter techniques. For instance, with the Random Forest classifier, the proposed method achieved 100 % accuracy with 11 selected genes, compared to 95.96 % and 83.91 % for the Extremely Randomized Tree and Variance Filter methods, respectively. Similar trends were observed with the other classifiers, where the proposed method achieved the highest accuracies, demonstrating its robustness and effectiveness. These findings underscore the potential of the proposed hybrid approach to significantly enhance classification accuracy and reliability in biomedical data mining applications, offering a powerful tool for gene selection and analysis in high-dimensional datasets.

Detection of sleep stages is crucial as a first step in the analysis and diagnosis of subjects with sleep disorders. However, the standard sleep staging methods are cumbersome and time-consuming, accurately determining the stages of wakefulness prior to NREM or REM periods through extensive but manual analysis of polysomnographic (PSG) data. In Chapter 10, we propose a new hybrid architecture using deep learning (DL) to study PSG sleep recording data in order to detect the sleep stages. We propose an approach to automatically detect sleep stages from PSG data using a model that uses convolutional neural networks (CNN), long short-term memory (LSTM), and gated recurrent units (GRU), called HySleep_Net. HySleep_Net is essentially a hybrid model, and this hybrid nature provides it with the ability to automatically perform data-driven feature selection that has not been possible with existing best-performing methods. HySleep_Net focuses on spatial and temporal dependencies of the PSG data that are important for appropriate sleep stage classification. The functionality of the model has been evaluated on 4 public datasets including Sleep-EDF, Sleep-EDF 78, Sleep Heart Health Study (SHHS) and ISRUC. The experimental results have concluded that our HySleep_Net method performs well with accuracies of 94 %, 89 %, 89 % and 90 % on the above datasets respectively. These results suggest that HySleep_Net is not only superior to the traditional methods, but also becomes a new state-of-the-art model for automatic sleep stage detection— enabling the use of an efficient tool in practice of clinical and research-based studies related with prospective applications regarding sleep medicine.

Chapter 11 presents an innovative portal of modern healthcare system such as ambulance booking and tracking website. MedWheels is a pioneering solution revolutionizing emergency medical transportation. Inspired by the seamless efficiency of ridesharing services like Uber and Ola. MedWheels offers an intuitive web application that connects individuals in need with prompt and professional ambulance services. Users can swiftly request an ambulance to their location by simply specifying their destination. Our platform ensures that every journey is performed by certified medical professionals, in state-of-the-art ambulances equipped with life-saving equipment. Real-time tracking provides users with transparency and peace of mind throughout the transport process. With options for specialized medical care, wheelchair accessibility, and efficient routing algorithms, MedWheels prioritizes user safety, comfort, and timely response. By leveraging technology and innovation, MedWheels aims to bridge the gap between medical assistance and those in need, making emergency healthcare more accessible and reliable for communities. Join us in our mission to create a safer, more efficient future of emergency medical transportation. Rescuers find it very challenging to select the ideal location for the rescue centers in order to conduct the rescue operation effectively during any emergency caused by natural disasters.

Chapter 12 develops an effective Emergency Rescue Decision Model (ERD) which is required to assist the rescuers to determine the optimal path for reaching the affected locations. The ERD model is crucial for emergency rescue management since it can lower the number of casualties and financial damage of a disaster. The EDR model consists of a set of rescue centres (RC) and a collection of demand points (DP). The RCs are used to schedule and distribute the resources among the DPs and DPs provide the service within the communities. Therefore, choosing the best location to build the RC is essential for dealing with the unpredictable travel times caused by congestion and breakdowns as well as the unpredictable demand for logistics among DPs. Principles of interval analysis and entropy measurement are taken into consideration in this proposed ERD model. The uncertainty of the RCs is estimated by the entropy, and the lower entropy value of the RC is selected for the final construction. The expected travel time from the uncertain interval travel time from RC to DP is extracted using interval analysis. The total cost of building a RC consists of a fixed established cost and uncertain transportation cost based on the distance and travel time between RC and DP. Finally, we give an example of our recommended approach for the locations where an emergency rescue center should be established with lowest cost. Moreover, a comprehensive sensitivity analysis is performed to verify the proposed stability and effectiveness of the methodology.

Sentiment analysis is a common task in natural language processing that aims to detect the polarity of a text document. In the simplest situation, we only distinguish between positive and negative sentiment, turning the task into a standard binary classification problem. Sentiment classification can be useful in business intelligence by quickly summarizing consumer sentiment as feedback for a particular product. Movie reviews are of great importance as they can help viewers get an overview of the movie and also provide the producers and directors feedback on their work based on the public's opinion. However, manually analyzing sentiments in reviews becomes tedious due to the large amount of corpus present across several movie review sites. In Chapter 13, we investigate various deep learning algorithms for sentiment classification and try to implement various ensemble models over three sequential models on the IMDb movie review dataset. The results of this research show that the ensemble models achieve higher accuracy than their base learners, the highest being 90.4 % on the IMDb dataset, which is on par with state-of-the-art research and our proposed model. These results demonstrate that ensemble learning methods can be used as a viable method for sentiment classification. Our results are easily reproducible, as we publish the code/notebooks of our experiment.

In the field of homoeopathy, maintaining the quality and consistency of medicinal plants is fundamental to ensuring effective treatment outcomes. However, the inherent variability among these plants poses a significant challenge to quality assurance efforts. Chemometric standardization offers a promising solution, harnessing statistical and mathematical methods to enhance data accuracy and refine analytical procedures. Chapter 14 presents a comprehensive approach that encompasses preprocessing techniques, calibration methods, and validation procedures, all aimed at improving product quality and safety. By adopting chemometric standardization, homeopathic practitioners can effectively address issues such as ensuring batch-to-batch consistency, authenticating botanicals, and detecting potential adulterants. Consequently, this strategy strengthens the reliability of medicines and provides patients with greater confidence in the efficacy of homeopathic treatments. Moreover, embracing chemometric standardization facilitates compliance with regulatory requirements, further enhancing patient safety and trust. The establishment of standardized protocols and guidelines requires collaborative effort between academia, industry, and regulatory bodies. By working together, stakeholders can ensure consistent implementation of chemometric standardization practices, ultimately elevating the credibility and efficacy of homeopathic medicines. In essence, embracing chemometric standardization represents a pivotal step towards enhancing product quality, regulatory compliance, and overall patient well-being in the field of homeopathy.

Rauvolfia serpentina (L.) Benth. ex Kurz is an endangered medicinal plant. Due to demand and scarcity, *R. serpentina* roots are adulterated or substituted with other Rauvolfia species, but in homeopathy only *Rauvolfia serpentina* species is used to prepare mother tincture or dilutions. For identification and discrimination based on genetic information among *R. serpentina, R. densiflora, R. tetraphylla, R. vomitoria*, and *R. micrantha*, DNA fingerprints were developed in Chapter 15 using RAPD analysis with 12 random primers according standard protocol. Genetic polymorphism was quantified by generating a similarity matrix based on the presence or absence of polymorphic bands. The dendrogram obtained represents the genetic relationships among the samples. According to the analysis, *R. serpentina* and *R. densiflora* are the most closely related species; whereas *R. tetraphyla* and *R. vomitoria* have maximum genetic distance, indicating their distant phylogenetic relation. These findings emphasize the importance of RAPD analysis in identifying genetic differences among various *Rauvolfia* species. Furthermore, DNA fingerprinting can hold the potential in supporting the pharmaceutical and nutraceutical industries by facilitating standardization and quality evaluation of medicinal plants.

1.4 Conclusion

The intersection of IoT, CV, AI, telemedicine, and drug discovery is changing the world and providing innovative solutions to critical issues. These interconnected domains are not only revolutionizing traditional workflows but also paving the way for a future driven by data, connectivity, and automation. The implications for healthcare, industry, and beyond are profound, setting the stage for a transformative era of progress and innovation.

Bibliography

[1] Rehman, A. U., Li, M., Wu, B., Ali, Y., Rasheed, S., Shaheen, S., Liu, X., Luo, R. & Zhang, J. (2024). Role of artificial intelligence in revolutionizing drug discovery. Fundam. Res., ISSN 2667-3258. https://doi.org/10.1016/j.fmre.2024.04.021.

[2] Yadav, S., Singh, A., Singhal, R. & Yadav, J. P. (2024). Revolutionizing drug discovery: the impact of artificial intelligence on advancements in pharmacology and the pharmaceutical industry. Intell. Pharm., 2(3), 367–380. ISSN 2949-866X. https://doi.org/10.1016/j.ipha.2024.02.009.

[3] Paul, D., Sanap, G., Shenoy, S., Kalyane, D., Kalia, K. & Tekade, R. K. (2021). Artificial intelligence in drug discovery and development. Drug Discov. Today, 26(1), 80–93. https://doi.org/10.1016/j.drudis.2020.10.010. Epub 2020 Oct 21. PMID: 33099022; PMCID: PMC7577280.

[4] Esteva, A., Chou, K., Yeung, S., et al. (2021). Deep learning-enabled medical computer vision. npj Digit. Med., 4, 5. https://doi.org/10.1038/s41746-020-00376-2.

[5] Sultana, A., Maseera, R., Rahamanulla, A., et al. (2023). Emerging of artificial intelligence and technology in pharmaceuticals: review. Future J. Pharm. Sci., 9, 65. https://doi.org/10.1186/s43094-023-00517-w.

[6] Kumar, S., Tiwari, P. & Zymbler, M. (2019). Internet of Things is a revolutionary approach for future technology enhancement: a review. J. Big Data, 6, 111. https://doi.org/10.1186/s40537-019-0268-2.

Siddhartha Roy
2 Machine learning transformations in drug discovery: a paradigm shift in development strategies

Abstract: The pharmaceutical industry is undergoing a massive transformative revolution by the integration of machine learning (ML) into drug discovery and development processes. This paper provides a comprehensive overview of the paradigm shift brought about by ML techniques, including predictive modeling, virtual screening, and de novo drug design. The applications of ML in target identification, compound screening, and lead optimization reveal its potential to significantly accelerate the drug development pipeline. Innovative ML-driven approaches are reshaping preclinical and clinical trials, leading to more efficient trial designs, patient stratification, and treatment response prediction. Moreover, advancements in explicable AI are addressing the interpretability concerns associated with complex ML models and building trust among researchers and clinicians.

The paper investigates successful case studies, including Atomwise's Ebola drug discovery and DeepMind's AlphaFold for protein folding, highlighting the tangible impact of ML on identifying new drug candidates. However, challenges such as limited data availability, interpretability, ethical considerations, and integration with traditional processes require collaborative efforts and strategic solutions to realize the full potential of ML. ML promises accelerated drug development timelines, precision medicine personalized to individual patient profiles, cost reduction through resource optimization, and the emergence of a collaborative ecosystem involving pharmaceutical companies, research institutions, and regulatory bodies. As ethical guidelines and regulatory frameworks evolve, the role of ML in drug discovery will be guided to revolutionize healthcare by addressing current challenges and advancing the frontiers of medical science.

Keywords: Pharmaceutical industry, machine learning (ML), drug discovery, predictive modeling, virtual screening, lead optimization, explainable AI

2.1 Background of drug discovery and development

Drug discovery and development constitute a multifaceted and resource-intensive endeavor dedicated to the identification and introduction of new therapeutic agents to the market. The conventional trajectory of this complex process involves a series

---

Siddhartha Roy, Dept. of Computer Science and Engineering (IoT, CS, BT), UEM, 5/10, Sevak Baidya Street, Kolkata 700029, West Bengal, India, e-mail: siddhartha_r24@yahoo.com

of stages beginning with target identification, progressing through lead compound discovery, traversing preclinical and clinical trials, and culminating in regulatory approval. Despite commendable advances in molecular biology, bioinformatics, and high-throughput screening technologies, the drug development pipeline faces formidable challenges, most notably exorbitant costs, protracted timelines, and a substantial attrition rate of potential candidate compounds.

The essence of this pursuit lies in comprehending the nuanced molecular mechanisms underlying diseases and identifying novel drug targets, which require an exhaustive and multidisciplinary approach. In recent years, a transformative shift with the integration of machine learning (ML) techniques has the ability to meet the tough challenges essential to drug discovery. ML algorithms, capable of examining vast and complex datasets, have the ability to expose hidden patterns and make predictive analyses. This ability represents a paradigm shift with transformative potential, capable of streamlining and enhancing various stages of the drug discovery process. The ML algorithm in drug discovery is shown in Figure 2.1.

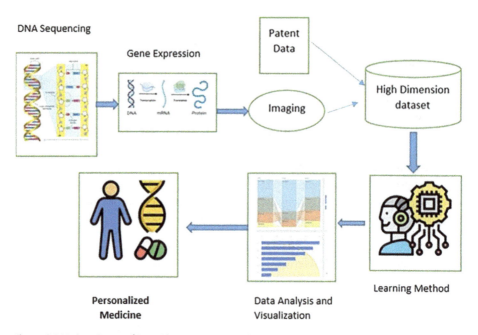

Figure 2.1: Various Stages of Drug Discovery Process using ML.

In this dynamic environment, the power of ML lies in its ability to integrate and deduce large-scale biological and chemical data sets. By interpreting the complex relationships within these datasets, ML algorithms can reveal hidden insights into the complex molecular entities associated with diseases. This data-driven approach enables the identification of potential drug targets with unique precision and efficiency, fostering a more targeted and accelerated drug development process.

Moreover, the integration of ML techniques provides a strategic advantage in optimizing the identification and validation of drug candidates. By leveraging predictive modeling, virtual screening [9], and de novo drug design [5], ML allows for an expanded chemical space with greater accuracy, thus improving the likelihood of identifying compounds with desired therapeutic properties. This not only accelerates the early stages of drug discovery, but also keeps the costs associated with experimental iterations in check.

The integration of drug discovery with ML [7] represents a new era in the pharmaceutical landscape. As ML algorithms continue to advance and prove their effectiveness across diverse applications, the prospect of a more effective, cost-effective, and successful drug development process is gradually gaining momentum. This merging of traditional biomedical approaches with cutting-edge machine learning methodologies motivates the field toward a future where the identification and introduction of therapeutic agents is characterized by unparalleled accuracy, speed, and success.

2.1.1 Motivation for integrating machine learning

The motivation to integrate machine learning into drug discovery and development stems from the need to accelerate the process, reduce costs, and increase the success rate of bringing new drugs to market. Traditional approaches to drug discovery often involve a trial-and-error methodology that can be time consuming and resource intensive. ML, with its ability to analyze massive datasets, extract significant information, and generate predictive models, provides an opportunity to accelerate the identification of potential drug candidates and optimize the drug development pipeline.

ML techniques can analyze biological and chemical data with unprecedented speed and precision, facilitating the identification of novel drug targets, predicting the efficacy and safety of candidate compounds, and optimizing lead compounds for further development. The motivation also stems from the increasing availability of diverse datasets, including genomics, proteomics, and clinical data, which provide an ideal environment for ML algorithms to learn and make informed decisions in the context of drug discovery.

2.1.2 Objectives of the paper

The objectives of this paper are to provide a comprehensive overview of the current landscape of drug discovery and development and to explore the role of machine learning in transforming this landscape. To review the traditional drug development process and identify challenges and limitations.

RO1: To examine the various machine learning techniques applied at different stages of drug discovery.
RO2: To highlight successful applications of machine learning in target identification, compound screening, and optimization.
RO3: To discuss the challenges and ethical considerations associated with the integration of machine learning into drug development.
RO4: To explore emerging trends and future directions in the field, including the potential impact on personalized medicine and patient stratification.

The methodology involved in this paper are literature review of existing research paper, analysis of ML, deep learning concepts and principles in drug discovery, examination of various real life use cases or examples of Atomwise's Ebola drug discovery and DeepMind's AlphaFold for protein folding, and a discussion of potential challenges and future directions.

2.2 Machine learning techniques in drug discovery

The application of machine learning (ML) to drug discovery has revolutionized the way researchers identify potential therapeutic compounds. This section explores into various ML techniques used at different stages of drug discovery, highlighting their roles and contributions.

2.2.1 Predictive modeling

Predictive modeling creates mathematical models to predict the activity or properties of molecules. This helps in narrowing down potential drug candidates and improving their characteristics.

2.2.1.1 Quantitative Structure-Activity Relationship (QSAR)

Quantitative Structure-Activity Relationship (QSAR) [11] stands as a basis in the domain of computational chemistry and drug discovery, offering a powerful predictive modeling technique that closely links the chemical structure of molecules to their biological activity. This approach is influential in understanding the complex relationship between molecular properties and biological responses, paving the way for informed decision-making in the selection and optimization of potential drug candidates.

At its core, QSAR involves a diverse set of molecular descriptors that capture various structural, electronic, and physicochemical properties of compounds. These descriptors serve as quantitative representations of a molecule's characteristics, enabling computational algorithms to discriminate patterns and relationships that may govern the observed biological activities.

Machine learning (ML) algorithms, with their ability to handle large and complex datasets, have become integral to the advancement of QSAR methodologies. These algorithms excel at decoding the complex relationships between molecular descriptors and biological responses by learning from diverse datasets containing information about the chemical structures of compounds and their corresponding biological activities. By discriminating hidden patterns within these datasets, ML algorithms contribute to the creation of robust predictive models.

In the context of QSAR, ML algorithms are proficient at separating complex relationships that are difficult in traditional analytical methods. These algorithms can identify subtle interactions and dependencies between molecular features and biological responses, enabling an understanding of structure-activity relationships.

The predictive power of QSAR models extends to various critical facets of drug discovery and development. Using ML-driven QSAR models, researchers can predict the biological activity, potency, or toxicity of a compound with a high degree of accuracy. This predictive capability significantly accelerates the early stages of drug development, enabling the prioritization of compounds with the most favorable properties for further experimental validation.

ML-enhanced QSAR models contribute to the optimization of lead compounds by guiding researchers toward chemical modifications that enhance desired biological activities while minimizing unwanted side effects. This iterative process of prediction [6] and validation accelerates the identification of promising drug candidates and provides a cost-effective and efficient approach to navigating the vast chemical space.

The integration of QSAR and machine learning stands as an evidence to the evolving landscape of drug discovery. This integration not only refines our understanding of the complicated relationship between molecular structures and biological activities, but also empowers researchers with predictive tools that have the potential to revolutionize the drug development pipeline.

2.2.1.2 Pharmacophore modeling

Pharmacophore modeling serves as a crucial technique in computational drug discovery, explaining the critical structural and chemical features that are essential for a molecule to manifest a specific biological activity. This method helps researchers in decoding the three-dimensional arrangement of functional groups and fractions that contribute to a compound's interaction with a biological target, such as a receptor or enzyme.

The process begins with the assembly of a dataset containing both active and inactive compounds, allowing the ML algorithm to distinguish patterns and correlations.

Molecular descriptors, representing various physicochemical and geometric properties, are extracted from these compounds to quantitatively characterize their properties. The ML algorithm then learns the distinctive features associated with the active compounds and identifies the critical elements that contribute to their biological activity.

Once trained, the ML algorithm helps to construct pharmacophore models by discriminating the three-dimensional arrangement of essential features within the active compounds. This model captures the 3D relationships between key molecular components, such as hydrogen bond donors, acceptors, hydrophobic regions, and aromatic rings. These features collectively define the pharmacophoric pattern necessary for a molecule to elicit the desired biological response.

The constructed pharmacophore model serves as a predictive tool, enabling researchers to screen virtual compound libraries for molecules that conform to the identified pharmacophoric pattern. This approach accelerates the identification of potential drug candidates by focusing on compounds that share structural and chemical similarities with known active molecules.

2.2.2 Virtual Screening

Virtual screening is a pivotal computational technique in drug discovery that harnesses the power of computational methods to efficiently assess large compound libraries. This approach serves as a strategic and cost-effective means of sifting through vast chemical spaces to narrow down the pool of potential drug candidates for subsequent experimental testing. Virtual screening accelerates the identification of molecules most likely to exhibit the desired biological activity, thereby streamlining the drug discovery process.

The fundamental objective of virtual screening is to prioritize and select compounds that are most likely to bind to a specific biological target, such as a protein associated with a disease. This process is analogous to a digital filter that rapidly evaluates a large number of compounds, distinguishing promising candidates from those less likely to exhibit the desired pharmacological effects.

The virtual screening workflow typically includes the following key steps (Fig. 2.2).

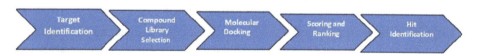

Figure 2.2: Steps of Virtual Screening Workflow.

Target identification

Clearly defining the biological target relevant to the disease of interest is the first step. This could be a protein, enzyme, receptor, or other biomolecular entity associated with the pathological process. Compounds for virtual screening are drawn from extensive chemical libraries, which may include commercially available compounds, natural products, or computationally generated molecules. These libraries represent a wide variety of chemical structures. Computational algorithms perform molecular docking simulations that predict how each compound in the library interacts with the three-dimensional structure of the target. This involves assessing potential binding modes, orientations, and attractions. The results of the molecular docking simulations are scored, and compounds are ranked based on their predicted binding affinity and interaction characteristics. Compounds with higher scores are considered more promising. Compounds that emerge as top hits in the virtual screening process are considered potential candidates for experimental validation. These hits are selected for further testing in vitro and in vivo assays to confirm their biological activity.

The advantages of virtual screening are evident in its ability to rapidly triage large numbers of compounds, significantly reducing the experimental workload and associated costs. By employing computational methods to preselect candidates, researchers can focus their resources on the most promising molecules, increasing the efficiency of the drug discovery pipeline.

While virtual screening is a powerful tool, it is essential to validate the computational predictions with experimental analyses to confirm the actual biological activity of the selected compounds.

2.2.2.1 Ligand-based virtual screening

In ligand-based virtual screening, the chemical properties of potential ligands are compared with known active compounds. ML algorithms, such as similarity search and machine learning classifiers, enhance the screening process by predicting ligand binding affinity and identifying compounds with similar pharmacological profiles.

2.2.2.2 Structure-based virtual screening

Structure-based virtual screening relies on the 3D structures of biological targets to identify potential ligands. ML algorithms analyze structural information, docking scores, and other parameters to predict the binding affinity and selectivity of molecules, helping to prioritize candidates for further exploration.

2.2.3 De novo drug design

De novo drug design represents an innovative and transformative approach to drug discovery that involves the creation of entirely new molecular structures tailored to exhibit specific desired properties. This method aims to design novel compounds with optimal pharmacological activities while minimizing adverse effects. Machine learning (ML) plays a pivotal role in accelerating and enhancing the de novo drug design process by leveraging computational algorithms to guide the generation of molecular structures.

2.2.3.1 Generative models

Generative models, a subset of ML techniques, are particularly useful in de novo drug design. These models are trained on large datasets of chemical structures and learn the underlying patterns and relationships within the chemical space. Notable generative models include variational autoencoders (VAEs) and generative adversarial networks (GANs).
- *Variational Autoencoders (VAEs)*: VAEs are capable of learning a probabilistic mapping of the chemical space. By encoding and decoding molecular representations, VAEs generate novel structures that exhibit similar patterns to those present in the training data. This allows for the creation of diverse and chemically relevant compounds.
- *Generative Adversarial Networks (GANs)*: GANs employ a generative and discriminative network to create realistic molecular structures. The generative network produces new compounds, while the discriminative network evaluates their similarity to existing molecules. This adversarial training process refines the generative capabilities, resulting in the creation of unique and chemically plausible structures.

2.2.3.2 Reinforcement learning in molecule generation

Reinforcement learning [10] provides another approach for de novo drug design. In this context, reinforcement learning algorithms are trained to optimize the generation of molecules based on specified objectives. These objectives may include desired pharmacological properties, bioavailability, or other criteria relevant to drug development.
- **Objective-Driven Molecule Generation:** Reinforcement learning models are trained to optimize a specific objective function. For instance, the model can be trained to generate molecules with high affinity for a target receptor or with specific physicochemical properties.
- **Iterative Optimization:** The reinforcement learning process is often iterative, with the model continuously learning and adapting its generative strategies based on

feedback from the objectives. This iterative optimization loop refines the generated structures over time.

Benefits of ML in de novo drug design:
1. **Efficient Exploration of Chemical Space:** ML models efficiently explore the vast chemical space, generating diverse and novel molecular structures that may not be readily apparent through traditional methods.
2. **Targeted Optimization:** ML-driven de novo drug design enables the optimization of molecular structures based on specific criteria, such as binding affinity, selectivity, or ADMET (absorption, distribution, metabolism, excretion, and toxicity) properties.
3. **Acceleration of Drug Discovery:** By guiding the creation of novel compounds, ML accelerates the early stages of drug discovery and provides a valuable tool for generating lead candidates.
4. **Data-Driven Innovation:** ML models learn from existing chemical data, allowing them to capture complex patterns and relationships. This data-driven innovation contributes to the generation of novel structures with improved chances of success in experimental validation.

De novo drug design, empowered by machine learning techniques, offers a paradigm shift in the creation of novel therapeutics. The synergy between generative models, reinforcement learning, and computational chemistry holds immense promise for accelerating the drug discovery process and unlocking new avenues for the development of innovative medicines.

2.3 Applications of machine learning in drug discovery

Machine learning (ML) has found many applications across various stages of drug discovery, enhancing efficiency, improving the success rate of identifying and developing new therapeutic agents.

2.3.1 Target identification and validation

ML plays a crucial role in identifying and validating of potential drug targets by analyzing biological data to identify molecules or pathways associated with disease.

Omics data analysis: ML algorithms analyze genomics, proteomics, and transcriptomics data to identify potential targets involved in disease.

Network biology: Predictive modeling helps understand complex biological networks, highlighting key nodes as potential drug targets.

2.3.2 Compound screening and prioritization

Efficient screening and prioritization of compounds are essential to focus resources on the most promising candidates. ML techniques contribute to this process through:

Virtual screening: ML algorithms predict the likelihood of compounds binding to a target, allowing for the prioritization of candidates prior to experimental testing.

Chemoinformatics: Quantitative structure-activity relationship (QSAR) models help predict the biological activity of compounds, aiding in the prioritization of lead compounds.

2.3.3 Optimization of lead compounds

Once lead compounds are identified, ML techniques help optimize their properties for improved efficacy and reduced side effects.

Structure-based design: ML models analyze 3D structures and predict modifications to enhance binding affinity and selectivity.

Pharmacokinetics and toxicity prediction: ML algorithms predict the pharmacokinetic profile and potential toxicity of a compound, guiding the optimization process.

2.3.4 Drug-drug interaction prediction

ML is employed to predict potential interactions between drugs, which are crucial for avoiding adverse effects and ensuring patient safety.
- Pharmacogenomics: ML models analyze genetic data to predict individual responses to drugs, minimizing the risk of adverse reactions.

2.3.5 Biomarker discovery

The identification of biomarkers associated with disease or treatment response is facilitated by ML:
- Pattern recognition: ML algorithms analyze large amounts of data to identify patterns that indicate disease presence, progression, or response to treatment.
- Diagnostic models: ML contributes to the development of diagnostic models that use biomarkers for early detection of disease.

2.3.6 Personalized Medicine and Patient Stratification

ML enables the development of personalized treatment strategies by considering individual variability:
- Predictive modeling: ML models predict individual responses to specific treatments, enabling tailored therapeutic interventions.
- Disease subtyping: Clustering techniques stratify patients based on molecular profiles, facilitating personalized treatment approaches.

The integration of ML into drug discovery is driving transformative changes across diverse applications, from target identification to personalized treatment strategies. These applications enhance the efficiency and success of the drug development process and offer promising avenues for the discovery of novel therapeutics.

2.4 Challenges in implementing machine learning in drug discovery

Despite the promising potential of ML in drug discovery, several challenges need to be addressed for effective integration. This section explores key challenges and considerations associated with implementing ML in drug development processes. The success of ML models depends heavily on the availability of high-quality, diverse, and well-annotated data. In drug discovery, obtaining comprehensive datasets with relevant biological, chemical, and clinical information can be challenging because integration data from various sources (genomics, proteomics, chemical databases) can be complex due to differences in formats and standards. Limited datasets or differences in data classes can hinder the training of robust and generalizable models. To overcome this, appropriate data sharing and collaboration between research institutions and pharmaceutical companies can address the issue of limited data availability. Applying data augmentation methods can increase the size and diversity of datasets and resolve issues related to imbalances.

Interpreting ML models in the context of drug discovery is crucial for gaining insight into the decision-making process. The complexity of certain ML algorithms, particularly deep learning models [1, 2], poses challenges in understanding the basis of predictions. Developing and adopting explainable AI techniques can provide interpretable insights into model predictions, ensuring transparency and trust. Combining complex models with interpretable ones strikes a balance between accuracy and explainability. The application of ML in drug discovery raises ethical concerns related to patient privacy, data security, and regulatory compliance. Ensuring that ML models meet ethical standards and regulatory requirements is essential for responsible implementation. Establish clear ethical guidelines for the collection, use, and sharing of patient data in

ML-driven drug discovery. Collaborate with regulatory bodies to develop frameworks that ensure ML models comply with existing regulations, such as data protection laws and patient rights. Integrating ML into traditional drug development processes poses challenges related to cultural shifts, acceptance by the scientific community, and alignment with existing workflows. Conduct workshops and training programs to educate researchers, clinicians, and stakeholders about the benefits and integration of ML in drug discovery. The gradual integration of ML tools and methodologies into existing processes minimizes disruptions and allows for adaptation over time.

Addressing these challenges requires collaboration, technological innovation, and the establishment of ethical and regulatory frameworks. Overcoming these challenges will pave the way for the successful integration of machine learning into drug discovery and unlock its full potential for transformative advances in pharmaceutical research and development.

Machine learning (ML) has been successfully applied in various drug discovery projects, leading to the identification of novel drug candidates and accelerating the drug development process. The following Table 2.1 shows some notable examples of ML-driven drug discovery.

These examples highlight the diverse applications of machine learning in drug discovery, from virtual screening and de novo drug design to personalized medicine. ML-driven approaches have demonstrated the potential to accelerate the identification of promising drug candidates, contributing to the efficiency and success of the drug development process.

2.5 Future directions and emerging trends

As machine ML continues to evolve, its application in drug discovery is expected to shape the future of pharmaceutical research. This section explores emerging trends and future directions in the integration of ML in drug discovery. Explainable AI (XAI) is gaining momentum to enhance the interpretability of ML models in drug discovery. As complex ML models, especially deep learning, are applied more extensively, understanding the decision-making process becomes crucial for gaining the trust of researchers, clinicians, and regulatory bodies. The ongoing development of techniques will provide transparent and interpretable insights into ML models, allowing researchers to understand how predictions are made. The adoption of model-agnostic methods that can be applied to various ML models will facilitate the broader application and standardization. Advances in XAI will lead to greater trust and adoption of ML models in drug discovery, as researchers gain deeper insights into the features that influence model predictions, leading to more informed decisions. ML will be increasingly integrated into preclinical and clinical trial processes to optimize trial design, patient recruitment, and treatment response monitoring. ML models will play a crucial role in identifying patient subgroups

Table 2.1: Example of ML Driven drug discovery system.

Name	Objective	ML Approach	Outcome
Atomwise – Ebola Drug Discovery	Identification of compounds for treating Ebola virus infection	Atomwise used deep learning [3] models for virtual screening of existing compounds against the Ebola virus	The ML model identified two existing drugs with the potential to inhibit Ebola infection, paving the way for further experimental validation
DeepMind – AlphaFold for Protein Folding [4]	Accurate prediction of protein structures [6] to understand their functions and interactions	DeepMind's AlphaFold has used deep learning techniques to predict 3D protein structures	AlphaFold has demonstrated remarkable accuracy in predicting protein structures, providing valuable insights for drug design by understanding the shape and function of proteins
In silico Medicine – Generative Models for Drug Design [8]	Discovery of novel molecules with anti-aging properties	In silico Medicine employed generative adversarial networks (GANs) for de novo drug design	The ML model generated a set of potential compounds with anti-aging effects. One of the compounds, subsequently named "DS-4420," is being pursued as a potential drug candidate
IBM Watson – Oncology Drug Discovery	Personalized treatment recommendations for cancer patients based on genetic information	IBM Watson for Oncology utilized machine learning to analyze medical literature, clinical trial data, and patient records	Watson for Oncology provided treatment recommendations aligned with expert oncologists, aiding in personalized cancer treatment decisions
Amyotrophic Lateral Sclerosis (ALS) Drug Discovery	Identification of novel drug candidates for ALS	BenevolentAI used natural language processing (NLP) and machine learning to analyze biomedical literature and databases	ML algorithms identified a previously overlooked molecule, and subsequent experimental validation demonstrated its potential as a treatment for ALS
AstraZeneca and Exscientia – Centaur Chemist AI	Accelerated drug discovery for cardiovascular and metabolic diseases	AstraZeneca collaborated with Exscientia, leveraging their AI platform, Centaur Chemist, for automated drug design	The collaboration resulted in the rapid discovery of a drug candidate for a metabolic disease, significantly reducing the time required for lead optimization

for more targeted and personalized clinical trials. ML algorithms will help predict clinical trial outcomes, helping researchers design more efficient trials and reduce costs. Efficient integration of ML into preclinical and clinical trials will accelerate drug development timelines, reduce costs, and increase success rates, ultimately bringing innovative therapies to patients more rapidly. AI-driven drug repurposing, where existing drugs are identified for new therapeutic indications, is gaining momentum as a cost-effective and time-efficient strategy. ML models will increasingly draw on diverse data sources, including real-world evidence, to identify potential drug repurposing candidates. Advances in modeling drug interactions and understanding the poly-pharmacology of existing compounds are enhancing the ability of researchers to predict drug efficacy and safety. AI-driven drug repurposing has the potential to accelerate the identification of new therapeutic uses for existing drugs, providing faster routes to clinical application and addressing unmet medical needs. As ML applications in drug discovery become more prevalent, regulatory bodies are working to establish frameworks and guidelines to ensure the responsible and ethical use of these technologies. Collaboration between pharmaceutical companies, researchers, and regulatory agencies is increasing, aiming to develop clear guidelines for the use of ML in drug discovery. Ethical considerations, data privacy standards, and transparency requirements in regulatory frameworks must be considered. A well-defined regulatory framework will provide clarity on the validation, approval, and deployment of ML models in drug discovery, promoting responsible innovation while addressing safety and ethical concerns.

These emerging trends and future directions represent a continued evolution in the application of ML in drug discovery. As technology advances, the integration of explainable AI, expanded use in clinical trials, drug repurposing strategies, and robust regulatory frameworks will collectively shape a more efficient, transparent, and responsible landscape for ML-driven drug discovery.

2.6 Conclusion

The integration of ML into drug discovery is a transformative shift in the pharmaceutical industry, offering innovative solutions. ML techniques, from predictive modeling to virtual screening, are enhancing effectiveness and increasing success rates throughout the drug discovery process. Examples such as Atomwise's Ebola drug discovery and DeepMind's AlphaFold demonstrate the power of ML in identifying new drugs and understanding biological processes. Challenges such as limited data, interpretability, ethics, and integration with traditional processes require collaborative efforts. Ongoing trends in explainable AI, AI-driven drug repurposing, and regulatory frameworks emphasize the evolution of ML in drug discovery. ML-driven approaches are accelerating drug development, which is critical to addressing global health challenges. ML's role in personalized medicine is transforming treatment by tailoring therapies, minimizing side effects, and optimizing outcomes. ML in drug discovery reduces costs through resource efficiency, optimized trials, and drug repurposing, promoting pharmaceutical companies and healthcare systems. Ethical considerations, data privacy, and regulatory compliance become crucial with the rising pervasiveness of ML applications. Collaboration between pharmaceutical companies, research institutions, AI developers, and regulators is essential for responsible innovation. In essence, the integration of ML into drug discovery is not just a technology, but a paradigm shift with far-reaching implications for the pharmaceutical industry. Stimulating possibilities lie ahead as we harness the potential of ML to address healthcare challenges, improve patient outcomes, and advance medical science.

Bibliography

[1] Angermueller, C., Pärnamaa, T., Parts, L. & Stegle, O. (2016). Deep learning for computational biology. Mol. Syst. Biol., 12(7), 878.

[2] Chen, H., Engkvist, O., Wang, Y., Olivecrona, M. & Blaschke, T. (2018). The rise of deep learning in drug discovery. Drug Discov. Today, 23(6), 1241–1250.

[3] Ching, T., Himmelstein, D. S., Beaulieu-Jones, B. K., et al. (2018). Opportunities and obstacles for deep learning in biology and medicine. J. R. Soc. Interface, 15(141), 20170387.

[4] Goh, G. B., Hodas, N. O. & Vishnu, A. (2017). Deep learning for computational chemistry. J. Comput. Chem., 38(16), 1291–1307.

[5] Hartenfeller, M. & Schneider, G. (2010). De novo drug design. In Chemoinformatics and Computational Chemical Biology (pp. 299–323). Berlin: Springer.

[6] Hubatsch, I., Ragnarsson, E. G. E. & Artursson, P. (2007). Determination of drug permeability and prediction of drug absorption in caco-2 monolayers. Nat. Protoc., 2(9), 2111. https://doi.org/10.1038/nprot.2007.303.

[7] Kandoi, G., Acencio, M. L. & Lemke, N. (2015). Prediction of druggable proteins using machine learning and systems biology: a mini-review. Front. Physiol., 6, 366. https://doi.org/10.3389/fphys.2015.00366.

[8] Schneider, P., Walters, W. P. & Plowright, A. T. (2017). SWEETLEAD: an in silico database of approved drugs, regulated chemicals, and herbal isolates for computer-aided drug discovery. PLoS ONE, 12(7), e0181204.

[9] Liew, C. Y., Ma, X. H., Liu, X. & Yap, C. W. (2009). Svm model for virtual screening of lck inhibitors. J. Chem. Inf. Model., 49(4), 877–885. https://doi.org/10.1021/ci800387z.

[10] Sridharan, B., Mehta, S., Pathak, Y. & Deva Priyakumar, U. (2022). Deep reinforcement learning for molecular inverse problem of nuclear magnetic resonance spectra to molecular structure. J. Phys. Chem. Lett., 13(22), 4924–4933. https://doi.org/10.1021/acs.jpclett.2c00624.

[11] Amin, S. A., Ghosh, K., Gayen, S. & Jha, T. (2020). Chemical-informatics approach to COVID-19 drug discovery: Monte Carlo based QSAR, virtual screening and molecular docking study of some in-house molecules as papain-like protease (PLpro) inhibitors. J. Biomol. Struct. Dyn., 39, 4764–4773. https://doi.org/10.1080/07391102.2020.1780946.

Debmitra Ghosh, Dharmpal Singh, and Biswarup Neogi

3 Explainable AI approaches in drug classification from biomarkers of epileptic seizure

Abstract: Explainable AI has emerged as a powerful tool for drug discovery and development. In this study, machine learning (ML) is used for drug classification which is a key task in drug discovery. The machine learning algorithms that are used for drug classification are Logistic Regression, Support Vector Machine (SVM), Decision Tree, Random Forest, XGBoost, and Stacking Logistics Regression Random Forest Decision Tree model (SLRD). This study primarily focuses on drug prediction. From some data provided by the user, such as age, gender, blood pressure, cholesterol and sodium levels, the model can classify the person to a certain disease, and then the model itself predicts which drug is the most suitable for the person or user. Finally, we discuss the challenges and opportunities of using ML for drug classification.

Keywords: Machine learning (ML), Logistic Regression, Support Vector Machine (SVM), Decision Tree, Random Forest, XGBoost, Stacking Logistics Regression Random Forest Decision Tree model (SLRD)

3.1 Introduction

In the field of drug discovery and development, machine learning (ML) has emerged as a transformative force, revolutionizing the way we identify, classify, and predict the efficacy of potential therapeutic agents. This paper explores the application of ML for drug classification, a pivotal task in the drug discovery pipeline. Drug classification, the

---

Acknowledgement: We thank JIS University for allowing us to carry out this project work.

Data availability: All data are collected from Kaggle and are publicly available https://www.kaggle.com/datasets/prathamtripathi/drug-classification.

Conflict of interest: The authors declare no competing interests.

Funding source: This work was not supported by any grants.

Authors' contributions: All authors contributed equally in this paper.

Debmitra Ghosh, CSE/JIS University, 36, B.M. Banerjee Road, Belghoria, Kolkata 700056, India, e-mail: debmitraghosh@jisuniversity.ac.in
Dharmpal Singh, CSE/JIS University, 81, Nilgunj Rd, Jagarata Pally, Deshpriya Nagar, Agarpara, Kolkata 700109, India
Biswarup Neogi, ECE, JISCE, 36, B.M. Banerjee Road, Belghoria, Kolkata 700056, India

https://doi.org/10.1515/9783111504667-003

process of assigning drugs to specific therapeutic categories, is a critical step in understanding their pharmacological properties and potential clinical applications. Traditionally, drug classification has relied on extensive laboratory testing and in vivo studies, a time-consuming and resource-intensive endeavor. ML, with its ability to analyze large amounts of data and identify complex patterns, offers a more efficient and scalable approach to drug classification. This study explores the potential of various ML algorithms, including Logistic Regression, Support Vector Machine (SVM), Decision Tree, Random Forest, XGBoost, and Stacking Logistics Regression Random Forest Decision Tree model (SLRD), in drug classification. These algorithms excel at extracting meaningful insights from diverse datasets, enabling them to accurately classify drugs based on their molecular structures, chemical properties, and biological activities. The focus of this study lies in drug prediction, where ML models are trained to predict the most appropriate drug for an individual patient based on their unique health profile. By analyzing user-provided data such as age, gender, blood pressure, cholesterol levels, and sodium levels, ML models can identify patterns associated with specific diseases and recommend appropriate drug treatments. This personalized approach holds immense promise for improving patient outcomes and optimizing drug efficacy. While ML presents a promising avenue for drug classification, challenges remain. Ensuring data quality and availability is paramount to training robust ML models, and addressing data biases is crucial to prevent unfair or discriminatory results. In addition, improving the interpretability of ML models is essential for understanding their decision-making processes, and fostering trust and acceptance among healthcare professionals and patients alike. Despite these challenges, ML offers transformative opportunities to revolutionize drug discovery and development. By leveraging ML's predictive capabilities, researchers can streamline the drug development process, identify promising drug candidates, and personalize treatment strategies for individual patients. As ML techniques continue to evolve, their impact on shaping the future of medicine will become even more profound.

The remainder of the paper is organized as follows. In Section 3.2 some existing state-of-the-art methods for drug classification are defined. Therefore, Section 3.3 describes the necessary methods that we have used in our research work. Section 3.4 discusses the result comparison, while Section 3.5 describes challenges and opportunities. A discussion on future description is added in Section 3.6. Finally, we conclude the paper in Section 3.7 by highlighting some of the future research areas.

3.2 Related work

[1] To improve productivity, effectiveness, and output quality in drug research and discovery, machine learning and deep learning (DL) techniques have been applied to generate new drug prospects, design drug targets, and improve drug discovery processes. Technological advancements such as high-throughput screening, high-throughput com-

putational analysis, and high-throughput database mining, machine learning, and deep learning techniques have become more reliable with the development and inclusion of big data. Virtual screening and comprehensive online information have also been addressed to establish lead synthesis pathways. In the study of L. Patel and other co-authors, various machine learning algorithms, such as random forest (RF), Naive Bayesian (NB), support vector machine (SVM), and deep learning (DL) methods, were used for drug classification and discovery.

[2] According to the author of the paper, virtual screening (VS) has evolved over the last decade from traditional similarity search using a single reference compound to a sophisticated application domain for machine learning and data mining techniques that require a large and representative training set of compounds to generate reliable decision rules. The amount of chemical and biological data in the public domain is growing exponentially, which has led to a massive effort to develop, evaluate, and use innovative learning approaches. In this work, the author focuses on machine learning methods related to ligand-based visual sensing (LBVS). Furthermore, some relevant VS research that has been published recently is reviewed, providing a thorough assessment of the state of the art in the field and emphasizing both the achievements and the room for improvement.

[3] R. Gupta presented in this paper that the pipelines for drug development and discovery are extensive, intricate, and dependent on many variables. When combined with large amounts of high-quality data and well-defined queries, machine learning (ML) techniques offer a set of tools that can improve discovery and decision-making. The main obstacle to using machine learning lies in the fact that the findings it generates are not always interpretable or repeatable, which can limit its usefulness. High-dimensional data that is thorough and methodical still needs to be generated in all domains.

[4] In this paper, the author stated that drug-drug interactions (DDIs) are a crucial factor to consider when developing new drugs and using them in clinical settings, particularly when drugs are administered together. Although it is vital to find every potential DDI during clinical trials, DDIs are often reported after drugs are approved for clinical use. They are a major contributor to adverse drug reactions (ADRs) and rising medical costs. In clinical studies, computational prediction could help to find possible DDIs.

[5] In this review paper, we summarize the most recent developments in the field of machine learning-driven categorization research on toxicity endpoints and ADME (absorption, distribution, metabolism, and excretion) over the past six years (2015–2021). Only large dataset classification models—those having more than a thousand compounds—are the subject of this study. Nine different targets were the subject of a thorough literature search and meta-analysis: acute oral toxicity, mutagenicity, carcinogenicity, respiratory toxicity, permeability glycoprotein (P-gp) substrate/inhibitor, blood-brain barrier penetration, cytochrome P450 enzyme family, hERG-mediated cardiotoxicity, and irritation/corrosion. The goal of the best classification model comparison was to highlight the differences in dataset size, validation processes, endpoint-specific performances, machine learning algorithms, and modeling types. The analysis

of the data indicates that consensus modeling is becoming more and more common in drug safety prediction, while tree-based methods are (still) the industry standard. These goals remain crucial to ADMET-related research efforts, although excellent classification models already exist for hERG-mediated cardiotoxicity and the isoenzymes of the cytochrome P450 enzyme family.

[6] Drug development and discovery pipelines are extensive, intricate, and dependent on many variables. When combined with large amounts of high-quality data and well-defined queries, machine learning (ML) techniques offer a suite of tools that can improve discovery and decision-making. ML can be applied to every step of the drug development process. Target validation, predictive biomarker discovery, and digital pathology data processing in clinical trials are just a few examples. The methodology and context of the applications have varied, and certain approaches have produced insightful and accurate predictions. The main obstacle to using machine learning (ML) is that the insights it generates are not always interpretable or repeatable, which can limit its usefulness. High-dimensional data that is thorough and methodical has yet to be created in all domains. The application of machine learning (ML) can promote data-driven decision-making and has the potential to accelerate and reduce failure rates in drug discovery and development with further efforts to address these difficulties and increase understanding of the elements required to verify ML techniques.

[7] In this work, nowadays, the amount of user-generated textual material on the website is rapidly increasing due to the development of new computer-based technologies. Among the most important and practical textual materials on social media are patient-written medical and healthcare reviews, which have not received much attention from academics in the fields of data mining and natural language processing (NLP). These reviews include information about how people interact with physicians, receive treatment, and express satisfaction or dissatisfaction with the delivery of healthcare. To evaluate the medication reviews in this study, we present two deep fusion models based on three-way decision theory. The first fusion model called the 3-way fusion of a deep model with a traditional learning algorithm (3W1DT), was created by using a traditional learning method as a backup method to be used when the confidence of the deep method in classifying test samples is low. The primary classifier in this model is a deep learning method. In the second proposed deep fusion model, a 3-way fusion of three deep models with a traditional model (3W3DT), three deep models and one traditional model are trained on the entire training data, and each model independently classifies the test sample. Subsequently, the test drug report is classified by the most confident classifier.

[8] According to the author, one of the most important tasks in the drug discovery process is the identification of potential pharmacological targets. Computational prediction approaches can speed up the process of successfully identifying prospective drug targets across the entire genome, which is highly beneficial. We have successfully identified and distinguished human drug target proteins from human non-drug target proteins using a sequence-based prediction approach that we have developed in this

study. To build prediction models, the training features include sequence-based information such as dipeptide composition, amino acid composition, and amino acid property group composition. A well-known example of class imbalance is the categorization of human therapeutic target proteins. To solve this problem, they balanced the training data with a 1:1 ratio between drug targets (minority samples) and non-drug targets (majority samples) using the Synthetic Minority Over-sampling Technique (SMOTE). The best model with selected features can achieve 87.1 % sensitivity, 83.6 % specificity, and 85.3 % accuracy with a Matthews Correlation Coefficient (MCC) of 0.71 in a tenfold stratified cross-validation test using the ensemble classification learning method—Rotation Forest and Relief feature-selection technique. The evaluation of the compositional patterns in human pharmacological targets can be facilitated by the subset of optimum characteristics found. The results of the model for further validation were 88.1 % sensitivity, 83.0 % specificity, 85.5 % accuracy, and 0.712 mcc using a stringent leave-one-out cross-validation test. A second dataset was used to evaluate the suggested approach, and the present process produced encouraging results. We propose that the present strategy may be effectively used as an adjunct to current techniques for predicting new pharmacological targets.

[9] The term "machine intelligence," often referred to as "artificial intelligence," describes the intelligence displayed by computers. Various machine intelligence techniques have been used throughout the history of rational drug development to guide costly and time-consuming conventional studies. Quantitative structure-activity relationship (QSAR) modeling is one of the machine learning techniques that has been developed over the past few decades. It can quickly and inexpensively identify possible biologically active molecules from millions of candidate compounds. Deep learning techniques, on the other hand, evolved from machine learning approaches as drug development entered the era of "big" data. These approaches provide a more potent and effective means of handling the enormous volumes of data produced by contemporary drug discovery techniques. They offer an overview of the recent development of deep learning techniques and their applications in logical drug discovery, as well as a summary of the history of machine learning. They argue that in the current era of big data, early-stage drug design and discovery may now be guided by this growth of machine intelligence.

[10] Throughout the early phases of drug development, computational tools have become increasingly important in recent decades. Machine learning (ML) techniques they have received particular attention because they can be applied at various stages of drug discovery, including prediction of target structures, prediction of biological activity of new ligands through model building, hit optimization and discovering, and prediction of pharmacokinetic and toxicological profiles. This article provides an overview of different ML approaches used in drug design. A variety of methods are used for these purposes, including similarity searches, building biological activity classification and/or prediction models, docking and virtual screening, and prediction of secondary structures and binding sites. Both structure-based drug design (SBDD) and ligand-based

drug design (LBD) can be performed using these tools. Machine learning techniques have been shown to be effective when used with conventional methods for investigating medicinal chemistry issues in the literature. Machine learning approaches such as support vector machines, random forests, decision trees, and artificial neural networks are used in drug design. The application of machine learning techniques to improve the prediction of binding sites and docking solutions for docking and virtual screening assays is now a significant use of ML techniques.

[11] With its remarkable outcomes, machine learning (ML) is becoming more and more popular in the field of drug development. As its use grows, its limitations become more apparent. These limitations include their inability to be interpreted and their requirement for large amounts of sparse data. Furthermore, it has become clear that even after deployment, the approaches need to be retrained because they are not fully independent. In this study, we provide examples from drug development and related fields that show how sophisticated strategies may be used to overcome these obstacles. The author also discusses new methods and how they can be used in drug development. It is expected that the methods discussed here will increase the use of machine learning in the drug development process.

[12] Using dependency analysis and event trimming, the author of this paper extracts 65 types of DDI events from the DrugBank database. To build a model for predicting DDI-associated events, they present the DDIMDL multimodal deep learning framework, which integrates deep learning with a variety of pharmacological characteristics. To learn cross-modal representations of drug-drug pairs and predict DDI events, DDIMDL first builds deep neural network (DNN)-based sub-models, respectively, using four different types of drug features: chemical substructures, targets, enzymes, and pathways. The sub-models are then combined using a common DNN framework. In computer trials, DDIMDL achieves high efficiency and high accuracy results. Furthermore, DDIMDL outperforms baseline and state-of-the-art DDI event prediction techniques. The molecular substructures of medications appear to be the most revealing feature of all. Targets, substructures, and enzymes work together to provide DDIMDL an accuracy of 0.8852 and an area under the precision-recall curve of 0.9208.

[13] Unexpected pharmacological effects, such as adverse drug events (ADEs), can be caused by drug interactions, including drug-drug interactions (DDIs) and drug-food ingredient interactions (DFIs), the causes of which are often unclear. Numerous computational techniques have been developed to improve our understanding of drug interactions, particularly for DDIs. However, these techniques lack sufficient information beyond the likelihood of DDI incidence and require precise drug information, which is frequently unavailable for DDI prediction. Here, J. Y. Ryu and other co-authors describe the creation of a computational framework called DeepDDI that correctly generates 86 significant DDI types as outputs of human-readable sentences using the names of drug-drug or drug-food component pairs and their structural characteristics as inputs. Using the gold-standard DrugBank DDI dataset, which includes 192,284 DDIs contributed by 191,878 drug combinations, DeepDDI estimates 86 DDI types with an aver-

age accuracy of 92.4 % using deep neural networks with optimized prediction performance.

[14] Clinical adverse drug reactions are often caused by drug-drug interactions (DDIs). Early efforts have been made to accurately identify DDIs for drug safety assessment, including improvements in silico prediction methods. In particular, machine learning techniques have been used to predict similar processes and similar computer-based methods have been developed to measure DDIs with good accuracy. However, the selection of different DDI training data and inadequate similarity metrics can lead to the creation of less effective machine learning systems than expected. Using the method developed to measure consistency and general teaching knowledge presented in the literature, D. In this study, Song and co-authors developed a machine learning model using support vector machines (SVMs). Similar measures have been taken by well-known databases such as Drug Information Services (SIDER) and DrugBank. These parameters include 2D molecular structure similarity, 3D pharmacophore similarity, interaction spectrum fingerprint (IPF) similarity, target similarity, and adverse drug reaction (ADE) similarity. The input vector of the support vector machine (SVM) is a combination table designed using five similarity measures of drug combination knowledge and skill.

[15] Finding drug-target interactions could be the crucial first step in the drug discovery process, since it will significantly reduce the number of potential drugs to search for. Drug-target interaction (DTI) prediction may benefit from the use of highly efficient computational prediction approaches, because in vitro testing is very expensive and time-consuming. Our objective in this review is to provide a thorough overview, focusing on machine learning techniques. R. Chan and other co-authors provide a synopsis of a short number of databases commonly used in drug research, implement a hierarchical classification framework, and give multiple representative approaches, particularly the latest state-of-the-art methods, for each category. They also contrast the benefits and drawbacks of the methods of each category. Finally, they discuss the remaining difficulties and prospects for machine learning in DTI prediction. Future researchers may find this paper useful as a reference and lesson on machine learning-based DTI prediction.

[16] In this research, A. Aliper shows how different drugs can be classified into therapeutic groups based only on their transcriptional profiles using deep neural networks (DNNs) trained on large transcriptional response datasets. They matched 12 therapeutic use categories generated from MeSH to 678 drug perturbation samples spanning the A549, MCF-7, and PC-3 cell lines from the LINCS Project. They also used a pooled dataset of samples perturbed with varying drug concentrations for 6 and 24 hours, along with gene-level transcriptomic data and transcriptomic data processed using a pathway activation scoring technique, to train the DNN. Models based on pathway-level data outperformed those based on gene-level data, although the DNN achieved excellent classification accuracy and greatly outperformed the support vector machine (SVM) model in every multiclass classification task. They showed for the first time how a deep learning

neural network trained on transcriptome data could identify pharmacological properties of different drugs in a variety of biological systems and environments. They also propose repositioning drugs using deep neural net confusion matrices. This research serves as a proof of concept for the use of deep learning in drug development.

[17] H. L. Gururaj's research employs three machine learning models: Multi-label K-Nearest Neighbors, a proprietary neural network, and Binary Relevance K Nearest Neighbors (Type A and Type B). The mean column-wise log loss is used to assess these machine-learning models. With a log loss of 0.01706, the custom neural network model had the highest accuracy. The Flask framework is used to integrate this neural network model into an online application. A custom test feature dataset containing gene expression and cell viability levels can be uploaded by the user. The web application outputs the top drug classes, along with the scatter plots for each of drug.

[18] With its remarkable outcomes, machine learning (ML) is becoming increasingly popular in the field of drug development. As its use grows, its limitations become more apparent. These limitations include their inability to be interpreted and their requirement for large amounts of sparse data. Furthermore, it has become clear that the approaches still need to be retrained after use. In this study, M. Elbadawi and other co-authors provide examples from drug development and related fields that show how sophisticated strategies can be used to overcome these obstacles. They also discuss new methods and their potential use in drug discovery. It is expected that the methods discussed here will increase the use of machine learning in the drug development process.

[19] Over the past decade, deep learning has made significant progress in many areas of cognitive science. This method draws from early research on neural networks and outperforms other machine learning algorithms in many areas such as natural language processing, and image and speech recognition. Recent years have seen the first wave of deep learning applications in pharmaceutical research; these applications have proven useful in solving many drug design problems, not just bioactivity prediction. Bioactivity prediction, new molecule design, synthesis prediction, and bioimaging analysis will be explained with examples.

3.3 Experimental method/procedure/design

This section details the methodology of the study. Several aspects of the study are discussed below.

3.3.1 Data collection and preprocessing

The dataset is collected from the official website of Kaggle. This dataset consists of different types of biological activities of patients which are used to map with different drugs. The study was conducted with 40 individuals. To ensure the quality and consistency of the data, a rigorous data preprocessing pipeline was implemented. This included data cleaning, missing value handling, and feature engineering. Data normalization was applied to ensure that all features were on a similar scale, and dimensionality reduction techniques were employed to reduce the number of features and avoid overfitting.

3.3.2 Feature representation

There are several features of this dataset like age, sex, blood pressure levels (BP), cholesterol levels, and Na to Potassium ratio. These features are very important and can be used to identify in advance for predicting drugs by analyzing the symptoms of the patients.

3.3.3 Model selection and prediction

A variety of machine learning algorithms were evaluated for drug classification, including supervised learning algorithms such as Logistic Regression, SLRD, Support Vector Machines (SVMs), Decision Trees, Random Forests, and XGBoost. The performance of each algorithm was assessed using various metrics, such as accuracy and the loss of the respective models are calculated. The optimal algorithm for each drug classification task was selected based on its performance on a validation dataset. Of the models used, SLRD had the best accuracy of 98.33 % and a loss of 11 %.

3.3.4 Drug prediction

These trained machine learning models were used to predict the most appropriate drug for individual patients based on their unique health profiles. User-provided data, such as age, gender, blood pressure, cholesterol levels, and sodium-potassium levels, were input into the models to generate personalized drug recommendations. The performance of the drug prediction system was evaluated using a separate test dataset to assess its accuracy and generalizability.

3.4 Results and discussion

This section presents the results and comparison of the proposed methodology and the models.

Table 3.1 briefly demonstrates the accuracy and loss of the applied machine learning classifiers like the Logistic Regression, Support Vector Machine, Decision Tree, Random Forest, XGBoost, SLRD. SLRD has given the best accuracy out of the rest.

Table 3.1: Accuracy and loss comparison of different classifiers.

Model	Accuracy	Loss
Logistic Regression	93 %	20 %
SVM	90 %	28 %
Decision tree	95 %	32.3 %
Random forest	95.6 %	21.2111 %
xgboost	94 %	18 %
SLRD	98.33 %	11 %

Figure 3.1 shows the accuracy and loss performance of various machine learning models used for drug classification. The models include Logistic Regression, Support Vector Machine (SVM), Decision Tree, Random Forest, XGBoost, and Stacking Logistics Regression Random Forest Decision Tree (SLRD). The accuracy and loss values of each model are compared. Table 3.2 explains the key differences of the model, accuracy, and drawback of the related studies and works against the model proposed by this work. The accuracy achieved by our proposed model and methodology is far better than the related work on drug classification as shown.

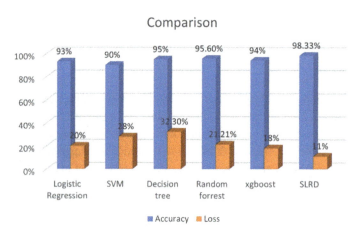

Figure 3.1: Accuracy and loss of used models.

Table 3.2: Comparison of related studies.

Author	Model	Accuracy	Drawbacks
Patel et al. [1]	QASR	90 %	Complex model, more computation time and less accuracy
Elbadawi et al. [2]	BNN	93 %	Less accuracy and more neural networks
Xinran et al. [3]	DDIMDL	88 %	Less accuracy
Proposed Model	SLRD	98.33 %	Complex architecture

3.5 Challenges and opportunities

Data quality and availability: Ensuring data quality and availability is critical to training robust ML models. Data biases must be addressed to prevent unfair or discriminatory results. Interpretability: Improving the interpretability of ML models is essential for understanding their decision-making processes, and fostering trust and acceptance among healthcare professionals and patients. Streamlining drug discovery: ML can streamline the drug discovery process by identifying promising drug candidates and predicting their efficacy.

Personalized medicine: ML can be used to develop personalized treatment strategies for individual patients.

Drug repurposing: ML can be used to identify new uses for existing drugs.

3.6 Future directions

As ML techniques continue to evolve, we can expect to see even more innovative applications of ML in drug discovery and development. Some of the future directions of ML in drug discovery include:
- The development of new ML algorithms for drug classification.
- The use of ML to predict drug-drug interactions.
- The use of ML to design new drugs.

ML has the potential to revolutionize drug discovery and development. By leveraging ML's predictive capabilities, researchers can identify promising drug candidates, personalize treatment strategies for individual patients, and develop new drugs that are more effective and less toxic. As ML techniques continue to evolve, their impact on shaping the future of medicine will become even more profound.

Here are some additional thoughts on the future of ML in drug discovery:
- ML will play an increasingly important role in the drug discovery process, from target identification to lead optimization.

- ML will be used to develop more personalized and effective treatments for patients.
- ML will help to reduce the time and cost of drug development.

ML has the potential to make a significant contribution to the development of new and better drugs for patients.

3.7 Conclusion

Machine learning (ML) is becoming an increasingly powerful tool for the discovery and development of new drugs. This paper aims to review the application of machine learning (ML) to drug classification, which is one of the most important tasks in drug discovery. It has reviewed various machine learning algorithms, as well as various data representations that have been applied to drug classification. The use of machine learning for drug classification has also been discussed in terms of its challenges and opportunities.

Bibliography

[1] Patel, L., Shukla, T., Huang, X., Ussery, D. W. & Wang, S. (2020). Machine learning methods in drug discovery. Molecules, 25(22), 5277.
[2] Lavecchia, A. (2015). Machine-learning approaches in drug discovery: methods and applications. Drug Discov. Today, 20(3), 318–331.
[3] Gupta, R., Srivastava, D., Sahu, M., Tiwari, S., Ambasta, R. K. & Kumar, P. (2021). Artificial intelligence to deep learning: machine intelligence approach for drug discovery. Mol. Divers., 25, 1315–1360.
[4] Cheng, F. & Zhao, Z. (2014). Machine learning-based prediction of drug-drug interactions by integrating drug phenotypic, therapeutic, chemical, and genomic properties. J. Am. Med. Inform. Assoc., 21(e2), e278–e286.
[5] Rácz, A., Bajusz, D., Miranda-Quintana, R. A. & Héberger, K. (2021). Machine learning models for classification tasks related to drug safety. Mol. Divers., 25(3), 1409–1424.
[6] Vamathevan, J., Clark, D., Czodrowski, P., Dunham, I., Ferran, E., Lee, G. ... & Zhao, S. (2019). Applications of machine learning in drug discovery and development. Nat. Rev. Drug Discov., 18(6), 463–477.
[7] Basiri, M. E., Abdar, M., Cifci, M. A., Nemati, S. & Acharya, U. R. (2020). A novel method for sentiment classification of drug reviews using fusion of deep and machine learning techniques. Knowl.-Based Syst., 198, 105949.
[8] Kumari, P., Nath, A. & Chaube, R. (2015). Identification of human drug targets using machine-learning algorithms. Comput. Biol. Med., 56, 175–181.
[9] Zhang, L., Tan, J., Han, D. & Zhu, H. (2017). From machine learning to deep learning: progress in machine intelligence for rational drug discovery. Drug Discov. Today, 22(11), 1680–1685.
[10] Lima, A. N., Philot, E. A., Trossini, G. H. G., Scott, L. P. B., Maltarollo, V. G. & Honorio, K. M. (2016). Use of machine learning approaches for novel drug discovery. Expert Opin. Drug Discov., 11(3), 225–239.

[11] Elbadawi, M., Gaisford, S. & Basit, A. W. (2021). Advanced machine-learning techniques in drug discovery. Drug Discov. Today, 26(3), 769–777. ISSN 1359-6446.
[12] Deng, Y., Xu, X., Qiu, Y., Xia, J., Zhang, W. & Liu, S. A multimodal deep learning framework for predicting drug–drug interaction events. RT Journal.
[13] Ryu, J. Y., Kim, H. U. & Lee, S. Y. (2018). Deep learning improves prediction of drug–drug, and drug–food interactions. Proc. Natl. Acad. Sci., 115(18). E4304–E4311.
[14] Song, D., Chen, Y., Min, Q., Sun, Q., Ye, K., Zhou, C., Yuan, S., Sun, Z. & Liao, J. (2019). Similarity-based machine learning support vector machine predictor of drug-drug interactions with improved accuracies. J. Clin. Pharm. Ther., 44(2), 268–275.
[15] Chen, R., Liu, X., Jin, S., Lin, J. & Liu, J. (2018). Machine learning for drug-target interaction prediction. Molecules, 23(9), 2208.
[16] Aliper, A., Plis, S., Artemov, A., Ulloa, A., Mamoshina, P. & Zhavoronkov, A. (2016). Deep learning applications for predicting pharmacological properties of drugs and drug repurposing using transcriptomic data. Mol. Pharm., 13(7), 2524–2530.
[17] Gururaj, H. L., Flammini, F., Chaya Kumari, H. A., Puneeth, G. R. & Sunil Kumar, B. R. (2021). Classification of drugs based on mechanism of action using machine learning techniques. Discov. Artif. Intell., 1, 1–14.
[18] Elbadawi, M., Gaisford, S. & Basit, A. W. (2021). Advanced machine-learning techniques in drug discovery. Drug Discov. Today, 26(3), 769–777.
[19] Chen, H., Engkvist, O., Wang, Y., Olivecrona, M. & Blaschke, T. (2018). The rise of deep learning in drug discovery. Drug Discov. Today, 23(6), 1241–1250.

Prateek Kumar, Vishal Pradhan, Vivek Panwar, and
Anjan Bandyopadhyay

4 Harnessing predictive analytics and machine learning in personalized medicine: patient outcomes and public health strategies

Abstract: In order to generate individualized risk scores, predictive analytics is essential for evaluating risk by examining lifestyle decisions, medical histories, and genetic predispositions. It facilitates proactive strategy optimization and the prioritization of high-risk patients. By analyzing proteomic and genetic data, finding susceptibility signs, and forecasting treatment outcomes, machine learning improves personalized medicine. Customized treatment strategies that enhance patient outcomes are the outcome of this. Machine learning in public health makes it possible to analyze health data in real-time for the early identification of disease outbreaks, enabling organizations to effectively allocate resources and respond proactively. Targeted safety precautions are supported by pharmacovigilance, which gives priority to adverse occurrences in the FDA Adverse Event Reporting System (FAERS). By predicting medication efficacy and identifying novel therapeutic targets, machine learning algorithms in drug discovery drastically cut down on development time and expenses. Clinical trial designs are optimized and the rate of discovery is accelerated via automated drug development processes. Notwithstanding these benefits, for wider use in the healthcare industry, problems including data quality, algorithmic bias, and regulatory compliance need to be resolved. Sequential learning and recommender systems are the main topics of this study since they are essential approaches in the ever changing biomedical field.

Keywords: FDA Adverse Event Reporting System (FAERS), Machine learning (ML), Drug discovery, Healthcare

4.1 Introduction

A subfield of advanced analytics called predictive analytics makes predictions about the future by analyzing both historical and present data. This procedure makes use of

---

Prateek Kumar, Vishal Pradhan, School of Applied Science, Kalinga Institute of Industrial Technology (KIIT-DU), Bhubaneswar, Odisha, India, 751024, e-mail: vishal.pradhanfma@kiit.ac.in
Vivek Panwar, School of Advanced Engineering, UPES, Dehradun, Uttarakhand, India, 248007
Anjan Bandyopadhyay, School of Computer Engineering, Kalinga Institute of Industrial Technology (KIIT-DU), Bhubaneswar, Odisha, India, 751024, e-mail: anjan.bandyopadhyayfcs@kiit.ac.in

methods from artificial intelligence, machine learning, data mining, and statistics [1]. To estimate the future, predictive analytics combines data science, business modeling procedures, and management techniques. Businesses may use big data to increase their revenues by putting predictive analytics into practice. With the use of data insights, this approach enables businesses to be proactive, forward-thinking, and able to predict trends or behaviors. As big data systems have grown, predictive analytics has made great strides [2]. Predictive analytics and machine learning (ML) have emerged as vital instruments in the healthcare industry, rethinking conventional approaches to illness detection, diagnosis, and treatment and bringing in a revolutionary age for disease prevention. These cutting-edge technologies have the power to drastically transform healthcare by facilitating the creation of more potent preventative strategies that may save lives. Healthcare workers may access and analyze massive datasets to find important insights and make well-informed decisions by utilizing the analytical capabilities of machine learning and predictive analytics. As a result, these technologies have had a significant influence on a number of important healthcare domains, indicating a significant change in the direction of the sector. Predictive analytics and machine learning are essential for enhancing early illness diagnosis and detection. These algorithms can spot trends and tiny indicators that doctors would miss by examining vast volumes of patient data, such as test results, genetic profiles, and medical records. Timely intervention can improve treatment success rates and perhaps save lives when illnesses including diabetes, cancer, and heart issues are detected early [3, 4]. By analyzing a number of variables, such as genetic characteristics, lifestyle decisions, and medical history, predictive analytics is essential in determining a person's chance of contracting specific diseases. Machine learning algorithms may provide individualized risk ratings by examining vast amounts of historical data as well as patterns within populations. This makes it possible for medical practitioners to carry out focused preventive measures. In addition to enhancing the effective use of healthcare resources, this proactive strategy prioritizes high risk patients, as they are more likely to gain from preventive measures. Disease onset may be decreased as a consequence, thereby lessening the strain on healthcare systems [5, 6].

Machine learning algorithms are able to provide customized risk scores by analyzing vast amounts of historical data as well as demographic patterns [7, 8].

Public health surveillance has changed as a result of the combination of predictive analytics and machine learning. Real-time analysis of massive datasets, including social media interactions, search patterns, and electronic health records, is possible using machine learning algorithms. This makes it possible to identify and track illness epidemics quickly [9].

This method helps public health organizations to spot early warning indicators and new trends by offering valuable insights into the dynamics of illness transmission and its effects. These groups are therefore able to take preemptive steps to control the spread of illness, more effectively distribute resources, and carry out focused interventions. A major development is the capacity to do real-time surveillance, which gives health authorities the means to respond quickly and efficiently to emerging public health risks [10].

Pharmacovigilance signal prioritization relies heavily on machine learning and predictive analytics. Machine learning algorithms may efficiently identify and rank possible adverse events by integrating data from the FDA Adverse Event Reporting System (FAERS) with other healthcare datasets, including electronic health records and claims data. To ascertain the relevance and possible impact of these occurrences, these models evaluate variables including severity, reporting frequency, and the characteristics of the impacted patient group [11]. These approaches improve pharmacovigilance efforts by concentrating resources on high-priority safety concerns and enabling prompt actions, thereby safeguarding the health and welfare of patients. Drug development and discovery are being advanced by machine learning algorithms. Through the analysis of extensive chemical and biological databases, these algorithms speed up the process of finding new drugs [12]. They accomplish this by determining novel therapeutic targets, estimating the efficacy of possible drug candidates, and improving pharmacological characteristics. This speedup cuts down on the time and expenses involved in bringing new medications to market. In the end, this increases access to better healthcare for marginalized communities by making it easier to discover therapies for uncommon diseases and ailments with few therapeutic alternatives [13].

It is critical to acknowledge the substantial obstacles that machine learning and predictive analytics must overcome. The quality and representativeness of the data, algorithmic bias, interpretability of the model, privacy issues, and legal constraints are some of the main drawbacks. Building widespread acceptance and confidence in healthcare applications requires addressing these problems. We require thorough legislative frameworks, rigorous algorithm evaluation, and ethical and transparent data management procedures in order to get over these obstacles. Machine learning and predictive analytics may realize their full potential by carefully putting these strategies into practice and continually improving them. This will result in significant improvements in illness prevention and better healthcare outcomes globally. To begin using predictive analytics in healthcare, a consistent and often de-identified dataset must be created (Fig. 4.1).

4.2 Present scenario of drug discovery

Limitations of traditional methods

Historically, drug discovery has largely relied on hit-and-trial strategies, in which scientists test unusual compounds to evaluate their healing effects. However, these conventional techniques are characterized by excessive failure rates and long development times. The introduction of a new drug regularly takes several years and enormous re-

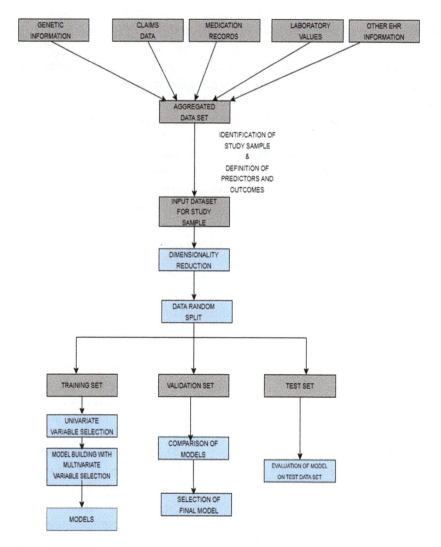

Figure 4.1: Predictive analytics-based population health management intervention implementation steps.

sources, as the serious applicants are not able to bypass scientific trials. Furthermore, traditional strategies often lack an in-depth knowledge of complex organic structures and the mechanisms of diseases [14–16].

Development of era in pharmaceutical research

High-throughput screening strategies permit researchers to unexpectedly compare massive libraries of compounds, accelerating the preliminary stages of drug discovery [17].

Advances in genomics, proteomics, and different omics technologies have increased our knowledge of organic structures and disease pathways. In addition, computational strategies have received significance, permitting researchers to simulate molecular interactions and appropriately expect the homes of capacity drug applicants [18, 19].

Rise of AI in drug discovery

Drug discovery has changed as a result of artificial intelligence (AI) techniques, especially machine learning (ML) and deep learning, which make it possible to analyze big data and predict molecular characteristics. The time and expense of experimental screening can be decreased by using AI algorithms to perform virtual screenings of compound libraries to find compounds that are most likely to bind to targets. In order to assist researchers in prioritizing candidates, AI models also forecast pharmacokinetic and pharmacodynamic features. They also help with the analysis of patient data in order to find biomarkers and customize treatments, which results in better outcomes. Although there is a lot of promise for using AI in drug discovery, issues including data quality, legal issues, and ethical issues must be resolved before its full advantages can be realized. While the combination of AI in drug discovery has remarkable potential, demanding situations like information quality, regulatory issues, and moral issues should be taken care of, to completely free up its benefits [20–23]. Fig. 4.2 lists the AI methods utilized in drug development along with their main advantages, application areas, and difficulties.

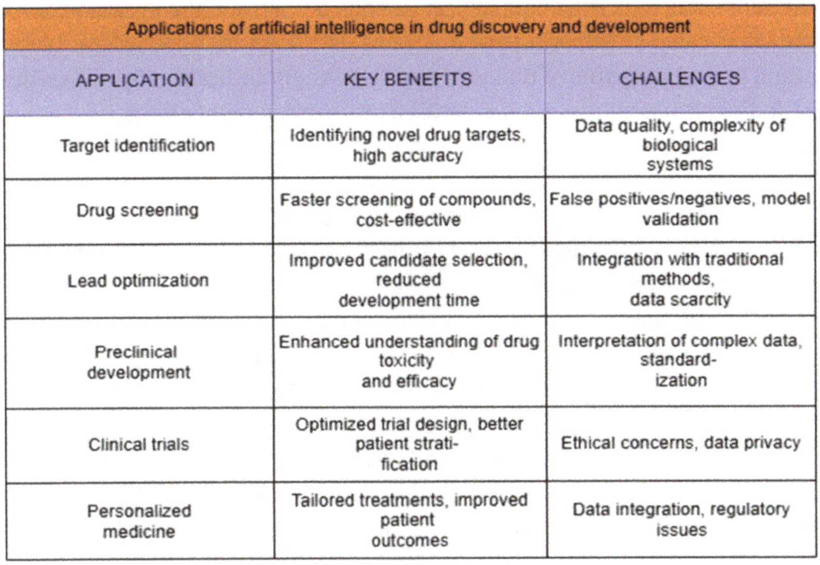

Applications of artificial intelligence in drug discovery and development		
APPLICATION	KEY BENEFITS	CHALLENGES
Target identification	Identifying novel drug targets, high accuracy	Data quality, complexity of biological systems
Drug screening	Faster screening of compounds, cost-effective	False positives/negatives, model validation
Lead optimization	Improved candidate selection, reduced development time	Integration with traditional methods, data scarcity
Preclinical development	Enhanced understanding of drug toxicity and efficacy	Interpretation of complex data, standardization
Clinical trials	Optimized trial design, better patient stratification	Ethical concerns, data privacy
Personalized medicine	Tailored treatments, improved patient outcomes	Data integration, regulatory issues

Figure 4.2: AI applications in medication research and discovery.

4.3 Detection & diagnosis

Machine learning algorithms confirmed the effectiveness of disease identification and prognosis by reading vast amounts of patient-related data, including clinical records, lab results, genetic information, and imaging studies. These algorithms are specifically professional at scrutinizing significant datasets, permitting them to find complicated styles and hit upon diffused symptoms and symptoms of contamination that would move overlooked through human practitioners. By taking gain of those analytical capabilities, device gaining knowledge of substantially improves early detection and prognosis for numerous conditions, such as the sluggish onset of most cancers in addition to the huge outcomes of cardiovascular illnesses, diabetes, and neurodegenerative disorders. Early identity of those illnesses is vital, because it permits healthcare specialists to behave swiftly, administering well timed and powerful remedies that could beautify affected person effects and, in a few scenarios, even do away with the disorder [24, 25].

The implementation of device gaining knowledge of algorithms in healthcare for early detection and prognosis affords large possibilities for improvement, outpacing the precision and accuracy of traditional diagnostic techniques. These algorithms are able to swiftly reading huge datasets of affected person information, uncovering complicated styles and relationships associated with diverse illnesses. This data-pushed approach now no longer simplest boosts the accuracy of diagnoses however additionally aids in spotting early caution symptoms and symptoms which can get away the eye of healthcare providers. By using this potential to perceive diffused signs and anomalies, device gaining knowledge of permits proactive healthcare measures that could intercept disorder development at its earliest stages, therefore improving affected person effects.

Furthermore, machine learning's impact extends beyond specific instances. These algorithms are capable of gathering and analyzing data from big populations, revealing important trends and patterns that are important for public health. Healthcare professionals and governments can develop focused programs to reduce the incidence and consequences of different diseases by identifying common risk factors and trends within particular areas. By promoting prevention, optimizing resource allocation, and significantly lowering the societal effect of diseases, this population-focused approach, supported by the analytical capabilities of machine learning, has the potential to completely transform healthcare systems [26–28].

Machine learning algorithms are essential to changing the healthcare industry from a reactive to a proactive approach. They assist in identifying people who are more likely to get specific diseases by examining past data and locating important predictive indicators. By offering individualized risk evaluations, these algorithms enable healthcare providers to take action before a disease manifests. In the end, this proactive approach lessens the effect of disease and enhances patient outcomes by supporting customized preventive measures including lifestyle modifications and focused screening. With its ability to evaluate risk based on genetic information, medical history, and lifestyle, machine learning is a potent tool in preventive medicine. It enables rapid action that may change the course of a disease and potentially save lives.

Beyond the identification of diseases, machine learning algorithms provide significant benefits. They are able to forecast the course of a disease and recognize different disease subtypes. These algorithms are able to identify distinct subgroups within impacted populations by combining many characteristics and examining a variety of data sources. This realization makes it easier to create individualized treatment programs and focused treatments. Furthermore, by predicting future illness trajectories, machine learning helps physicians foresee possible issues and modify treatment plans appropriately. By facilitating well-informed clinical decision-making, this innovative method not only enhances patient outcomes but also revolutionizes disease management [29, 30]. We present an outline of AI usage in drug improvement in Fig. 4.3.

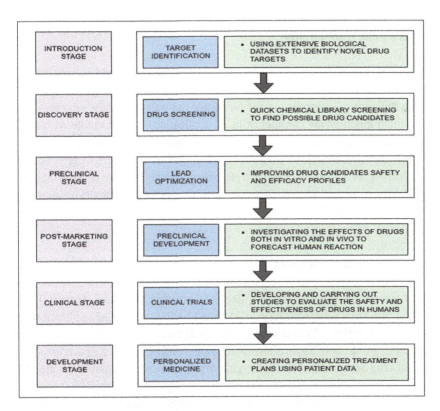

Figure 4.3: A comprehensive workflow of AI applications in drug development and discovery that illustrates the various phases and the associated AI methods employed.

4.4 Challenges & ethics

Data quality and bias

To generate precise forecasts and facilitate wise decision-making, it is crucial to preserve the quality and dependability of the data used to train AI models. Because AI models may inherit and magnify the biases in the training data, biases, errors, and missing data might produce erroneous results. This may lead to inaccurate forecasts or judgments. Biases based on socioeconomic position, gender, or skin color can have a detrimental effect on patient outcomes, making this issue especially important in the healthcare industry. Therefore, promoting ethical AI applications in drug discovery requires the development of methods to identify and reduce biases in AI models as well as making sure that training datasets are representative and diverse [31–33].

Interpretability and transparency

Due to the complexity of their internal architecture, deep learning models in particular are sometimes referred to as "black boxes", since they are challenging for humans to understand. This lack of openness may cause people to doubt how these systems make decisions, which might erode confidence in AI applications. Interpretable AI models that enable domain experts and regulatory bodies to comprehend the reasoning behind forecasts or recommendations are therefore becoming more and more in demand. Upholding ethical norms in drug development requires the establishment of accountability measures for AI-driven decisions, such as guaranteeing openness in model training and validation processes [34–36].

Regulatory and ethical implications

Regulations established by organizations like the European Medicines Agency (EMA) and the Food and Drug Administration (FDA) must be followed by AI applications in drug research. Given the unique characteristics of AI technology, there are particular difficulties in aligning these applications with frameworks that were first created for conventional drug development. Getting regulatory clearance for AI-generated medication candidates or treatment suggestions requires proving their safety and effectiveness. Implementing strict validation and testing procedures is essential to reducing threats to patient safety. Furthermore, it is crucial to protect private patient information and sensitive medical data used in AI applications. Upholding ethical norms and preserving public trust depend on compliance with data protection laws, such as the General Data Protection Regulation (GDPR) and the Health Insurance Portability and Accountability Act (HIPAA) [37–39].

4.5 Risk assessment

Evaluating risk is critical for successful disease prevention, and predictive analytics serves as a powerful technique for estimating an individual's probability of developing particular health issues. Successful disease prevention requires assessing risk, and predictive analytics is a useful tool for calculating a person's likelihood of acquiring particular health problems. A thorough assessment of several aspects associated with illness risk, including genetics, lifestyle decisions, and medical history, may be carried out by utilizing machine learning algorithms that are capable of analyzing massive datasets. To create individualized risk ratings, these machine learning algorithms analyze past data and identify patterns across big population groups. With the use of this data, healthcare professionals may concentrate their resources and efforts on patients who are more vulnerable. This focused strategy enables medical practitioners to carry out proactive, customized therapies that can lower the risk of illness development and promote early treatment. Healthcare professionals can improve preventive tactics and patient health outcomes by promptly recognizing and treating risk factors.

Predictive analytics provides a thorough approach to risk assessment by looking at a variety of factors influencing the onset of disease. This comprises genetic elements including inherited features and genetic markers that aid in more precisely identifying a person's vulnerability to particular illnesses. Lifestyle decisions including food, physical exercise, and exposure to environmental variables are also included in the analysis. By including a person's medical history, prior diagnoses, treatments, and family medical history, predictive models may produce a thorough health profile. This extensive collection of information is used by machine learning algorithms to generate risk scores, which provide a comprehensive picture of an individual's susceptibility to specific illnesses [40, 41].

Accurately identifying a person's risk of contracting a disease is a major leap forward in healthcare that enables for a shift from reactive to proactive methods. Through the usage of custom designed danger ratings, healthcare vendors can discover high-danger people and put early, targeted preventative measures into place. These approaches should contain nutritional and hobby modifications in addition to habitual checking out to discover early signs of disease development whilst cures are maximum effective. In addition to maximizing healthcare aid allocation with by giving precedence to people who need it most, this proactive contamination prevention technique has the ability to noticeably reduce the weight of disease on each person and society.

Additionally, machine learning and predictive analytics methods improve risk assessment by analyzing big data. Through the analysis of past data from sizable population groups, these models are able to pinpoint trends, patterns, and risk factors linked to the onset of disease. Because risk evaluations are more accurate thanks to this data-centric approach, medical practitioners are better equipped to make educated, evidence-based decisions. The analysis of population data facilitates the creation of targeted preventive measures by offering insightful information about the similarities and differences in disease risk across various demographic groups. By utilizing the power of big data, machine learning models enhance our knowledge of disease risk factors and assist risk assessment efforts.

Accurately determining a person's risk of illness allows for a proactive approach rather than a reactive one, which is a significant improvement in healthcare. Healthcare providers can identify high-risk people using individualized risk ratings to conduct early, focused preventive intervention. Along with routine tests to identify early indicators of disease development when it is more curable, these therapies may involve lifestyle modifications such as improvements in diet or physical activity. This proactive approach to illness prevention has the potential to maximize healthcare resource allocation and lessen the total burden of disease on people and society by giving priority to those who are most in need.

Predictive analytics and machine learning models further improve risk assessment through the use of comprehensive data analysis. By examining past data from big population samples, these models are able to pinpoint patterns, trends, and risk factors associated with the onset of disease. By increasing the accuracy of risk assessments, this data-driven approach enables medical practitioners to base their judgments on solid evidence. The development of tailored preventive treatments is made possible by the study of population data, which offers important insights into the similarities and variances in disease risk across demographic groups. Using big data, machine learning algorithms provide a deeper knowledge of disease risk factors and improve risk assessment skills [42, 43].

Risk assessment in disease prevention has been transformed by predictive analytics. Healthcare practitioners may create personalized risk ratings by integrating variables like genetics, lifestyle choices, and medical history into machine learning algorithms. These exact ratings make it possible to identify high-risk individuals and implement focused preventive measures. Proactive steps can be made to lessen the overall effect of illnesses and enhance health outcomes by precisely identifying disease risks. Continuous improvements in data analysis and machine learning are improving the accuracy of risk assessment, which is changing the healthcare industry and resulting in more successful disease preventive tactics.

4.6 Precision medicine

Machine learning algorithms have greatly improved precision medicine, a contemporary approach to healthcare. These algorithms are excellent at deciphering intricate proteomic and genomic data, making it possible to find genetic markers associated with therapy response and illness risk. With the use of this crucial information, medical professionals may create individualized treatment programs that are specific to each patient's genetic composition, departing from the conventional one-size-fits-all approach and taking into account various genetic variances.

Predictive skills, which may significantly enhance therapeutic treatments, are machine learning's primary benefit in precision medicine. Machine learning produces a strong prediction framework by examining big data and finding patterns and connections that human practitioners would miss. By assessing the efficacy of different treatment choices, these algorithms enable medical practitioners to make well-informed, data-driven decisions that improve patient outcomes. Furthermore, by anticipating possible side effects, healthcare professionals may proactively manage risks and modify treatment strategies to maximize patient safety and well-being.

With the potential to completely transform the healthcare system and usher in a new age of customized medicine marked by accuracy, efficacy, and individualized treatment, machine learning is having a significant impact on precision medicine. Healthcare providers can investigate innovative therapeutic approaches by taking into account an individual's unique genetic profile when establishing a course of therapy. Targeted therapies have made it possible to manage diseases that were previously thought to be difficult to treat, greatly improving patient care. Delivering genuinely individualized treatment that takes into account each patient's unique demands is made possible by the use of machine learning in precision medicine [44, 45].

The great chance to improve clinical decision-making is presented by the application of machine learning algorithms in precision medicine. For human doctors, the size and complexity of the proteomic and genomic information processed by these algorithms might be daunting. Healthcare workers may effectively manage these massive amounts of data by using machine learning, which enables them to identify trends and derive important insights. In the end, this improves patient care and makes it possible for patients to get life-saving treatments more quickly by allowing doctors to make more accurate and faster judgments. Furthermore, machine learning is essential to the expansion of scientific understanding. Researchers can find new connections, relationships, and genetic markers that could otherwise go undetected by analyzing large and complex genomic and proteomic data. This abundance of data promotes the development of ground-breaking drugs by expanding our knowledge of illnesses and aiding in the identification of new therapeutic targets. Each patient encounter advances the discipline of precision medicine and eventually improves patient outcomes worldwide by adding to the body of knowledge [46, 47].

One significant development in healthcare is the use of machine learning algorithms into precision medicine. These algorithms enable the development of individualized treatment plans by examining intricate genomic and proteomic data to find genetic markers linked to treatment effectiveness and illness risk. Additionally, they are able to predict treatment outcomes and detect possible adverse effects, leading to better treatment regimens that enhance patient outcomes. This innovative tool advances our scientific knowledge while streamlining clinical decision-making. A new age in healthcare is being ushered in by the combination of contemporary technology with individualized care, where treatment regimens are created tailored to each patient, improving their efficacy, safety, and general quality of care.

4.7 Drug discovery and development

There are several advantages to using machine learning algorithms in the areas of medication research and discovery. The drug development process is greatly streamlined by these algorithms, which are excellent at processing big biological and chemical datasets. Researchers may more quickly identify promising compounds and eliminate the need for expensive and time-consuming experimental testing by using machine learning to estimate the likelihood that medication candidates will succeed. The time and cost associated with introducing new medications to the market are reduced by this increased efficiency. This method therefore has great potential, especially for rare diseases and situations for which there have been few available treatments in the past [48, 49].

Finding new treatment targets has been made incredibly easy by machine learning techniques. These algorithms can identify new molecular pathways and processes linked to a variety of illnesses by examining large biological datasets. This enhanced comprehension aids in the creation of novel treatments by giving researchers vital information about possible pharmacological intervention sites. These methods might change the field of therapeutic treatments and meet important unmet medical needs.

Optimizing drug characteristics at every stage of the drug development process also requires machine learning. Through the analysis of extensive chemical datasets, these algorithms are able to spot trends and connections between desirable pharmacological properties and molecular structures. Researchers can improve medicine formulations using this skill, increasing their efficacy, decreasing adverse effects, and eventually improving patient outcomes. The pharmaceutical business might undergo a revolution if machine learning is included into drug property optimization. This would increase the efficiency of developing safe and effective treatments for a variety of disorders [50].

Machine learning is driving the fast improvement of drug discovery, which holds great promise for developing medicines for uncommon illnesses and ailments. Historically, a lack of information and data has hindered efforts to discover treatments for uncommon diseases. However, researchers can reveal insights about these disorders by analyzing large biological and chemical datasets using machine learning. Machine learning algorithms may find therapeutic targets, identify viable drug candidates, and optimize medication attributes especially suited for uncommon disorders by extensively examining this enormous amount of data. By opening the door for new treatment choices and enhancing general quality of life, this innovative method gives people and families impacted by such disorders fresh hope.

Using machine learning in medication research and discovery has the potential to drastically change the pharmaceutical industry. Machine learning has the potential to significantly cut down on the time and expenses involved in introducing new drugs to the market by speeding up the discovery of promising drug candidates, identifying new therapeutic targets, and improving pharmacological characteristics. Additionally, unusual and previously untreated diseases now have more treatment options because of this technology. It is anticipated that machine learning will have a significant influence on the pharmaceutical sector as it develops further, providing new hope and better opportunities for patient care and results [51–53].

4.8 Conclusion

In order to improve disease prevention in healthcare, machine learning and predictive analytics are becoming more and more important. The detection, diagnosis, and treatment of illnesses are being completely transformed by these technologies, leading to better health outcomes and more successful preventative measures. Early illness identification and diagnosis is one of the main advantages of machine learning and predictive analytics. In order to enable prompt therapies and better prognoses for problems including cancer, cardiovascular diseases, diabetes, and neurodegenerative disorders, these algorithms analyze enormous volumes of patient data in order to find tiny patterns and early symptoms that could otherwise go overlooked. Furthermore, by analyzing variables like genetics and medical history to provide customized risk ratings, predictive analytics improves risk assessment. This makes it possible to halt the progression of illness in high-risk patients by implementing tailored therapies. Additionally, predictive analytics complements danger evaluation via way of means of analyzing elements like genetics, lifestyle, and clinical records to create customized danger scores, making an allowance for focused interventions for people at excessive danger, that can assist save you sickness from developing.

Additionally, by combining data from several sources to recognize and rank safety signals, machine learning improves pharmacovigilance. These models assist in drawing attention to significant safety problems by evaluating the frequency and severity of adverse events and taking impacted populations into account. This allows for prompt and focused action to safeguard patient health. By examining enormous biological and chemical databases, machine learning also speeds up the process of finding and developing new drugs. By predicting the effectiveness of possible drug candidates, finding novel therapeutic targets, and optimizing pharmacological characteristics, these algorithms can drastically cut down on the time and expense required to introduce new drugs to the market, particularly for rare illnesses with few available treatments. Data quality, representativeness, algorithmic bias, model interpretability, privacy concerns, and regulatory compliance are just a few of the obstacles that still need to be overcome in spite of these developments. Achieving wider acceptability and moral integration into healthcare systems requires addressing these issues with meticulous improvement and responsible application.

Furthermore, machine learning improves pharmacovigilance by synthesizing records from numerous datasets to identify and prioritize protective signals. By comparing the severity and frequency of adverse occasions even when thinking about affected populations, these fashions assist recognition sources on huge protection problems, permitting well-timed and focused movements to protect the health of affected people. Additionally, machine learning accelerates drug discovery and improvement by means of studying enormous organic and chemical datasets. These algorithms can anticipate the effectiveness of capacity drug candidates, pick out new healing targets, and improve drug characteristics, thereby lowering the time and price related to bringing new drugs to market, particularly for uncommon diseases with limited remedy options.

To sum up, predictive analytics and machine learning offer revolutionary potential to improve healthcare outcomes and disease prevention. Their wide-ranging influence is demonstrated by their capacities in early detection, customized risk assessment, individualized therapy formulation, public health monitoring, safety signal prioritizing, and medication discovery. These technologies are in a strong position to help make healthcare throughout the world more robust and healthy in the future by addressing current issues and encouraging further development. In conclusion, machine learning and predictive analytics have a transformative capacity to improve sickness prevention and healthcare outcomes. Their competencies in early disease detection, customized risk evaluation, tailored remedy improvement, public health tracking, safety signal prioritization, and drug improvement underscore their huge influence. By addressing these challenges and inspiring ongoing progress, these technologies can contribute to a more resilient and effective healthcare system.

Bibliography

[1] Elkan, C. (2013). Predictive Analytics and Data Mining (Vol. 600). San Diego: University of California.
[2] Reddy, A. R. & Kumar, P. S. (2016). Predictive big data analytics in healthcare. In 2016 Second International Conference on Computational Intelligence & Communication Technology (CICT). (pp. 623–626). IEEE.
[3] Nithya, B. & Ilango, V. (2017). Predictive analytics in health care using machine learning tools and techniques. In 2017 International Conference on Intelligent Computing and Control Systems (ICICCS). (pp. 492–499). IEEE.
[4] Muniasamy, A., Tabassam, S., Hussain, M. A., Sultana, H., Muniasamy, V. & Bhatnagar, R. (2020). Deep learning for predictive analytics in healthcare. In The International Conference on Advanced Machine Learning Technologies and Applications (AMLTA2019) 4 (pp. 32–42). Springer International Publishing.
[5] Passos, I. C., Mwangi, B. & Kapczinski, F. (2016). Big data analytics and machine learning: 2015 and beyond. Lancet Psychiatry, 3(1), 13–15.
[6] Dev, S., Wang, H., Nwosu, C. S., Jain, N., Veeravalli, B. & John, D. (2022). A predictive analytics approach for stroke prediction using machine learning and neural networks. Healthc. Anal., 2, 100032.

[7] Ahmed, Z., Mohamed, K., Zeeshan, S. & Dong, X. (2020). Artificial intelligence with multi-functional machine learning platform development for better healthcare and precision medicine. Database, 2020, baaa010.

[8] Uyyala, P. & Yadav, D. C. (2023). The advanced proprietary AI/ML solution as AntifraudTensorlink4cheque (AFTL4C) for Cheque fraud detection. Int. J. Anal. Exp. Modal Anal., 15(4), 1914–1921.

[9] Poulin, C., Thompson, P. & Bryan, C. (2016). Public health surveillance: predictive analytics and big data. In Artificial Intelligence in Behavioral and Mental Health Care (pp. 205–230). Academic Press.

[10] Kim, E., Kim, J., Park, J., Ko, H. & Kyung, Y. (2023). TinyML-based classification in an ECG monitoring embedded system. Comput. Mater. Continua, 75(1), 1751–1764.

[11] Trifirò, G., Sultana, J. & Bate, A. (2018). From big data to smart data for pharmacovigilance: the role of healthcare databases and other emerging sources. Drug Safety, 41, 143–149.

[12] Veronin, M. A., Schumaker, R. P., Dixit, R. R. & Elath, H. (2019). Opioids and frequency counts in the US Food and Drug Administration Adverse Event Reporting System (FAERS) database: a quantitative view of the epidemic. Drug Healthc. Patient Saf., 65–70.

[13] Arnaud, M., Bégaud, B., Thurin, N., Moore, N., Pariente, A. & Salvo, F. (2017). Methods for safety signal detection in healthcare databases: a literature review. Expert Opin. Drug Saf., 16(6), 721–732.

[14] Harvey, A. (2010). The role of natural products in drug discovery and development in the new millennium. IDrugs: Invest. Drugs J., 13(2), 70–72.

[15] Begley, C. G. & Ellis, L. M. (2012). Raise standards for preclinical cancer research. Nature, 483(7391), 531–533.

[16] Korinek, M., Hsieh, P. S., Chen, Y. L., Hsieh, P. W., Chang, S. H., Wu, Y. H. & Hwang, T. L. (2021). Randialic acid B and tomentosolic acid block formyl peptide receptor 1 in human neutrophils and attenuate psoriasis-like inflammation in vivo. Biochem. Pharmacol., 190, 114596.

[17] Tingaud-Sequeira, A., Carnevali, O. & Cerdà, J. (2011). Cathepsin B differential expression and enzyme processing and activity during Fundulus heteroclitus embryogenesis. Comp. Biochem. Physiol., Part A, Mol. Integr. Physiol., 158(2), 221–228.

[18] Wingender, E. (2008). The TRANSFAC project as an example of framework technology that supports the analysis of genomic regulation. Brief. Bioinform., 9(4), 326–332.

[19] Baig, M. H., Ahmad, K., Rabbani, G., Danishuddin, M. & Choi, I. (2018). Computer aided drug design and its application to the development of potential drugs for neurodegenerative disorders. Curr. Neuropharmacol., 16(6), 740–748.

[20] Dana, D., Gadhiya, S. V., St. Surin, L. G., Li, D., Naaz, F., Ali, Q., ... & Narayan, P. (2018). Deep learning in drug discovery and medicine; scratching the surface. Molecules, 23(9), 2384.

[21] Urban, G., Bache, K., Phan, D. T., Sobrino, A., Shmakov, A. K., Hachey, S. J., ... & Baldi, P. (2018). Deep learning for drug discovery and cancer research: automated analysis of vascularization images. IEEE/ACM Trans. Comput. Biol. Bioinform., 16(3), 1029–1035.

[22] Lim, J., Ryu, S., Park, K., Choe, Y. J., Ham, J. & Kim, W. Y. (2019). Predicting drug–target interaction using a novel graph neural network with 3D structure-embedded graph representation. J. Chem. Inf. Model., 59(9), 3981–3988.

[23] Chen, Z., Liu, X., Hogan, W., Shenkman, E. & Bian, J. (2021). Applications of artificial intelligence in drug development using real-world data. Drug Discov. Today, 26(5), 1256–1264.

[24] Dixit, R. R. (2022). Predicting fetal health using cardiotocograms: a machine learning approach. J. Adv. Anal. Healthc. Manag., 6(1), 43–57.

[25] Kim, E., Lee, J., Jo, H., Na, K., Moon, E., Gweon, G., ... & Kyung, Y. (2022). SHOMY: detection of small hazardous objects using the you only look once algorithm. KSII Trans. Int. Inf. Syst., 16(8), 2688–2703.

[26] Waljee, A. K., Weinheimer-Haus, E. M., Abubakar, A., Ngugi, A. K., Siwo, G. H., Kwakye, G., ... & Saleh, M. N. (2022). Artificial intelligence and machine learning for early detection and diagnosis of colorectal cancer in sub-Saharan Africa. Gut, 71(7), 1259–1265.

[27] Jiang, F., Jiang, Y., Zhi, H., Dong, Y., Li, H., Ma, S., ... & Wang, Y. (2017). Artificial intelligence in healthcare: past, present and future. Stroke Vasc. Neurol., 2(4).

[28] Kim, E., Lee, Y., Choi, J., Yoo, B., Chae, K. J. & Lee, C. H. (2023). Machine learning-based prediction of relative regional air volume change from healthy human lung CTS. KSII Trans. Int. Inf. Syst., 17(2), 576–590.

[29] Alloghani, M., Al-Jumeily, D., Aljaaf, A. J., Khalaf, M., Mustafina, J. & Tan, S. Y. (2019). The application of artificial intelligence technology in healthcare: a systematic review. In International Conference on Applied Computing to Support Industry: Innovation and Technology (pp. 248–261). Cham: Springer International Publishing.

[30] da Silva, D. B., Schmidt, D., da Costa, C. A., da Rosa Righi, R. & Eskofier, B. (2021). DeepSigns: A predictive model based on Deep Learning for the early detection of patient health deterioration. Expert Syst. Appl., 165, 113905.

[31] Makinson, K., Pearce, D., Hodgson, D. A., Bentley, M. J., Smith, A. M., Tranter, M., ... & Siegert, M. J. (2016). Clean subglacial access: prospects for future deep hot-water drilling. Philos. Trans. R. Soc., Math. Phys. Eng. Sci., 374(2059), 20140304.

[32] Househ, M. S., Aldosari, B., Alanazi, A., Kushniruk, A. W. & Borycki, E. M. (2017). Big data, big problems: a healthcare perspective. Inform. Empowers Healthc. Transform., 36–39.

[33] Mehrabi, N., Morstatter, F., Saxena, N., Lerman, K. & Galstyan, A. (2021). A survey on bias and fairness in machine learning. ACM Comput. Surv., 54(6), 1–35.

[34] Zachary, C. L. (2016). The mythos of model interpretability. Commun. ACM, 1–6.

[35] Zitnik, M., Nguyen, F., Wang, B., Leskovec, J., Goldenberg, A. & Hoffman, M. M. (2019). Machine learning for integrating data in biology and medicine: principles, practice, and opportunities. Inf. Fusion, 50, 71–91.

[36] Wachter, S., Mittelstadt, B. & Russell, C. (2017). Counterfactual explanations without opening the black box: automated decisions and the GDPR. Harv. J. Law Technol., 31, 841.

[37] Zhavoronkov, A. (2018). Artificial intelligence for drug discovery, biomarker development, and generation of novel chemistry. Mol. Pharm., 15(10), 4311–4313.

[38] Cohen, S. (Ed.). (2020). Artificial Intelligence and Deep Learning in Pathology. Elsevier Health Sciences.

[39] Hiwale, M., Walambe, R., Potdar, V. & Kotecha, K. (2023). A systematic review of privacy-preserving methods deployed with blockchain and federated learning for the telemedicine. Healthc. Anal., 3, 100192.

[40] Passos, I. C., Mwangi, B. & Kapczinski, F. (2016). Big data analytics and machine learning: 2015 and beyond. Lancet Psychiatry, 3(1), 13–15.

[41] Chen, M., Hao, Y., Hwang, K., Wang, L. & Wang, L. (2017). Disease prediction by machine learning over big data from healthcare communities. IEEE Access, 5, 8869–8879.

[42] Sarwar, M. A., Kamal, N., Hamid, W. & Shah, M. A. (2018). Prediction of diabetes using machine learning algorithms in healthcare. In 2018 24th International Conference on Automation and Computing (ICAC) (pp. 1–6). IEEE.

[43] Kaur, P., Sharma, M. & Mittal, M. (2018). Big data and machine learning based secure healthcare framework. Proc. Comput. Sci., 132, 1049–1059.

[44] Sahu, M., Gupta, R., Ambasta, R. K. & Kumar, P. (2022). Artificial intelligence and machine learning in precision medicine: a paradigm shift in big data analysis. Prog. Mol. Biol. Transl. Sci., 190(1), 57–100.

[45] Ahmed, Z. (2020). Practicing precision medicine with intelligently integrative clinical and multi-omics data analysis. Hum. Genomics, 14(1), 35.

[46] Hassan, M., Awan, F. M., Naz, A., deAndrés-Galiana, E. J., Alvarez, O., Cernea, A., ... & Kloczkowski, A. (2022). Innovations in genomics and big data analytics for personalized medicine and health care: a review. Int. J. Mol. Sci., 23(9), 4645.

[47] Wilkinson, J., Arnold, K. F., Murray, E. J., van Smeden, M., Carr, K., Sippy, R., ... & Tennant, P. W. (2020). Time to reality check the promises of machine learning-powered precision medicine. Lancet Digit. Health, 2(12), e677–e680.

[48] Dixit, R. R., Schumaker, R. P. & Veronin, M. A. (2018). A decision tree analysis of opioid and prescription drug interactions leading to death using the FAERS database. In IIMA/ICITED Joint Conference 2018 (pp. 67–67). International Information Management Association.
[49] Bhardwaj, R., Nambiar, A. R. & Dutta, D. (2017). A study of machine learning in healthcare. In 2017 IEEE 41st Annual Computer Software and Applications Conference (COMPSAC) (Vol. 2, pp. 236–241). IEEE.
[50] Schumaker, R. P., Veronin, M. A., Dixit, R. R., Dhake, P. & Manson, D. (2017). Calculating a severity score of an adverse drug event using machine learning on the FAERS database. In IIMA/ICITED UWS Joint Conference (pp. 20–30). International Information Management Association.
[51] Kumari, J., Kumar, E. & Kumar, D. (2023). A structured analysis to study the role of machine learning and deep learning in the healthcare sector with big data analytics. Arch. Comput. Methods Eng., 30(6), 3673–3701.
[52] Patel, L., Shukla, T., Huang, X., Ussery, D. W. & Wang, S. (2020). Machine learning methods in drug discovery. Molecules, 25(22), 5277.
[53] Zhavoronkov, A., Vanhaelen, Q. & Oprea, T. I. (2020). Will artificial intelligence for drug discovery impact clinical pharmacology? Clin. Pharmacol. Ther., 107(4), 780–785.

Edeh Michael Onyema, Sharanya S, Karthikeyan S, Prabukavin B, and Deepak Arun Annamalai

5 A data-driven framework for future healthcare diagnosis through predictive analytics

Abstract: The swift development of technological advances, along with the continuing explosion of healthcare data, has ushered in a new era of precision medicine and intelligent diagnostics. Traditional diagnostic procedures, which are frequently based on clinical skill and limited datasets, are increasingly being supplemented and, in some cases, transformed by advanced data-driven methodologies. Predictive analytics is at the center of this revolution, a powerful tool that uses historical and real-time data to forecast health outcomes, detect illnesses earlier, and tailor patient care. This paper outlines an extensive approach for using predictive analytics into future healthcare diagnostics based on machine learning algorithms, deep learning and real-time observation of patients. This approach intends to increase decision-making accuracy, reduce diagnostic mistakes, and hopefully enhance outcomes for patients. As medical systems throughout the world deal with increasing bills, elderly patients, and complex disease profiles, the shift to data-driven diagnostics will be more than just a novelty, but vital to quality healthcare service delivery.

Keywords: Artificial intelligence, deep learning, CNN, RNN, healthcare delivery, predictive analytics, telemedicine

5.1 Introduction

Predictive analytics is rapidly gaining momentum in the modern data driven era. Researchers now leverage the power of AI to diagnose diseases or future occurrences based on available data [1]. AI driven solutions are changing the nature of healthcare [2, 3]. In

---

Edeh Michael Onyema, Department of Mathematics and Computer Science, Coal City University, Enugu, Nigeria; and Adjunct Faculty, Saveetha School of Engineering, Saveetha Institute of Medical and Technical Sciences, Chennai 602105, India, e-mail: mikedreamcometrue@gmail.com, https://orcid.org/0000-0002-4067-3256
Sharanya S, Prabukavin B, Department of Data Science and Business Systems, SRM Institute of Science and Technology, Kattankulathur, India, e-mails: sharanys1@srmist.edu.in, ceaserkavin@gmail.com
Karthikeyan S, Department of Aerospace Engineering, BS Abdur Rahman Crescent Institute of Science and Technology, Vandalur, India
Deepak Arun Annamalai, Saveetha School of Engineering, Saveetha Institute of Medical and Technical Sciences, Chennai, India, e-mail: deepakarun@saveetha.com

https://doi.org/10.1515/9783111504667-005

the past few years, the medical field has experienced a paradigm change, transitioning from reactive treatment methods to more proactive and preventative measures. Predictive analytics, a sophisticated approach based on machine learning and data science techniques that can identify probable health consequences before they become urgent conditions, lies at the heart of this shift. The massive amount of healthcare data created by electronic health records (EHRs), wearable devices, genomic sequencing, medical imaging, and remote patient monitoring systems is hastening this transition. As the volume and complexity of this data increases, the challenge and opportunity is to translate it into practical knowledge that might improve patient outcomes, streamline resource allocation, and, eventually, cut expenses related to healthcare [4].

The use of predictive analytics in healthcare is not a novel idea; it is already making substantial progress in fields such as chronic illness management, hospitalization prediction, and clinical decision support systems (CDSS). However, this opportunity remains largely untapped because to disparate data systems, interoperability challenges, ethical concerns about patient privacy, and a lack of scalable frameworks that can be widely implemented. This study addresses these challenges by presenting an integrated, adaptable framework that can be tailored to a variety of clinical settings while adhering to regulatory standards [5]. Fig. 5.1 highlights the increasing market of healthcare in India.

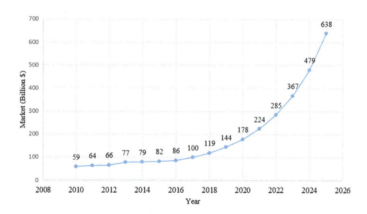

Figure 5.1: Indian healthcare market analysis (OECD Analysis).

At its core, the framework consists of five important components: data collecting, preliminary processing, predictive modeling, validation, and decision support. Each module contributes significantly to the accuracy, relevance, and usability of the predicted insights generated. Data collection is the structured collecting of heterogeneous datasets such as lab results, demographic data, lifestyle knowledge, and unorganized clinical notes. Data preparation ensures the inputs' integrity by addressing missing values, standardizing formats, and anonymizing sensitive identifiers. Predictive modeling detects trends and forecasts health hazards using statistical and machine learning approaches such as logistic regression and decision trees, as well as more complicated deep learning architectures. Flexible thinking is a fundamental feature of this framework. Healthcare institutions differ greatly in terms of data maturity, technical infrastructure, and clinical operations. As a result, an effective structure must be adaptable enough to be adopted in stages, enabling companies to increase capacity over time. Cloud computing, federated learning, and edge analytics are platforms that enable scalable, secure, and dispersed health data processing across several sites, hence supporting adaptation.

The paper proposes an extensive data-driven architecture for future healthcare diagnostics, with predictive analytics serving as the cornerstone. The goal is to demonstrate how new developments in technology may work together to create a smart system capable of early disease detection, individualized treatment planning, and real-time health tracking. By using previous patient data and powerful algorithms, healthcare professionals can get closer to the ideal of precise medicine: giving the right medication to the right patient at the appropriate moment in time.

5.1.1 Data analytics in health care

Data analytics plays a pivotal role in the healthcare sector. It assists in the detection of anomalies in patient's records or condition. The application of emerging technologies for data analysis helps hospitals or physicians to base their decisions on accurate data. Fig. 5.2 shows the different kind of data analytics relating to the healthcare sector.

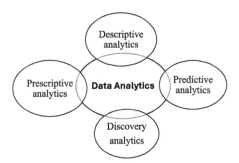

Figure 5.2: Types of data analytics in the healthcare sector.

Descriptive analytics focuses on understanding the patient's past records while predictive analytics deals with modeling the patient's future health outcomes. Prescriptive analytics opens new doors by uncovering new strategies and methods of treatment. Discovery analytics focuses on the next steps of exploration into the medical data. Some of the potential application areas which provide ample scope for the deployment of predictive analytics in the healthcare sector are shown in Fig. 5.3.

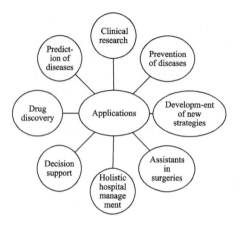

Figure 5.3: Applications of predictive analytics in healthcare.

5.1.2 Predictive modeling in healthcare

The prediction of health conditions or diseases is now possible through the use of machine learning algorithms. The models rely on historical data to diagnose diseases and also predict likely occurrence of illnesses. The use of intelligent algorithms facilitates the early detection of potential diseases and reduces mortality. This is due to the fact that early detection can lead to timely and more efficient treatment. Developing predictive models in healthcare applications is a multistage process. Fig. 5.4 shows the various stages in the development of the predictive analytics model for healthcare applications.

The first phase is the collection of data from various health sensors and sources. The collected data is later preprocessed by removing noise, redundant data, missing data and data imputation. The quality of the data determines the efficiency or accuracy of the algorithm. The reliability of data can be improved via data cleaning, classification and validation. The second step is to perform the analysis on the preprocessed data [6], which includes visualizing the data to understand the primary correlations and variance among them. The accuracy of prediction by algorithms is largely dependent on the quality of data and the viability of the model.

The next important phase is the development of a healthcare predictive analytical model. The detailed analysis in the previous phase would leave a hint to the developer in choosing the right model or algorithm. The next phase is the integration of the developed predictive analytical model into the healthcare business process. This is a crucial step as it involves bridging the virtual and physical resources to improve patient care and the overall hospital management. When incorporated into real world environment, the proposed models are expected to function based on their specification and training. The successful implementation of predictive analytical models could be helpful to physicians to explore deeper insights from medical data and emerging health issues [7]. This

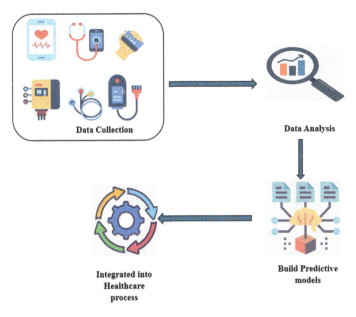

Figure 5.4: Stages in the development of a predictive analytics model for healthcare applications.

goes a long way to reduce the risk associated with emerging health threats and facilitate proactive interventions [8].

5.2 Literature review

The combination of artificial intelligence and big data analytics is transforming customized medicine. AI-driven algorithms can personalize treatment strategies according to distinct patient profiles by evaluating large datasets such as genomic records and real-time data from mobile devices. This technique increases the precision of diagnosis and treatments, resulting in better outcome for patients and greater effectiveness in administration of healthcare.

The use of federated learning and deep generative models has proved effective in accurate health predictions [9]. Researchers have also found the use of machine learning algorithms to be very reliable in improving treatment outcomes [10]. It is clear that the healthcare sector creates a considerable amount of big data, requiring the use of numerous sophisticated algorithms to create predictive analytic models. A Naïve Bayes technique for predicting cardiac illnesses is created using Hadoop-Spark as a large data computing tool to gain deeper insights. The model proved successful in predicting the future health states of several patients after training on data from the UCI machine learning repository [11]. A new disease risk assessment technique based on Bayesian multitask learning is offered for clinical use. This strategy works by coordinating several basic models that communicate with each other. These models are used to generate complex disease risk profiles [12].

Experts are leveraging the power of AI models to forecast health situations and also to track patient's progress and response to treatments. For instance, Faizan Zafar et al. [14] developed a model for predicting type 2 diabetes and their results were promising. Similarly, Glenn Cohen et al. studied the challenges encountered at each phase while developing the predictive analytical models [15]. Also [16] advocated for more studies regarding the implementation of health related models into clinical settings. The study by [17] raised concern about the issue of privacy in the use of AI in the medical field. Kolasa et al. [18] provided examined ethical compliance by stakeholders when using ML models to build tailored treatment strategies. Yi Zheng et al. [19] and [20] asserted that global mortality rate can be reduced if supporting infrastructures and more investments are made to harness the possibilities of AI models in medicine.

Despite its potentials, the use of AI techniques has also attracted criticism. A holistic approach would be to ensure the confidentiality and also address other ethical concerns that accompany the use of AI models in clinical settings. Addressing these issues is pivotal for the widespread usage of predictive analytical models in the healthcare sector [5]. Stakeholders need to do more to bridge the gap between modeling health issues in simulated environments and in the real world [13], in order to truly realize the enormous potential of AI in practice.

Natural Language Processing (NLP)

Natural Language Processing (NLP) is a subset of AI that uses ML algorithms to help computers understand human languages. From the perspective of healthcare, digital devices are made to recognize the prescriptions and observations of physicians to gain insight into the diagnosis process. The sequence of activities carried out in handwritten prescription and observation recognition is given in Fig. 5.6.

NLP in healthcare prediction is a new and effective field of artificial intelligence that leverages text and speech data from medical records to forecast health outcomes, enhance diagnosis, and aid in medical decision-making [21].

Convolutional Neural Networks

A Convolutional Neural Network (CNN) is a deep learning method that excels at processing grid-structured input like images or time series. CNNs are commonly employed in health prediction because they can extract complex information from input information [22]. They are very useful in image classification and analysis thereby improving the quality of medical image scans and interpretation. CNNs are helping physicians to enhance diagnosis and also improve the management of patients.

5 A data-driven framework for future healthcare diagnosis through predictive analytics — 65

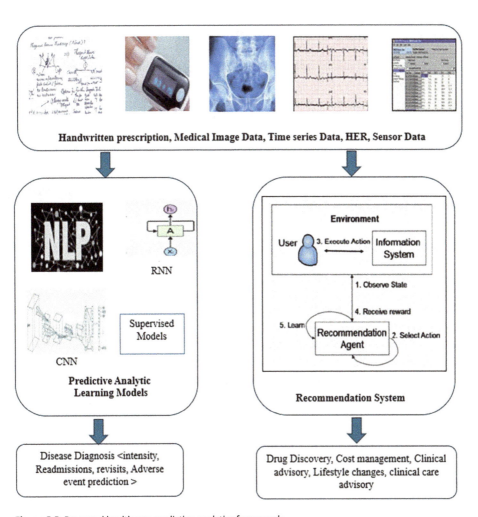

Figure 5.5: Proposed healthcare predictive analytics framework.

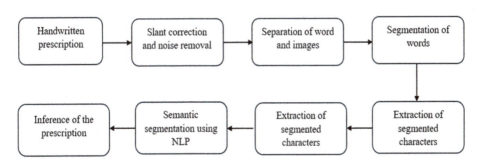

Figure 5.6: Sequence of activities for handwritten prescription and observations for healthcare analytics.

Recurrent Neural Networks (RNN)

Recurrent Neural Networks (RNN) are used for learning sequential and temporal data. Their inherent memory cell permits the remembering of previous cell states and their use to predict the current output. The time-based medical signals like ECG, EEG and the EHR data can be converted into medical concept vectors [23]. Though RNNs work similar to CNNs, they have many advantages. Firstly, RNNs can work with variable length medical data. Also, they can give better accuracy even with small number of datasets. The computation of gradients in RNNs occur in more effective manner so that it avoids most of the unit saturation problems. This is claimed to be an effective model in learning temporal dependencies among the data, which is crucial for health care applications.

Recommendation systems

The proposed predictive analytics framework encompasses a recommendation system. Almost all healthcare providers maintain the EHRs of patients. The analysis the historic data from these records can be done efficiently using recommendation systems. A healthcare-based recommendation system works by filtering the information that is more relevant to the patients and healthcare providers. These systems observe the current scenario and recommend the most appropriate action to be taken by the stakeholders. Some of the common tasks that can be addressed by the healthcare-based recommendation systems are listed below:

Drug Discovery: Artificial intelligence (AI) is transforming the pharmaceutical industry, notably in terms of medication discovery. Traditionally, developing a new medicine is a time-consuming, expensive, and frequently risky process that might take more than a decade and cost billions of dollars. AI, with its ability to analyze large datasets and detect patterns, provides a strong tool for accelerating and improving this process. Predictive modeling is one of the most important ways AI helps with drug discovery. Machine learning algorithms can use data from biomedical literature, clinical trials, and chemical databases to anticipate how various substances would interact with biological targets. This enables researchers to find new medication candidates more rapidly and accurately than conventional techniques [24]. AI is also helpful in medicine development. Generative models can generate novel molecular structures with the needed features while optimizing for efficacy, safety, and manufacturability. Deep learning approaches, such as deep neural networks, can assist refine these predictions and develop compounds that will perform better in clinical trials.

Furthermore, AI simplifies the developmental and clinical testing steps. By assessing patient data and past trial outcomes, AI can identify appropriate patient demographics, forecast side effects, and even recommend optimal dosages, resulting in greater effectiveness and targeted trials.

Cost Management: Cost management in healthcare providers is primarily about reducing the costs. However, a more strategic spending by the healthcare providers may help them deliver excellent patient experience. The behavioral, clinical and operational sources of expenditure need to be audited, and the recommendation engine can suggest a more appropriate plan [25, 26].

Clinical Advisory: The recommendation engine can aid the non-clinical staff by assessing the local health condition [27]. This may be helpful to maintain healthcare infrastructure, pharmaceutical companies and other related organizations.

5.3 Discussion about the framework

The proposed framework covers many parts of the healthcare sector. The primary objective was to use the intelligent and smart methods to fasten the clinical processes without compromising accuracy or ethics. The proposed framework shown in Figure 5.5 has some salient and noteworthy features which include:
- The proposed framework is very inclusive. It facilitates the gathering of health data in versatile formats. The framework enhances the comprehension of handwritten prescriptions and observations, which are very common in mid-level healthcare providers.
- Also, by tracking the previous and present health records, the proposed framework facilitates the prediction of adverse events like epidemics, pandemic or any deviant symptoms of a chronic or acute disease.
- The model does not suggest a specific prediction algorithm. Instead, it enumerates list of common DL and ML algorithms that can handle different medical data.
- The secondary information derived from the prediction outcomes is first of its kind and can assist hospitals to plan their activity.
- The recommendation engine is incorporated as a part of the predictive analytic model with potential to strengthen medical referrals and emergencies.

Thus, it can be observed that the proposed predictive analytics model offers a multitude of advantages. Its robust and versatile nature permits its deployment into any kind of healthcare infrastructure. Processing the predictions will also help integrate the model with the already existing healthcare business processes. Nevertheless, some of the design constraints and challenges of the proposed predictive analytics framework are listed below:
- Data gathering and storage is the foundational step in realizing the predictive analytics framework. To ensure its smooth functioning, the healthcare organizations must focus on developing secure protocols for data storage and transmission.
- As each type of medical data requires a unique data processing system, it can be difficult to adopt one single model for all types of tasks.

- Managing healthcare systems is a multifaceted task with lot of systems, operations, domains, sub-domains and unfamiliar medical protocols. These factors must be considered before building a model.
- Also the legal and ethical frameworks for healthcare not the same all over the world. This imposes access restrictions on the collection and processing of medical data.
- There is a lot of demand for skilled labor for data collection and processing tasks.
- Setting up infrastructure like GPUs, network connectivity, servers and computers may incur high costs.

Despite of these limitations, the proposed work will be a milestone in building a futuristic, next-generation healthcare system.

5.4 Conclusions and future work

In an era characterized by digital change, using advanced analytics in medical diagnostics represents a paradigm shift from reactionary to proactive patient care. This study provides a complete data-driven paradigm for increasing diagnosis accuracy, increasing patient outcomes, and maximizing healthcare resources. The suggested paradigm, which makes use of large-scale datasets, techniques for machine learning, and real-time analytics, not only allows for early disease identification but also individualized treatment options. As the volume and variety of data grows, the potential future of healthcare lies on clever, adaptable, and deeply data-informed systems. Continued multidisciplinary cooperation, responsible data governance, and investment in technical infrastructure will be key in making this goal a solid, long-term reality for international healthcare systems. In conclusion, the potential future of healthcare depends on its ability to forecast rather than react. This paper lays out a clear, extensible, and morally sound data-driven paradigm for employing predictive analytics within healthcare diagnostics.

Bibliography

[1] Muniasamy, A., Tabassam, S., Hussain, M. A., Sultana, H., Muniasamy, V. & Bhatnagar, R. (2020). Deep learning for predictive analytics in healthcare. In The International Conference on Advanced Machine Learning Technologies and Applications (AMLTA2019) (pp. 32–42). Springer International Publishing.

[2] Sharanya, S., Venkataraman, R. & Murali, G. (2024). Predicting remaining useful life of turbofan engines using degradation signal based echo state network. Int. J. Turbo Jet-Engines, 40(s1), s181–s194.

[3] Edeh, M. O., Otto, E. E., Richard-Nnabu, N. E., Ugboaja, S. G., Umoke, C. C. & Omachi, D. (2021). Potential of Internet of Things and semantic web technologies in the health sector. Niger. J. Biotechnol., 38(2), 73–83.

[4] Hassan, M. M., Billah, M. A., Rahman, M. M., Zaman, S., Shakil, M. M. & Angon, J. H. (2021). Early predictive analytics in healthcare for diabetes prediction using machine learning approach. In 2021 12th International Conference on Computing Communication and Networking Technologies (ICCCNT) (pp. 01–05). IEEE.
[5] Ibrahim, M. S. & Saber, S. (2023). Machine learning and predictive analytics: advancing disease prevention in healthcare. J. Contemp. Healthc. Anal., 7(1), 53–71.
[6] Boukenze, B., Mousannif, H. & Haqiq, A. (2016). Predictive analytics in healthcare system using data mining techniques. Comput. Sci. Inf. Technol., 1, 1–9.
[7] Liu, V. X., Bates, D. W., Wiens, J. & Shah, N. H. (2019). The number needed to benefit: estimating the value of predictive analytics in healthcare. J. Am. Med. Inform. Assoc., 26(12), 1655–1659.
[8] Van Calster, B., Wynants, L., Timmerman, D., Steyerberg, E. W. & Collins, G. S. (2019). Predictive analytics in health care: how can we know it works? J. Am. Med. Inform. Assoc., 26(12), 1651–1654.
[9] Zhang, A., Xing, L., Zou, J. & Wu, J. C. (2022). Shifting machine learning for healthcare from development to deployment and from models to data. Nat. Biomed. Eng., 6(12), 1330–1345.
[10] Park, D. J., Park, M. W., Lee, H., Kim, Y. J., Kim, Y. & Park, Y. H. (2021). Development of machine learning model for diagnostic disease prediction based on laboratory tests. Sci. Rep., 11(1), 7567.
[11] Venkatesh, R., Balasubramanian, C. & Kaliappan, M. (2019). Development of big data predictive analytics model for disease prediction using machine learning technique. J. Med. Syst., 43(8), 272.
[12] Lin, Y. K., Chen, H., Brown, R. A., Li, S. H. & Yang, H. J. (2017). Healthcare predictive analytics for risk profiling in chronic care. MIS Q., 41(2), 473–496.
[13] Naqishbandi, T. A. & Ayyanathan, N. (2019). Clinical big data predictive analytics transforming healthcare: an integrated framework for promise towards value based healthcare. In International Conference on E-Business and Telecommunications (pp. 545–561). Cham: Springer.
[14] Zafar, F., Raza, S., Khalid, M. U. & Tahir, M. A. (2019). Predictive analytics in healthcare for diabetes prediction. In Proceedings of the 2019 9th International Conference on Biomedical Engineering and Technology (pp. 253–259).
[15] Cohen, I. G., Amarasingham, R., Shah, A., Xie, B. & Lo, B. (2014). The legal and ethical concerns that arise from using complex predictive analytics in health care. Health Aff., 33(7), 1139–1147.
[16] Hassan, S., Dhali, M., Zaman, F. & Tanveer, M. (2021). Big data and predictive analytics in healthcare in Bangladesh: regulatory challenges. Heliyon, 7(6).
[17] Amarasingham, R., Patzer, R. E., Huesch, M., Nguyen, N. Q. & Xie, B. (2014). Implementing electronic health care predictive analytics: considerations and challenges. Health Aff., 33(7), 1148–1154.
[18] Kolasa, K., Admassu, B., Hołownia-Voloskova, M., Kędzior, K. J., Poirrier, J. E. & Perni, S. (2024). Systematic reviews of machine learning in healthcare: a literature review. Expert Rev. Pharmacoecon. Outcomes Res., 24(1), 63–115.
[19] Zheng, Y. & Hu, X. (2020). Healthcare predictive analytics for disease progression: a longitudinal data fusion approach. J. Intell. Inf. Syst., 55(2), 351–369.
[20] Sangeetha, D., Rathnam, M. V., Vignesh, R., Chaitanya, J. S. & Vaidehi, V. (2020). Medidrone—a predictive analytics-based smart healthcare system. In Proceedings of 6th International Conference on Big Data and Cloud Computing Challenges: ICBCC 2019, UMKC, Kansas City, USA (pp. 19–33). Singapore: Springer.
[21] Thirunavukarasu, A. J., Ting, D. S., Elangovan, K., Gutierrez, L., Tan, T. F. & Ting, D. S. (2023). Large language models in medicine. Nat. Med., 29(8), 1930–1940.
[22] Fourcade, A. & Khonsari, R. H. (2019). Deep learning in medical image analysis: a third eye for doctors. J. Stomatol. Oral Maxillofac. Surg., 120(4), 279–288.
[23] Lin, J., Niu, J. & Li, H. (2017). PCD: A privacy-preserving predictive clinical decision scheme with E-health big data based on RNN. In 2017 IEEE Conference on Computer Communications Workshops. (INFOCOM WKSHPS) (pp. 808–813). IEEE.
[24] Blanco-Gonzalez, A., Cabezon, A., Seco-Gonzalez, A., Conde-Torres, D., Antelo-Riveiro, P., Pineiro, A. & Garcia-Fandino, R. (2023). The role of AI in drug discovery: challenges, opportunities, and strategies. Pharmaceuticals, 16(6), 891.

[25] Tran, T. N., Felfernig, A., Trattner, C. & Holzinger, A. (2021). Recommender systems in the healthcare domain: state-of-the-art and research issues. J. Intell. Inf. Syst., 57(1), 171–201.

[26] Selvaraj, S., Alsayed, A. O., Ismail, N. A., Balasubramanian, P. K., Onyema, E. M., Gan, H. S. & Uchechi, A. Q. (2024). Super learner model for classifying leukemia through gene expression monitoring. Discov. Oncol., 15, 499. https://doi.org/10.1007/s12672-024-01337-x.

[27] Tran, T. A., Onyema, E. M. & Abougreen, A. N. (2024). Leveraging the Potential of Artificial Intelligence in the Real WorldSmart Cities and Healthcare (1st edn.). Taylor and Francis. ISBN 9781032667485. https://doi.org/10.1201/9781032667508.

Songita Sett, Soumita Seth, and Saurav Mallik
6 Revolutionizing home healthcare: telemedicine, predictive analytics, and AI-driven drug discovery

Abstract: The adoption of modern technologies such as telemedicine, predictive analytics, and artificial intelligence (AI) has significantly altered the home healthcare (HHC) scene. This chapter examines how new technologies can revolutionize patient care, increase accessibility, and improve health outcomes.

The significance of telemedicine in facilitating timely treatments and reducing the need for hospital visits is highlighted, especially in the context of remote consultations and continuous monitoring for patients with chronic illnesses.

With the help of artificial intelligence (AI) and machine learning, predictive analytics analyzes vast amounts of patient data to forecast the disease progression, improve treatment regimens, and prevent complications. Additionally, sophisticated genomics opens up new possibilities for personalized care by tailoring therapies to an individual's genetic profile, thereby increasing medication efficacy and reducing risk. The significance of blockchain technology in securing private telemedicine interactions and protecting sensitive health data is also covered in this chapter. Furthermore, by lowering the carbon footprint of healthcare delivery systems, green logistics—which includes the use of electric vehicles (EVs) and optimized routing algorithms—contribute to the sustainability of HHC. Through case studies in emergency response, diabetes management, and cancer treatment, this chapter demonstrates how these technologies are currently applied in practical contexts to improve patient outcomes, reduce healthcare costs, and increase the overall effectiveness of home-based care. As the demand for home healthcare continues to grow, these developments will be crucial in shaping the future of healthcare systems, making them more sustainable, patient-centered, and efficient.

Keywords: Home healthcare (HHC), telemedicine, predictive analytics, artificial intelligence, personalized medicine, genomics, blockchain technology, operations research, green logistics, remote monitoring, healthcare optimization, AI models, healthcare sustainability, disease management

---

Songita Sett, Department of Management and Business Administration in Business Analytics, Maulana Abul Kalam Azad University of Technology, Haringhata, Nadia 741249, West Bengal, India, e-mail: songita.sett@gmail.com
Soumita Seth, Department of Computer Science and Engineering, Future Institute of Engineering and Management, Narendrapur, Kolkata 700150, West Bengal, India; and Department of Computer Science and Engineering, Aliah University, Kolkata 700160, West Bengal, India, e-mail: soumita.seth@teamfuture.in
Saurav Mallik, Department of Pharmacology and Toxicology, University of Arizona, Tucson, AZ 85721, USA; and Department of Environmental Health, Harvard T. H. Chan School of Public Health, Boston, MA 02115, USA, e-mail: smallik@arizona.edu

6.1 Introduction

Recent technological breakthroughs and the growing demand for personalized and accessible care have significantly transformed the global healthcare landscape. To meet these demands, home healthcare (HHC), which delivers medical services in the comfort of patients' homes, has emerged as a viable option. HHC provides convenience and reduces hospital readmissions, supporting post-operative recovery and chronic disease management, all aligned with the objectives of patient-centric care (Goodarzian et al., 2023 [1]).

The importance of telemedicine in HHC cannot be overstated. Telemedicine, enabling real-time consultations, remote monitoring, and even virtual treatment sessions, proved to be a lifesaver for patients requiring continuous medical care during the COVID-19 pandemic. Healthcare practitioners can now maintain close contact with patients through devices such as wearable ECGs, smart pulse oximeters, and continuous glucose monitors (CGMs), which help bridge the gap between patient outcomes and care delivery (Grenouilleau et al., 2019 [4]).

Furthermore, HHC has advanced by enabling personalized therapy through the incorporation of predictive analytics. AI-driven models evaluate patient data to minimize adverse medication reactions, optimize treatment regimens, and predict disease progression. Pharmacogenomics, for example, customizes medication schedules according to the unique genetic profile of each patient, reducing adverse effects and improving therapeutic efficacy (Weiping et al., 2023 [28]).

Lastly, AI and machine learning have significantly contributed to drug discovery. These tools anticipate patient-specific efficacy, simulate drug interactions, and accelerate the identification of treatment candidates, especially in chronic conditions such as cancer and diabetes. Together with telemedicine, predictive analytics ensures timely medication delivery, adherence, and optimization, providing a comprehensive home-based care solution.

The intersection of telemedicine, predictive analytics, and drug discovery within the context of HHC is the focus of this chapter. It examines the methodologies, applications, challenges, and future trends, illustrating how these innovations are reshaping healthcare delivery in the modern world.

6.2 Fundamental terms and preliminaries

6.2.1 Home healthcare systems

The delivery of medical services is undergoing a paradigm shift with home healthcare (HHC), which transfers treatment from clinics and hospitals to patients' homes. Comfort, accessibility, and personalized care are given top priority in this approach, serving patients with chronic conditions, the elderly, and those looking affordable alternatives to inpatient care.

6.2.2 Categories of HHC services

According to Grenouilleau et al. (2019) [4], HHC services can be broadly classified into three main categories:
1. Medical Services:
   - Routine medical examinations and follow-up consultations.
   - Medication administration, including intravenous treatment.
   - Chronic condition monitoring, including diabetes and hypertension.
2. Patient-Centric Services:
   - Rehabilitation therapies, including physiotherapy and speech therapy.
   - Palliative care and hospice support for terminally ill patients.
   - Support for patients with mobility-impairments through specialized equipment.
3. Support Services:
   - Provision and maintenance of medical devices such as oxygen concentrators.
   - Laboratory sample collection and delivery.
   - Patient education and teleconsultation support.

6.2.3 The workflow of HHC services

The delivery of HHC services requires coordinated collaboration among healthcare providers, patients, and enabling technology. The typical workflow includes:
- **Patient Enrolment**: Patients register for HHC services, often through hospital referrals or telemedicine platforms.
- **Needs Assessment**: A personalized care plan is developed based on the patient's medical history and individual requirements.
- **Service Delivery**: This stage includes home visits by healthcare professionals, telemedicine interactions, and device-based monitoring.
- **Data Collection**: IoT devices and mobile applications monitor patient vitals and progress, sending updates to healthcare providers.
- **Follow-up and Adjustments**: Healthcare providers analyze collected data to adjust treatment plans, ensuring continuous care optimization.

Below is an illustrative diagram of the workflow for HHC services:

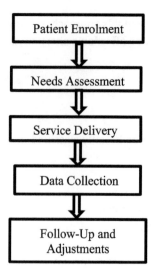

Figure 6.1: Workflow of HHC services.

The workflow in Figure 6.1 demonstrates how HHC integrates human services with technology, creating a seamless patient care experience.

6.2.4 Global adoption and challenges

The adoption of HHC varies significantly across countries. Developed countries such as the USA and Japan have well-established HHC systems, supported by advanced telemedicine technologies and robust insurance infrastructures. In contrast, developing countries face challenges including limited access to technology, high service costs, and a lack of trained healthcare professionals (Goodarzian et al., 2023 [1]).

For example:
- **USA**: HHC plays a significant role i chronic disease management, supported by IoT devices and reimbursement policies.
- **India**: While HHC is expanding, the cost remains prohibitive for many patients, and telemedicine adoption is still in its early stages.

Comparative studies indicate that countries with strong technological infrastructure and government support experience better outcomes in HHC implementation. This disparity underscores the need for scalable and cost-effective solutions, especially in resource-constrained settings.

6.3 Telemedicine in HHC

Telemedicine has become a cornerstone of modern home healthcare (HHC), enabling patients to access quality care remotely. By integrating advanced communication technologies, IoT devices, and data analytics, telemedicine helps bridge the gap between patients and healthcare providers. It ensures timely interventions, continuous monitoring, and improved health outcomes, particularly for individuals with chronic conditions or mobility limitations (Warner 1997 [9]).

6.3.1 Enabling technologies for telemedicine in HHC

Several technological innovations have made telemedicine indispensable in HHC:
- **IoT Devices**: Wearable sensors such as smartwatches, continuous glucose monitors (CGMs), and ECG patches collect real-time patient data, providing actionable insights.
- **Cloud Computing**: Secure cloud platforms store and process patient data, facilitating seamless communication between healthcare providers and patients.
- **Mobile Health Applications**: Apps enable video consultations, appointment scheduling, and medication adherence reminders.
- **AI-Powered Analytics**: Predictive algorithms identify anomalies in patient data, allowing early clinical interventions.

6.3.2 Workflow of telemedicine in HHC

The telemedicine-driven HHC workflow consists of the following steps:
- **Data Acquisition**: IoT devices collect data on vitals such as heart rate, glucose levels, and blood pressure.
- **Data Transmission**: The collected data is securely transmitted to cloud servers via mobile or Wi-Fi networks.
- **Analysis and Alerts**: AI algorithms analyze the data to identify trends or anomalies. Alerts are sent to healthcare providers in case of anomalies.
- **Teleconsultation**: Providers interact with patients through video calls or messaging platforms, adjusting care plans as needed.
- **Follow-Up and Documentation**: The interaction is documented, and patients receive instructions for further care.

6.3.3 System architecture diagram for telemedicine in HHC

Below Figure 6.2 is a simplified system architecture for telemedicine-driven HHC services:

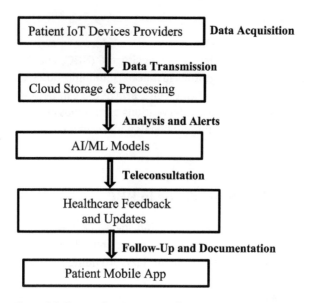

Figure 6.2: The seamless integration of IoT, cloud computing, and AI analytics in delivering efficient telemedicine services.

6.3.4 Benefits and limitation of telemedicine in HHC

Comparative benefits of telemedicine in HHC

– Improved Accessibility: Telemedicine removes geographic barriers, allowing patients in remote areas to access specialists.
– Real-Time Monitoring: Continuous data tracking enables early detection of potential health issues.
– Cost-Effectiveness: Telemedicine reduces hospital visits and readmissions, thereby lowering healthcare costs.
– Patient Engagement: Interactive platforms empower patients to take an active role in managing their health.

Limitations and challenges

While telemedicine has revolutionized HHC, several challenges persist:
– Technological Barriers: Patients in rural or underserved areas often lack access to reliable internet connections or advanced devices.
– Data Privacy Concerns: Ensuring secure transmission and storage of sensitive health data is critical.
– Provider Training: Healthcare professionals must adapt to new technologies, which requires time and financial investment.

- Initial Costs: Implementing telemedicine infrastructure can be cost-prohibitive for smaller healthcare organizations.

6.3.5 Application of telemedicine

- **Chronic Disease Management:** Patients with diabetes use CGMs to monitor glucose levels. The data is analyzed by AI models, which alert healthcare providers to irregularities, prompting timely adjustments in insulin dosages.
- **Post-Surgical Care:** Post-operative patients attend virtual follow-up appointments via mobile health applications, reducing travel while ensuring effective recovery monitoring.
- **Cancer Care:** Telemedicine platforms support oncologists in remotely monitoring chemotherapy patients, ensuring that side effects are managed effectively (Xiang et al., 2023 [8]).

6.4 Predictive analytics and drug discovery in home healthcare

Predictive analytics has revolutionized personalized medicine in home healthcare (HHC), enabling tailored treatments that address individual patient needs. By analyzing historical and real-time data, predictive models can forecast disease progression, optimize treatment plans, and improve adherence to prescribed regimens. This approach significantly enhances patient outcomes, particularly in managing chronic and complex conditions such as cancer, diabetes, and cardiovascular diseases (Calster et al. 2019 [10]).

6.4.1 Key techniques in predictive analytics

Predictive analytics employs a variety of artificial intelligence (AI) and machine learning (ML) techniques (Kumar & Grag 2018 [11]), including:
- **Regression Models:**
    - Linear and logistic regression models predict health outcomes based on patient data.
    Example: Estimating the likelihood of hospital readmissions in patients with chronic illnesses.
- **Decision Trees and Random Forests:**
    - Tree-based models classify patients into risk categories and suggest optimal interventions.

- **Neural Networks:**
  - Deep learning models analyze complex data, such as genomics, to detect patterns associated with drug efficacy.
- **Clustering Techniques:**
  - Algorithms such as k-means clustering group patients based on health profiles, supporting personalized treatment planning (Belhor et al., 2023 [27]).
- **Time-Series Analysis:**
  - Recurrent neural networks (RNNs) predict changes in patient vitals over time, enabling proactive care.

6.4.2 Applications in drug discovery

- **Drug Adherence Monitoring**
  Predictive models identify patients at risk of non-adherence by analyzing behavioral and demographic data. Tailored interventions, such as reminders or teleconsultations, can improve adherence rates.
- **Disease Management**
  Predictive analytics can forecast disease progression, allowing timely adjustments to treatment plans. For instance, patients with heart failure benefit from AI models that predict decompensation based on daily monitoring data.
- **Optimizing Drug Dosages**
  Models such as pharmacokinetics simulators adjust drug dosages to individual metabolic rates, reducing side effects.

6.4.3 Workflow of predictive analytics in HHC

The typical workflow (Figure 6.3) for predictive analytics in HHC includes the following steps:
- **Data Collection**:
  - Patient data is collected through IoT devices (e. g., wearable ECGs, CGMs) and electronic health records (EHRs).
- **Data Preprocessing**:
  - Data is cleaned, normalized, and structured to remove errors and inconsistencies.
- **Model Training and Testing**:
  - Historical data is used to train machine learning (ML) models to detect patterns and predict outcomes.
- **Real-Time Monitoring**:
  - Deployed models analyze live data streams, detect anomalies and flag potential health risks.

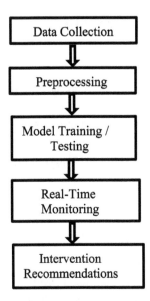

Figure 6.3: Workflow of predictive analytics in HHC.

– **Intervention Recommendations:**
  – Alerts are sent to healthcare providers, offering actionable insights and enabling timely interventions.

6.4.4 Application of predictive analytics

– **Chemotherapy Optimization**
  A cancer treatment center implemented a predictive model to optimize chemotherapy regimens. Based on patient genetics, vital signs, and treatment response history, the model adjusted drug dosages, reducing adverse effects and improving treatment efficacy (Xiang et al., 2023 [8]).
– **Diabetes Management**
  Predictive analytics combined with IoT devices such as CGMs monitored patients' glucose levels in real time. The system alerted providers to deviations, enabling timely insulin adjustments and preventing emergencies.
– **Cardiovascular Risk Prediction**
  AI-based models identified early signs of arrhythmias by analyzing ECG data from wearable devices. These proactive interventions reduced hospitalizations by 25 % in high-risk patients.

6.4.5 Benefits and limitations of predictive analytics in HHC

Benefits of predictive analytics in HHC

- Improved Accuracy: Predictive models outperform traditional methods by identifying subtle patterns in patient data.
- Proactive Interventions: Early detection reduces complications and improves survival rates.
- Cost Savings: By minimizing hospitalizations and adverse events, predictive analytics lowers healthcare costs (Jamarani et al. 2024 [12]).

Limitations and future scope

While predictive analytics holds immense potential, challenges remain:
- Data Quality: Inconsistent or incomplete patient data can reduce model accuracy.
- Model Interpretability: Healthcare providers often struggle to understand complex ML models.
- Integration Barriers: Integrating predictive systems with existing telemedicine platforms requires significant investment.

Emerging technologies such as explainable AI (XAI) and blockchain technology for secure data sharing could address these limitations, paving the way for widespread adoption in HHC.

6.5 Operations research in HHC optimization

Operations Research (OR) provides systematic methods for addressing logistical and operational challenges in home healthcare (HHC). By applying mathematical models, optimization algorithms, and simulation techniques, OR improves the efficiency of resource allocation, scheduling, and routing. This is critical for managing the complexity of HHC services, where timely delivery and coordination are vital for achieving patient outcomes (Goodarzian et al., 2023 [1]; Braekers et al., 2016 [3]; Demirbilek et al. 2019 [5]).

6.5.1 Key OR techniques in HHC

The important OR techniques in HHC as follows (Grieco et al. (2020) [13]):
1. **Mixed-Integer Linear Programming (MILP):**
    - MILP models solve problems involving discrete decisions, such as scheduling caregiver visits or allocating resources.

- Example: Optimizing nurse assignments to minimize travel time while meeting patient care requirements.
2. **Metaheuristics:**
   - Algorithms such as Particle Swarm Optimization (PSO) and Ant Colony Optimization (ACO) address large-scale, complex problems where exact solutions are infeasible.
   - Example: Routing ambulances or medical supply deliveries in real time.
3. **Stochastic Programming:**
   - This technique accounts for uncertainty in patient demand, ensuring robust solutions under variable conditions.
4. **Constraint Programming (CP):**
   - CP is used for scheduling tasks with strict constraints, such as caregiver availability and time windows for patient visits.
5. **Simulation Models:**
   - Simulations evaluate HHC scenarios, testing various strategies prior to implementation.

6.5.2 Applications of OR in HHC

1. **Caregiver Scheduling**
   - OR models optimize the assignment of caregivers based on location, patient needs, and time constraints (Nikzad et al., 2023 [7]).
   - Example: A study by Trautsamwieser and Hirsch (2011) [6] used Variable Neighborhood Search (VNS) to minimize nurse travel time and maximize patient satisfaction.
2. **Routing and Logistics**
   - Algorithms determine the most efficient routes for delivering medical supplies or transporting caregivers.
   - Example: Grenouilleau et al. (2019) [4] proposed a set partitioning heuristic for HHC routing, reducing overall costs.
3. **Inventory Management**
   - OR techniques maintain optimal stock levels of medical equipment at patients' homes, avoiding shortages or excess.
4. **Emergency Response**
   - Stochastic models improve response times for urgent medical needs, such as delivering medications to critically ill patients.

6.5.3 Workflow of OR-based logistics in HHC

The typical workflow for logistics optimization using OR techniques includes the following steps:

- **Data Input:** Collect data on caregiver availability, patient locations, service requirements, and estimated travel times.
- **Model Formulation:** Define objectives (e. g., minimizing cost or travel time) and constraints (e. g., time windows, resource limits).
- **Optimization Algorithm:** Apply MILP, metaheuristics, or other OR techniques to determine the optimal solution.
- **Implementation:** Deploy the optimized plan, such as caregiver schedules or delivery routes.
- **Monitoring and Adjustment:** Use real-time data to refine and adjust plans dynamically.

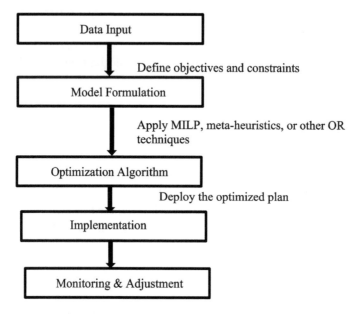

Figure 6.4: Workflow of OR-based logistics optimization.

This workflow (Figure 6.4) highlights how OR techniques systematically optimize complex logistics in HHC.

6.5.4 Application of OR techniques

- **Nurse Scheduling in Urban Areas:** A MILP model optimized nurse scheduling in a metropolitan HHC network, reducing travel time by 20 % and improving patient satisfaction (Trautsamwieser & Hirsch, 2011 [6]).

- **Routing Medical Supplies During COVID-19:** A metaheuristic algorithm enabled efficient delivery of oxygen cylinders to COVID-19 patients, ensuring timely availability despite high demand (Goodarzian et al., 2021 [2]; Oladzad-Abbasabady et al., 2023 [29]).
- **Hybrid Algorithms for Rural HHC:** In rural areas, where distances between patients are significant, hybrid algorithms combining ACO and genetic algorithms optimized caregiver routes, reducing costs by 15 %.

6.5.5 Benefits of OR in HHC

- **Efficiency Gains:** Optimized scheduling and routing reduce operational costs and caregiver fatigue.
- **Scalability:** OR models adapt to increasing patient demand, making them suitable for large-scale HHC systems.
- **Flexibility:** Stochastic models accommodate uncertainties such as last-minute patient requests or caregiver unavailability.

6.5.6 Challenges and future directions of OR techniques in HHC

While OR has proven its value in HHC, several challenges persist:
- **Data Integration:** OR models require accurate and comprehensive data, which can be difficult to collect in fragmented healthcare systems.
- **Computational Complexity:** Large-scale problems often require significant computational resources, particularly in real-time scenarios.
- **Adoption Barriers:** Smaller HHC providers may lack the expertise or resources to implement advanced OR models.

Future research should focus on developing hybrid OR-AI models that combine the robustness of OR with the adaptability of AI, enabling real-time, scalable solutions for HHC logistics.

6.6 Case studies and real-world applications

The integration of telemedicine, predictive analytics, and operations research in home healthcare (HHC) has led to measurable improvements in patient outcomes, operational efficiency, and cost-effectiveness. Below are detailed real-world examples that demonstrate the effectiveness of these technologies in various healthcare domains (Chabouh et al. 2023 [14]).

Case study 1. Cancer care at home: optimizing chemotherapy regimens

Providing cancer care at home presents significant challenging. Chemotherapy often requires frequent hospital visits, causing inconvenience and exposure to infections, especially during the COVID-19 pandemic (Nipp et al. 2022 [15]). Patients with cancer benefit from a model that allows them to undergo treatments at home, closely monitored through telemedicine and predictive analytics.

Virtual consultations with oncologists enable continuous monitoring of patients. AI models predict the effectiveness of chemotherapy drugs based on genetic data and patient history. These models adjust the chemotherapy dosage in real-time, minimizing side effects and improving treatment outcomes. IoT devices are used to track key patient metrics such as temperature, heart rate, and oxygen saturation, sending alerts to healthcare providers for timely interventions. Proper implementation of cancer care model in home healthcare offers significant advantages. Real-time adjustments to drug dosages significantly reduced the need for hospital visits. Patients reported an improved quality of life due to the convenience of home treatment and continuous virtual monitoring. Fewer hospital visits translated into reduced healthcare costs for both patients and providers.

Case study 2. Diabetes management: real-time glucose monitoring

Diabetes management involves constant monitoring of blood glucose levels, which can be difficult for patients to manage on their own, especially in rural or underserved areas. Inconsistent blood sugar levels can lead to complications such as diabetic ketoacidosis, affecting patient health. Doctors provide virtual consultations and continuous patient support, adjusting insulin dosages as required (Rghioui et al. 2020 [16]). Continuous glucose monitors (CGMs) collect real-time data on blood sugar levels, which are transmitted to healthcare providers for analysis. Using predictive analytics AI models predict glucose fluctuations based on diet, activity levels, and insulin usage, providing real-time suggestions to patients. Such a diabetes management model can enrich the healthcare system with multiple benefits. Patients received timely reminders and guidance for insulin adjustment, improving adherence to treatment protocols. Predictive models identified glucose anomalies before they became severe, preventing diabetic emergencies. Patients became more proactive in managing their health, with personalized interventions based on real-time data.

Case study 3. Emergency response: rapid medical intervention for heart attacks

Timely intervention is critical in emergency situations such as heart attacks, where every minute counts (Thomas et al. 2019 [17]). Delays in receiving treatment can lead to severe complications or death. Real-time video consultations and diagnostic support are required for patients experiencing symptoms of a heart attack (Hubert et al. 2023 [18]). IoT devices such as wearable ECG monitors detect signs of heart attacks, such as arrhythmias or irregular heart rates, and alert both patients and healthcare providers. AI models, analyzing data from IoT devices and medical histories, predict the likelihood of heart failure or other emergencies, facilitating rapid medical intervention. This model delivered several positive outcomes. It made the response time faster. Predictive analytics reduced the time between symptom onset and medical intervention, saving lives. Early interventions led to more effective treatments, reducing the need for extended hospital stays. The model was cost-effective, as reduced emergency room visits and shorter hospital stays saved significant healthcare costs.

Case study 4. Post-operative care: optimizing recovery at home

Post-operative patients often require frequent check-ups and monitoring to ensure proper recovery, leading to unnecessary hospital visits and extended stays (Nilsson et al. 2020 [19]). This burden can be reduced by allowing patients to communicate with healthcare providers via video consultations to assess their recovery. Smart bandages and sensors monitor wound healing, body temperature, and other vital signs, transmitting data to doctors for assessment. AI models predict potential complications, such as infections or blood clots, by analyzing real-time patient data and medical history. This model improved healthcare delivery in several ways. Virtual consultations and remote monitoring enabled post-operative recovery at home, reducing hospital readmissions. Patients experienced greater comfort recovering at home, with continuous support from healthcare professionals. Early detection of complications allowed for quicker interventions, improving overall recovery (Bell et al. 2019 [20]).

6.7 Future trends and emerging technologies in home healthcare

The future of home healthcare (HHC) is poised to be shaped by groundbreaking technologies that promise to enhance care delivery, ensure data security, and contribute to environmental sustainability. As the demand for HHC increases, these innovations will address the challenges of cost, scalability, and patient safety, while opening new avenues for improving patient outcomes (Chabouh et al. 2023 [14]). Below, we explore three emerging trends that are set to revolutionize HHC in the coming years.

6.7.1 Blockchain technology for secure telemedicine data management

The growing use of telemedicine in HHC has raised concerns regarding the privacy and security of sensitive patient data. Ensuring that data remains protected against breaches, while enabling seamless sharing among healthcare providers, is critical for the widespread adoption of telemedicine solutions (Ahmad et al. 2021 [21]). Blockchain technology offers a decentralized and immutable ledger system that ensures data security and transparency (refer Figure 6.5). Each patient's health data, including telemedicine interactions, can be stored in a distributed ledger, ensuring that the data cannot be altered or accessed by unauthorized parties. Smart contracts automatically enforce terms between patients, healthcare providers, and insurers, reducing administrative overhead and improving efficiency. Blockchain technology enables patients to own and control their data, sharing it only with authorized parties and ensuring that their privacy is maintained (Kushwaha et al. 2024 [22]). The benefits of such trend are as follows:
– Blockchain technology ensures secure, encrypted storage and transmission of health data, enhancing data security
– It maintains transparency by allowing patients and providers to trace the access and modification history of data, fostering trust.
– Blockchain technology enables seamless data sharing between different healthcare systems, improving care coordination.

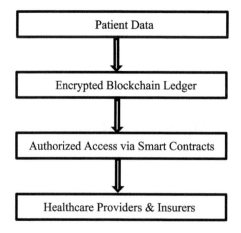

Figure 6.5: Blockchain for Telemedicine Data Security.

6.7.2 Advanced genomics in personalized medicine

Personalized medicine has emerged as a solution to optimize treatment plans for patients based on their genetic structure. However, integrating genomic data with HHC platforms and making it actionable for telemedicine services remains a challenge, particularly in resource-limited settings (Brunicardi et al. 2011 [23]). Advanced genomic sequencing techniques, such as CRISPR and next-generation sequencing (NGS) (Mallik et al. 2024 [25]), allow for deeper insights into the genetic profiles of patients. This information can be used to predict responses to specific drugs, tailor treatment regimens, and avoid adverse reactions. Pharmacogenomics examines how genetic variations influence individual responses to medications. Integrating pharmacogenomics with predictive analytics enables precise dosing and drug selection for patients, optimizing therapeutic outcomes. AI models analyze genomic data alongside clinical records to predict disease risk and treatment responses (Dhayalan et al. 2024 [24]). These models help healthcare providers make data-driven decisions about personalized therapies (refer Figure 6.6). The advantages of such technology include:
- Genomic data enables precise, patient-specific treatment plans, reducing adverse reactions and improving efficacy.
- Genetic risk factors can be identified, enabling earlier intervention for diseases such as cancer or cardiovascular diseases.
- Genomic data accelerates the identification of new drug candidates by pinpointing genetic factors related to disease progression.

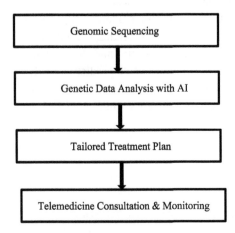

Figure 6.6: Advanced Genomics in Personalized Medicine.

6.7.3 Emerging trends of AI in real-time decision making

The ongoing evolution of AI will play a central role in real-time decision-making for HHC (Yang, et al., 2023 [26]). As AI models become more advanced, they will process vast amounts of patient data from telemedicine consultations, wearables, and predictive analytics in real time. This will enable instant recommendations for treatment adjustments, emergency interventions, and patient care optimization.
   Emerging AI Technologies:
- **Deep Learning:** Advanced neural networks will identify complex patterns in health data, enabling proactive disease management.
- **Natural Language Processing (NLP):** NLP will allow healthcare providers to analyze unstructured data, such as patient communication and medical records, in real time.

These technologies will work synergistically with telemedicine platforms, ensuring that care delivery is always timely, personalized, and data-driven. This integration improves patient outcomes and reduces healthcare costs.

6.8 Conclusion and vision for the future

The future of home healthcare (HHC) will be driven by innovative technologies that integrate telemedicine, predictive analytics, genomic data, and sustainable logistics. As these technologies evolve, they will make HHC more efficient, personalized, and accessible. By leveraging AI, blockchain technology, and advanced genomics, the healthcare system can provide better care at lower costs, especially for chronic and elderly patients. In future, we plan to develop and optimize such AI models using predictive analytics, deep learning, NGS technology, blockchain technology to enhance critical disease monitoring and treatment in home healthcare, improving efficiency while reducing healthcare costs and patient inconvenience.

Bibliography

[1] Goodarzian, F., Shokri Garjan, H. & Ghasemi, P. (2023). A state-of-the-art review of operation research models and applications in home healthcare. Healthc. Anal., 4, 100228. https://doi.org/10.1016/j.health.2023.100228.
[2] Goodarzian, F., Abraham, A. & Fathollahi-Fard, A. M. (2021). A bi-objective home healthcare logistics considering the working time and route balancing: a self-adaptive social engineering optimizer. J. Comput. Des. Eng., 8(1), 452–474.
[3] Braekers, K., Hartl, R. F., Parragh, S. N. & Tricoire, F. (2016). A bi-objective homecare scheduling problem: analyzing the trade-off between costs and client inconvenience. Eur. J. Oper. Res., 248(2), 428–443.

[4] Grenouilleau, F., Legrain, A., Lahrichi, N. & Rousseau, L. M. (2019). A set partitioning heuristic for the home healthcare routing and scheduling problem. Eur. J. Oper. Res., 275(1), 295–303.
[5] Demirbilek, M., Branke, J. & Strauss, A. (2019). Dynamically accepting and scheduling patients for home healthcare. Healthc. Manag. Sci., 22(1), 140–155.
[6] Trautsamwieser, A. & Hirsch, P. (2011). Optimization of daily scheduling for home healthcare services. J. Appl. Oper. Res., 3(3), 124–136.
[7] Nikzad, E., Bashiri, M. & Abbasi, B. (2023). Home healthcare staff dimensioning problem for temporary caregivers: a metaheuristic solution approach. Comput. Oper. Res., 106126.
[8] Xiang, T., Li, Y. & Szeto, W. Y. (2023). The daily routing and scheduling problem of home health care: based on costs and participants' preference satisfaction. Int. Trans. Oper. Res., 30(1), 39–69. 2021.
[9] Warner, I. (1997). Telemedicine applications for home health care. J. Telemed. Telecare, 3(Suppl. 1), 65–66. https://doi.org/10.1258/1357633971930427. PMID: 9218389.
[10] Van Calster, B., Wynants, L., Timmerman, D., Steyerberg, E. W. & Collins, G. S. (2019). Predictive analytics in health care: how can we know it works? J. Am. Med. Inform. Assoc., 26(12), 1651–1654. https://doi.org/10.1093/jamia/ocz130. PMID: 31373357; PMCID: PMC6857503.
[11] Kumar, V. & Garg, M. L. (2018). Predictive analytics: a review of trends and techniques. Int. J. Comput. Appl., 182(1), 31–37. https://doi.org/10.5120/ijca2018917434.
[12] Jamarani, A., Haddadi, S., Sarvizadeh, R., et al. (2024). Big data and predictive analytics: a systematic review of applications. Artif. Intell. Rev., 57, 176. https://doi.org/10.1007/s10462-024-10811-5.
[13] Grieco, L., Utley, M. & Crowe, S. (2020). Operational research applied to decisions in home health care: a systematic literature review. J. Oper. Res. Soc., 72(9), 1960–1991. https://doi.org/10.1080/01605682.2020.1750311.
[14] Chabouh, S., El-Amraoui, A., Hammami, S. & Bouchriha, H. (2023). A systematic review of the home health care planning literature: emerging trends and future research directions. Decis. Anal. J., 7, 100215, ISSN 2772-6622. https://doi.org/10.1016/j.dajour.2023.100215.
[15] Nipp, R. D., Shulman, E., Smith, M., et al. (2022). Supportive oncology care at home interventions: protocols for clinical trials to shift the paradigm of care for patients with cancer. BMC Cancer, 22, 383. https://doi.org/10.1186/s12885-022-09461-z.
[16] Rghioui, A., Lloret, J., Harane, M. & Oumnad, A. (2020). A smart glucose monitoring system for diabetic patient. Electronics, 9(4), 678. https://doi.org/10.3390/electronics9040678.
[17] Thomas, R. J., Beatty, A. L., Beckie, T. M., Brewer, L. C., Brown, T. M., Forman, D. E., Franklin, B. A., Keteyian, S. J., Kitzman, D. W., Regensteiner, J. G., Sanderson, B. K. & Whooley, M. A. (2019). Home-based cardiac rehabilitation: a scientific statement from the American Association of Cardiovascular and Pulmonary Rehabilitation, the American Heart Association, and the American College Of Cardiology. J. Cardiopulm. Rehabil. Prev. 39(4), 208–225. https://doi.org/10.1097/HCR.0000000000000447. PMID: 31082934; PMCID: PMC7530797.
[18] Haywood, H. B., Fonarow, G. C., Khan, M. S., Van Spall, H. G. C., Morris, A. A., Nassif, M. E., Kittleson, M. M., Butler, J. & Greene, S. J. (2023). Hospital at home as a treatment strategy for worsening heart failure. Circ. Heart Fail. J., 16(10), e010456. https://www.ahajournals.org/doi/abs/10.1161/CIRCHEARTFAILURE.122.010456.
[19] Nilsson, U., Gruen, R. & Myles, P. S. Postoperative recovery: the importance of the team, 05 January 2020, Wiley. https://doi.org/10.1111/anae.14869.
[20] Bell, M., Eriksson, L. I., Svensson, T., Hallqvist, L., Granath, F., Reilly, J. & Myles, P. S. (2019). Days at home after surgery: an integrated and efficient outcome measure for clinical trials and quality assurance. eClinicalMedicine, 27(11), 18–26. https://doi.org/10.1016/j.eclinm.2019.04.011. PMID: 31317130; PMCID: PMC6610780.
[21] Ahmad, R. W., Salah, K., Jayaraman, R., Yaqoob, I., Ellahham, S. & Omar, M. (2021). The role of blockchain technology in telehealth and telemedicine. Int. J. Med. Inform., 148, 104399, ISSN 1386-5056. https://doi.org/10.1016/j.ijmedinf.2021.104399.

[22] Kushwaha, A., Chauhan, R., Rawat, R., Aluvala, S. & Singh, R. (2024). Role of blockchain in tele-health and tele-medicine. In 2024 IEEE 9th International Conference for Convergence in Technology (I2CT), Pune, India (pp. 1–6). https://doi.org/10.1109/I2CT61223.2024.10543999.

[23] Brunicardi, F. C., Gibbs, R. A., Wheeler, D. A., Nemunaitis, J., Fisher, W., Goss, J. & Chen, C. (2011). Overview of the development of personalized genomic medicine and surgery. World J. Surg. 35(8), 1693–1699. https://doi.org/10.1007/s00268-011-1056-0. PMID: 21424870; PMCID: PMC3281749.

[24] Dhayalan, M., Wang, W., Mohammed Riyaz, S. U., Dinesh, R. A., Shanmugam, J., Irudayaraj, S. S., Stalin, A., Giri, J., Mallik, S. & Hu, R. (2024. Advances in functional lipid nanoparticles: from drug delivery platforms to clinical applications. 3 Biotech, 14(2): 57. https://doi.org/10.1007/s13205-023-03901-8.

[25] Mallik, S., Gaur, L., Seth, S., Bhadra, T. & Wang, M. (2024). 1 Introduction: fundamentals of next-generation sequencing, pattern recognition, and biomedical images. In Landscape of Next Generation Sequencing Using Pattern Recognition: Performance Analysis and Applications (pp. 1–28). River Publishers.

[26] Yang, C.-H., Chen, Y.-C., Hsu, W. & Chen, Y.-H. (2023). Evaluation of smart long-term care information strategy portfolio decision model: the national healthcare environment in Taiwan. Ann. Oper. Res. (in press).

[27] Belhor, M., El-Amraoui, A., Jemai, A. & Delmotte, F. (2023). Multi-objective evolutionary approach based on K-means clustering for home health care routing and scheduling problem. Expert Syst. Appl., 213, 119035.

[28] Weiping, X., Liu, T., Li, X. & Zheng, C. (2023). Robust homecare service capacity planning. Comput. Oper. Res., 154, 106155.

[29] Oladzad-Abbasabady, N., Tavakkoli-Moghaddam, R., Mohammadi, M. & Vahedi-Nouri, B. (2023). A bi-objective home care routing and scheduling problem considering patient preference and soft temporal dependency constraints. Eng. Appl. Artif. Intell., 119, 105829.

Saboor Uddin Ahmed, Preetam Suman, Akshara Makrariya, and
Rabia Musheer Aziz

7 AI-driven insights: a machine learning approach to lung cancer diagnosis

Abstract: Lung discomfort emerges as a prevalent early symptom in cancer treatment, posing significant diagnostic challenges due to delays in radiologist assessments. To address this, we propose an advanced computational framework designed to assist radiologists in the precise detection of lung cancer. This study introduces a multi-tiered prognostic model leveraging cutting-edge machine learning (ML) techniques. The segmentation process employs a threshold-based and marker-controlled watershed algorithm, coupled with a dual-classifier system, to enhance data refinement and accuracy. Detecting lung cancer demands exceptional sensitivity, achieved through training on a curated dataset using sophisticated algorithms including Support Vector Machine (SVM), K-Nearest Neighbors (KNN), Decision Tree (DT), Logistic Regression (LR), Naive Bayes (NB), and Random Forest (RF). Notably, the Random Forest algorithm delivers a superior performance metric, achieving an accuracy of 88.5 %. This innovative approach underscores the transformative potential of integrating advanced ML methodologies with radiological expertise to revolutionize early lung cancer diagnosis and improve patient outcomes.

Keywords: Lung cancer, machine learning, computational diagnostics, segmentation, watershed algorithm, Random Forest, SVM, KNN, Decision Tree, Logistic Regression, Naive Bayes, radiologist assistance

7.1 Introduction

Lung cancer remains a major global health challenge, contributing to approximately 1.8 million deaths annually, making it the leading cause of cancer-related mortality worldwide (WHO, 2023). The disease often manifests through early symptoms such as respiratory discomfort, fatigue, and chest pain, which are frequently overlooked or misdiagnosed due to their non-specific nature. Risk factors for lung cancer are multifaceted,

---

Saboor Uddin Ahmed, Preetam Suman, School of Computing Science and Engineering, VIT Bhopal University, Kothrikalan, Sehore, Madhya Pradesh – 466114, India, e-mails: saboor.ahmed2021@vitbhopal.ac.in, preetam.suman@vitbhopal.ac.in
Akshara Makrariya, School of Advanced Sciences and Language, VIT Bhopal University, Kothrikalan, Sehore, Madhya Pradesh – 466114, India, e-mail: akshara.makrariya@vitbhopal.ac.in
Rabia Musheer Aziz, Researcher Officer, State Planning Institute, Planning Department, Lucknow, Utter Pradesh – 226001, India, e-mail: rabia.aziz2010@gmail.com

encompassing demographic variables like age and gender, physiological markers such as blood pressure and obesity, and lifestyle factors including smoking, alcohol consumption, and irregular heart rates. Smoking, in particular, stands out as a predominant risk factor, with smokers being 15–30 times more likely to develop lung cancer compared to non-smokers (CDC, 2023). The disease primarily presents in two forms: Non-Small Cell Lung Cancer (NSCLC), which accounts for 85 % of cases, and Small-Cell Lung Cancer (SCLC), a more aggressive subtype. Both types originate from the uncontrolled growth of aberrant cells in the lung tissue, often forming tumors in the bronchi that metastasize rapidly, leading to high mortality rates, especially among individuals over 60. Early detection is critical, as the five-year survival rate for lung cancer drops from 59 % at localized stages to 6 % once metastasis occurs (American Cancer Society, 2023) [1–5].

Traditional diagnostic methods, such as imaging (e. g., CT scans) and biopsy, rely heavily on radiologist expertise, often leading to delays in diagnosis and treatment. Moreover, the complexity of lung cancer exacerbated by its association with comorbidities like chronic diseases, allergies, and anxiety demands more sophisticated approaches for accurate risk stratification and prognosis. Recent advancements in data mining and machine learning (ML) have opened new avenues for addressing these challenges by enabling the analysis of complex, multidimensional datasets to uncover hidden patterns associated with lung cancer risk. Previous studies have explored ML techniques for lung cancer prediction, employing algorithms such as K-Nearest Neighbors (KNN), Decision Trees (DT), Naive Bayes (NB), Logistic Regression (LR), and Support Vector Machines (SVM) to classify patients based on imaging or clinical data (Smith et al., 2022; Jones & Lee, 2021) [6, 7]. However, these studies often focus on a limited set of features, neglecting the broader spectrum of risk factors that contribute to lung cancer development. There are some modern methods for analyzing lung cancer. The dataset includes features such as thalassemia, constrictive pericarditis, smoking, peer pressure, gender, age, smoking, yellow_fingers, anxiety, chronic disease, fatigue, allergy, wheezing, alcohol consuming, coughing, shortness of breath, swallowing difficulty, and chest pain. The dataset was split into 75 % for training and 25 % for testing to build and evaluate the prediction model.

This study aims to bridge this gap by developing a comprehensive ML-based framework for the early detection of lung cancer, leveraging an extensive set of predictive features. These features include demographic factors (age, gender), behavioral factors (smoking, alcohol consumption, peer pressure), clinical symptoms (coughing, shortness of breath, chest pain, swallowing difficulty, wheezing, fatigue), and health conditions (thalassemia, constrictive pericarditis, chronic diseases, allergies, yellow fingers, anxiety). By employing data mining techniques, such as clustering, we preprocess the dataset to enhance feature segmentation and improve model performance. The dataset was split into 75 % for training and 25 % for testing, ensuring robust validation of the proposed models. A suite of ML algorithms—KNN, DT, NB, LR, and SVM—is applied to classify patients and identify metabolic patterns linked to lung cancer risk. This research seeks not only to improve diagnostic accuracy but also to provide actionable insights for clinicians, ultimately reducing the burden of lung cancer mortality through timely and precise interventions.

7.2 Literature survey

7.2.1 Bronchi failure prediction by applying ML models

Lung cancer, characterized by the uncontrolled proliferation of abnormal cells leading to malignant tumors, is one of the most prevalent and lethal cancers affecting both men and women globally. Recent advancements in machine learning (ML) have significantly improved the predictive modeling of bronchial failure, offering new opportunities for early diagnosis and intervention. This section reviews key methodologies and algorithms employed in the literature to address this critical health challenge.

A fundamental approach to ML-based cancer prediction leverages neural network models, often rooted in qualitative data analysis. Central to this approach is the back-propagation algorithm, which optimizes multilayer perceptrons (MLPs) through the gradient descent technique. In this process, initial weights are randomly assigned, and the network iteratively propagates inputs through hidden layers, computing the weighted contributions of each neuron. Activation functions at each neuron generate outputs, which are propagated forward until the output layer is reached. The resulting output is then compared to the target, calculating the error at the output layer. This error is back propagated to adjust weights, minimizing discrepancies through iterative updates. Such models excel in real-world prediction tasks, offering robust solutions for complex optimization problems in cancer diagnostics [8–10].

Another significant advancement lies in the application of Long Short-Term Memory (LSTM) networks, a specialized form of recurrent neural networks (RNNs), for time-series analysis and predictive tasks in lung cancer detection. LSTMs are designed with a sophisticated architecture comprising memory cells, input gates, output gates, and forget gates, enabling them to selectively retain or discard information over extended sequences. The forget gate plays a pivotal role by filtering out irrelevant data, while the input gate regulates the assimilation of new information. The output gate, utilizing a sigmoid activation function, determines the final output based on the cell state. By maintaining a memory of past events through weighted connections, LSTMs effectively capture temporal dependencies, reducing network errors and enhancing predictive accuracy in bronchial failure analysis [11, 12].

Additionally, Support Vector Regression (SVR), an extension of Support Vector Machines (SVMs), has emerged as a powerful tool for tackling regression-based prediction challenges in lung cancer prognosis. SVR aims to preserve the integrity of the original data values in dual-format prediction scenarios by minimizing the margin of error between observed and predicted outcomes. This is achieved by constructing support vectors—subsets of training examples—that define the decision boundary and optimize the model's generalization performance. By reducing the deviation between actual and predicted values, SVR ensures high-fidelity predictions, making it an invaluable asset in the computational diagnosis of lung cancer.

Collectively, these methods underscore the transformative potential of ML in predicting bronchial failure, paving the way for more accurate, data-driven diagnostic tools. This study builds on this foundation by integrating advanced ML techniques to further improve the precision and reliability of lung cancer detection systems.

7.2.2 Multiple phase lung failure detection by SVM model

Advances in lung cancer diagnostics have increasingly relied on sophisticated image enhancement techniques to generate high-resolution images that improve detection accuracy. This subsection explores methods that utilize computed tomography (CT) scans to identify lung cancer through a multi-phase approach. A critical step in this process involves the application of selective median filtering to preprocess masked CT images, which effectively reduces noise and enhances contrast to highlight anatomical structures essential for cancer detection. This preprocessing technique significantly improves the clarity of CT images, facilitating the subsequent stages of image processing and malignancy prediction [13].

A pivotal aspect of this methodology is the delineation of hydrological lines through marker-based edge detection, which compares marker boundaries to establish precise contours. This approach remains robust against challenges posed by low-contrast edges and neighborhood minima, ensuring that subtle tissue variations are accurately captured without interference from surrounding artifacts. This is followed by the feature extraction phase, which requires the systematic organization of extensive pixel data into a descending order of relevance to isolate significant diagnostic markers. This process distinguishes normal tissue patterns from abnormal deviations, leveraging pixel intensity arrangements to quantify textural and structural features indicative of lung cancer [14].

The extracted features are then classified using the Support Vector Machine (SVM) algorithm, a powerful machine learning tool renowned for its efficacy in distinguishing cancer cells from healthy tissue. SVM operates by constructing an optimal hyperplane that maximizes the margin between classes, enabling precise categorization of cancer stages within both localized damaged lung cells and broader affected regions. This multi-phase approach—integrating image enhancement, robust edge detection, feature extraction, and SVM-based classification—offers a comprehensive framework for lung cancer detection, enhancing diagnostic precision and supporting early intervention strategies.

7.2.3 Effects of race and smoking history on the ability of an electronic nose to detect lung cancer early in heavy smokers

Early detection of lung cancer in its nascent stages is a critical frontier in respiratory health, with breath analysis emerging as a promising non-invasive diagnostic tool. Exhaled breath serves as a reliable biomarker for respiratory diseases, including chronic obstructive pulmonary disease (COPD) and asthma, reflecting the dynamic equilibrium between oxygen levels and volatile organic compounds (VOCs) in respiratory plasma during disease monitoring. This approach has gained traction for lung cancer detection, leveraging electronic nose (e-nose) technology equipped with an array of sensors designed to detect synthetic VOCs. These sensors, coated with reactive compounds, generate electrical impulses through chemical interactions that produce measurable changes in resistance that are highly sensitive to molecular composition. This capability enables real-time chemical analysis of breath samples, offering a rapid and non-invasive method to screen for lung cancer [15].

The e-nose system typically integrates 32 polymeric sensors, each exhibiting a unique resistance pattern that collectively forms a distinctive olfactory fingerprint. This technology has proven effective in assessing advanced lung cancer, evaluating smoking-related complications, and monitoring high-risk current smokers. Pattern recognition algorithms are employed to process the sensor data and identify specific breath signatures associated with lung cancer. Research has explored the design of integrated case studies, focusing on individuals diagnosed with lung cancer, with demographic data indicating an age range of 45–79 years for both sexes. The study emphasizes the interplay between race and smoking history, key variables influencing lung cancer risk, particularly among heavy smokers. Detection efforts often rely on low-dose computed tomography (LDCT), which complements e-nose findings by providing anatomical validation of lung tumors. This synergistic approach underscores the potential of e-nose technology to enhance early detection strategies by tailoring interventions to high-risk populations defined by racial and smoking profiles [16].

7.3 Suggestive methodology

The development of an effective lung cancer detection system relies on a structured methodological framework that integrates comprehensive data handling and advanced machine learning techniques. The process begins with the acquisition of a robust dataset containing a wide range of patient-specific attributes, including smoking status, peer influence, age, gender, and family medical history. This dataset is meticulously preprocessed to eliminate inconsistencies, standardize variable scales, and achieve a balanced representation of lung cancer-positive and -negative cases, thereby mitigating potential biases in subsequent analyses. Figure 7.1 shows all features of data.

age	sex	cp	trtbps	chol	fbs	restecg	thalachh	exng	oldpeak
63	1	3	145	233	1	0	150	0	2.:
37	1	2	130	250	0	1	187	0	3.!
41	0	1	130	204	0	0	172	0	1.⟨
56	1	1	120	236	0	1	178	0	0.⟨
57	0	0	120	354	0	1	163	1	0.⟨
57	1	0	140	192	0	1	148	0	0.⟨
56	0	1	140	294	0	0	153	0	1.:
44	1	1	120	263	0	1	173	0	(
52	1	2	172	199	1	1	162	0	0.!
57	1	2	150	168	0	1	174	0	1.⟨
54	1	0	140	239	0	1	160	0	1.:
48	0	2	130	275	0	1	139	0	0.:
49	1	1	130	266	0	1	171	0	0.⟨
64	1	3	110	211	0	0	144	1	1.⟨
58	0	3	150	283	1	0	162	0	:
50	0	2	120	219	0	1	158	0	1.⟨
58	0	2	120	340	0	1	172	0	(
66	0	3	150	226	0	1	114	0	2.⟨
43	1	0	150	247	0	1	171	0	1.!
69	0	3	140	239	0	1	151	0	1.⟨
59	1	0	135	234	0	1	161	0	0.!

Figure 7.1: The dataset used in the above models.

Following preprocessing, feature engineering is employed to derive meaningful predictors from the dataset. Quantitative features such as lung tissue density, lesion size, and morphological characteristics are extracted alongside qualitative factors such as smoking intensity and peer pressure exposure. These engineered features are then integrated into a machine learning pipeline using robust classifiers such as Decision Tree or Random Forest algorithms, known for their interpretability and predictive power in medical diagnostics.

The training phase involves fitting the selected model to the pre-processed dataset, with optimization achieved through cross-validation techniques to prevent overfitting and enhance generalization across different patient cohorts. Model performance is rigorously assessed using a number of evaluation metrics, including accuracy, precision, recall, and F1-score, providing a comprehensive view of the model's diagnostic efficacy. To establish its competitiveness, the proposed model is benchmarked against leading state-of-the-art models documented in the literature, ensuring that it meets or exceeds contemporary standards in lung cancer detection.

In conclusion, this methodology outlines a systematic approach to lung cancer detection that leverages machine learning through sequential stages of data collection and preprocessing, feature engineering, model training with optimization, performance evaluation, and feature importance analysis. This framework aims to harness the interplay of lifestyle and genetic factors to improve early detection and inform clinical decision-making.

7.4 Design modules

The design of the lung cancer detection system is structured around a series of interconnected modules that facilitate efficient data handling, analysis, and visualization. The dataset, consisting of 303 records, is obtained from Kaggle.com and stored in CSV format for streamlined processing. To support data manipulation and visualization, essential Python libraries—pandas, matplotlib, and seaborn—are imported. Pandas enables robust data management, while matplotlib and seaborn provide advanced visualization capabilities, transforming numerical data into insightful graphical representations.

A key module focuses on exploratory data analysis (EDA), where statistical measures such as percentage distributions, mean, and standard deviation are computed to characterize the dataset. Using seaborn's visualization functions, the module generates plots to illustrate the average prevalence of lung cancer across affected and unaffected populations, offering a clear depiction of class distributions. Statistical analysis reveals that approximately 70 % of the normalized data values lie within the range of –1 to 1, indicating a standardized distribution suitable for subsequent modeling. Additionally, a target identification module leverages pandas' functionality to locate and isolate the target variable (lung cancer presence/absence), ensuring accurate labeling for supervised learning tasks.

This modular design provides a solid foundation for data preprocessing and analysis, enabling the seamless integration of machine learning models in later stages while providing a comprehensive understanding characteristics of the dataset through statistical and visual insights.

7.4.1 Data classification

The classification phase of the lung cancer detection framework is a pivotal step that ensures the robustness and reliability of machine learning models through systematic data partitioning and preparation. To facilitate this process, the train_test_split function from the sklearn.model_selection module of the scikit-learn library is employed. This method is a cornerstone in evaluating the performance of machine learning algorithms, providing a standardized approach to assessing model generalization on unseen data. The procedure begins with the acquisition and initial refinement of the dataset, which consists of 303 records sourced from Kaggle.com, described in the design modules.

The dataset undergoes a meticulous cleaning process to address missing values, inconsistencies, and outliers to ensure high quality input for model training. Following this, the train_test_split function is used to split the dataset into two distinct subsets: a training set and a test set. This split is strategically designed to allocate 203 records (approximately 67 %) for training purposes, enabling the model to learn intricate patterns and relationships within the data, while the remaining 100 records (approximately 33 %) are reserved for testing to evaluate the model's predictive accuracy on unseen data. This proportional partitioning follows to common practices in machine learning, balancing the need for sufficient training data with the requirement for a robust evaluation set.

The partitioning process is essential to address both the regression and classification challenges inherent in lung cancer detection. By training the model on a substantial portion of the dataset, it can effectively capture the underlying features—such as smoking status, peer influence, age, and clinical symptoms—that differentiate lung cancer cases from healthy cases. The test subset, meanwhile, serves as a benchmark to quantify the model's performance through metrics such as accuracy, precision, recall, and F1-score, ensuring that the model generalizes well beyond the training data. This methodology not only enhances the reliability of the predictive model but also aligns with machine learning best practices and lays a solid foundation for subsequent stages of model development and validation.

7.4.2 Machine learning algorithms

7.4.2.1 K-Nearest Neighbor algorithm (KNN)

The K-Nearest Neighbor (KNN) algorithm represents a cornerstone of supervised learning methods, known for its simplicity and effectiveness in classifying new data instances based on their similarity to existing cases within a dataset. This algorithm operates by leveraging the intrinsic relationships among data points, making it an intuitive choice for predictive modeling in lung cancer detection. At its core, KNN relies on the principle of "feature similarity," where the proximity of data points in a feature space determines their classification. The process begins by selecting the K nearest neighbors to a given unclassified data point, where proximity is typically measured using the Euclidean distance metric, which quantifies the geometric separation between points across multiple dimensions [17, 18].

Once the K nearest neighbors are identified—often set within a range such as 20 neighbors in practical implementations—the algorithm categorizes the target data point based on the majority class among these neighbors. This majority voting mechanism assigns the new data point to the class most prevalent among its K nearest neighbors, ensuring a data-driven decision-making process. The algorithm's strength lies in its nonparametric nature, allowing it to adapt to complex, non-linear patterns in datasets such as those containing smoking status, peer influence, and clinical symptoms. Visualization of the classification outcomes, often presented as graphical representations, further enhances interpretability by showing the distribution and clustering of data points across the feature space. This approach not only facilitates accurate classification, but also offers a transparent framework for understanding the underlying dynamics of lung cancer risk factors, making KNN a compelling tool in this study's analytical arsenal. Figure 7.2 illustrates the ROC curve obtained using the K-Nearest Neighbors (KNN) algorithm for lung cancer detection.

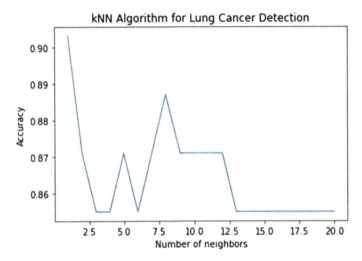

Figure 7.2: Roc curve for lung cancer detection using KNN algorithm.

7.4.2.2 Random Forest algorithm

Random Forest is considered as a widely recognized algorithm in the field of machine learning, renowned for its versatility in tackling classification, regression, and other complex predictive tasks. As an ensemble learning technique, Random Forest harnesses the collective power of multiple decision trees constructed during the training phase using distinct strategies. For classification tasks, the algorithm aggregates the mode of the class predictions from individual trees to yield a final output, while for regression tasks, it computes the mean of the predicted values, ensuring a robust consensus-driven result. This multi-tree architecture enhances the predictive capability of the model, making it particularly effective for applications such as lung cancer detection, where diverse features such as smoking history, peer influence, and clinical symptoms are analyzed [19, 20].

A distinctive feature of Random Forest lies in its training methodology, where each decision tree is built on a randomly sampled subset of the dataset and a randomly selected subset of features. This bagging approach, coupled with the randomness of the features, mitigates the risk of overfitting a common pitfall in single-tree models—thereby elevating the overall accuracy and generalizability of the model. The algorithm also incorporates sophisticated mechanisms to manage missing data, a critical advantage when handling real-world datasets that often contain incomplete or noisy records. By imputing missing values based on the proximity of available data points within the ensemble, Random Forest ensures robust performance even under challenging data conditions. This blend of ensemble diversity, overfitting prevention, and data imputation positions Random Forest as a powerful and reliable tool, offering a sophisticated framework for advancing diagnostic precision in medical research and beyond.

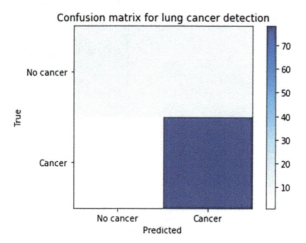

Figure 7.3: Confusion matrix for lung cancer detection using Random Forest algorithm.

Figure 7.3 presents the confusion matrix generated for lung cancer detection using the Random Forest classifier.

7.4.2.3 Decision Tree algorithm

Decision Tree is a widely adopted supervised learning technique used for solving both classification and regression tasks. It operates by learning decision rules inferred from prior data features and corresponding labels. The primary goal of a decision tree is to create a model that predicts the target variable by learning simple decision rules derived from historical data patterns.

The construction of a decision tree begins at the root node, which represents the feature that best splits the dataset based on a specific criterion—commonly Gini impurity, information gain (based on Entropy), or variance reduction (in regression problems). The tree is then recursively partitioned into branches, each representing a subset of the data that satisfies certain conditions defined by the decision node. Internal nodes (decision nodes) perform evaluations on selected features, while terminal nodes (leaf nodes) correspond to the predicted output or class label [21, 22].

The hierarchical structure of decision trees allows them to model non-linear decision boundaries, making them interpretable and suitable for domains requiring transparent decision-making processes. Model training involves recursively selecting the best feature to partition the dataset at each node, optimizing for homogeneity within the resulting branches. The prediction phase involves traversing the tree from the root to a leaf by evaluating the feature-based conditions at each decision node.

In practice, decision tree performance is evaluated using metrics such as accuracy, precision, recall, F1-score (for classification), and mean squared error (for regression).

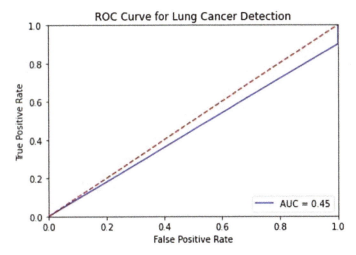

Figure 7.4: Roc curve for lung cancer detection using DT algorithm.

Overfitting is a common challenge with decision trees, often mitigated by techniques such as pruning, setting maximum tree depth, or using ensemble methods such as Random Forests or Gradient Boosted Trees for better generalization. Figure 7.4 shows the ROC curve illustrating the performance of the Decision Tree (DT) algorithm in detecting lung cancer.

7.4.2.4 Logistic Regression

Logistic regression (LR) is a fundamental supervised learning algorithm that is widely used for binary classification problems. Unlike linear regression, which predicts continuous values, logistic regression estimates the probability that a given input point belongs to a particular class. It is particularly useful when the dependent variable is categorical typically binary such as "yes or no," "true or false," or "positive or negative."

The logistic regression model is based on fitting a logistic (sigmoid) function to a linear combination of input features. The sigmoid function maps the predicted value to a range between 0 and 1, effectively providing a probabilistic interpretation of the classification [23, 24]. Figure 7.5 presents the ROC curve for lung cancer detection using the Logistic Regression algorithm, achieving an accuracy of 0.99.

Logistic regression is particularly effective in medical diagnostics (e. g., predicting whether a tumor is malignant or benign), credit scoring, and many other domains that require a probabilistic framework for decision-making. Although the underlying model is linear in the log-odds, its output is nonlinear due to the sigmoid transformation, allowing it to robustly handle real-world binary classification tasks.

One of the strengths of logistic regression lies in its simplicity, interpretability, and ability to work well with both continuous and discrete input variables. Despite the rise

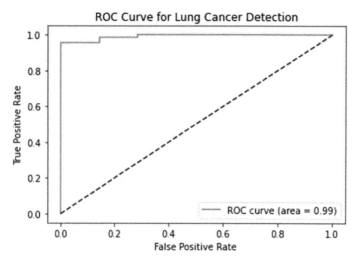

Figure 7.5: Roc curve for lung cancer detection using logistic algorithm.

of more complex machine learning models, logistic regression remains a critical tool, particularly when model tractability and computational efficiency are important considerations.

7.4.2.5 Naïve Bayes algorithm

Probably one of the easiest classification algorithms for building quick models for machine learning, the Naïve Bayes algorithm is known as a supervised learning method based on its application of the Bayes theorem to solve its classification tasks. Its probabilistic classifier is used to predict the probability of an object based on its data. It is composed of Naïve and Bayes, and based on its recognized color, shape, and taste, it has some features that are independent of other features [25–27]. Figure 7.6 shows the confusion matrix generated using the Naïve Bayes algorithm for lung cancer detection.

7.4.2.6 Support Vector Machine

Support Vector Machine (SVM) is a widely used machine learning algorithm, primarily designed for classification and regression tasks. The fundamental principle behind SVM is the construction of a hyperplane in a high-dimensional feature space that separates data points into distinct classes. The goal of the algorithm is to identify the optimal hyperplane that maximizes the margin between the two classes. By maximizing this margin, SVM improves the generalization ability of the model, ensuring better performance on unseen data. To handle nonlinear relationships between data points, SVM

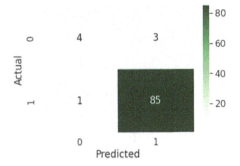

Figure 7.6: Confusion matrix by using Naïve Bayes algorithm for lung cancer detection.

employs kernel functions that transform the data into a higher-dimensional space. In this transformed space, it becomes more feasible to find a linear hyperplane that effectively divides the data into the desired classes. This flexibility makes SVM particularly effective in scenarios where the data is not linearly separable in the original feature space [27–30]. Figure 7.7 illustrates the average fitness per iteration and the ROC curve for lung cancer detection using the Support Vector Machine (SVM) algorithm.

7.5 Result

To detect lung failure at an early stage, several supervised machine learning algorithms were implemented and evaluated on a structured clinical dataset. The applied algorithms include decision tree, logistic regression, and others, as described in previous sections. Each model was trained using historical patient health data and validated based on classification accuracy and other performance metrics.

Among the models tested, Logistic Regression achieved the highest accuracy, demonstrating superior predictive performance for the early detection of lung failure. The comparative accuracies of all applied algorithms are visualized in the form of a bar graph, which clearly illustrates the performance variance between models. This visual representation confirms the effectiveness of logistic regression in this medical classification task. As shown in Figure 7.8, the accuracy performance varies significantly across different.

7.6 Conclusion

Lung cancer remains one of the leading causes of cancer-related mortality worldwide, with approximately 60 % of patients dying to the disease within one year of diagnosis. Despite advances in the molecular pathology of lung tumors and the development

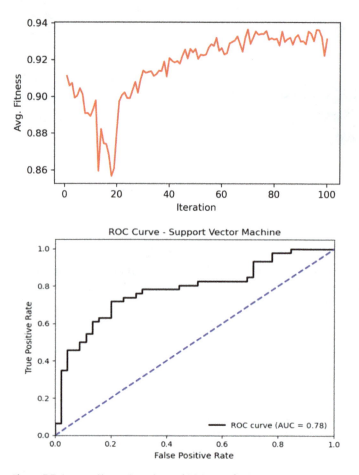

Figure 7.7: Average Fitness/Iteration and ROC curve for SVM.

of targeted therapies, accurate and early diagnosis is crucial to determine the most effective non-invasive or curative treatments. Non-invasive diagnostic techniques, such as positron emission tomography (PET) and thoracic computed tomography (CT), are widely used in clinical settings for early detection.

In this research work, machine learning techniques were applied to raw clinical data, leading to the development of a novel approach for early lung cancer detection. The use of these advanced algorithms offers promising potential for more precise and timely diagnosis. However, it is essential that lung cancer management continues to evolve, with continuous research into more effective diagnostic strategies.

Looking ahead, further improvements in the application of machine learning to lung cancer prediction will rely on enhanced feature selection techniques and the validation of the models using diverse datasets. Future studies should explore the integra-

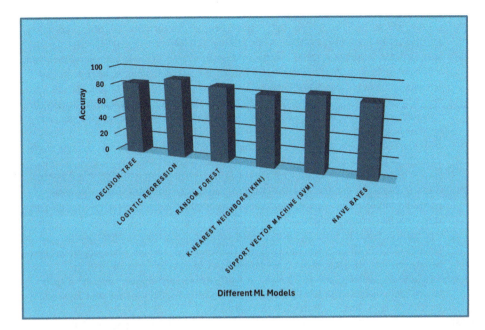

Figure 7.8: Accuracy bar chart of different ML models.

tion of these machine learning models with existing diagnostic tools to provide more accurate and reliable predictions for early-stage lung failure and cancer.

Bibliography

[1] Yaqoob, A., Verma, N. K. & Aziz, R. M. (2024). Improving breast cancer classification with mRMR+ SSO+ WSVM: a hybrid approach. Multimed. Tools Appl., 1–26.
[2] Amutha, A. & Wahidabanu, R. S. D. (2013). Lung tumor detection and diagnosis in CT scan images. In 2013 International Conference on Communication and Signal Processing (pp. 1108–1112). https://doi.org/10.1109/iccsp.2013.6577228.
[3] Afreen, S., Bhurjee, A. K. & Aziz, R. M. (2024). Feature selection using Game Shapley improved grey wolf optimizer for optimizing cancer classification. Knowl. Inf. Syst., 1–32.
[4] Raoof, S. S., Jabbar, M. A. & Fathima, S. A. (2020). Lung cancer prediction using machine learning: a comprehensive approach. In 2020 2nd International Conference on Innovative Mechanisms for Industry Applications (ICIMIA) (pp. 108–115). https://doi.org/10.1109/ICIMIA48430.2020.9074947.
[5] Sharma, A., Kumar, P., Ben, D., Bikhani, M. & Aziz, R. M. (2025). Improved GA based clustering with a new selection method for categorical dental data. In Swarm Optimization for Biomedical Applications (pp. 172–192).
[6] Smith, H. B., Schneider, J. S. & Tanner, N. T. (2022). An evaluation of annual adherence to lung cancer screening in a large national cohort. Am. J. Prev. Med., 63(5), 615–618. https://doi.org/10.1016/j.amepre.2022.06.013.

[7] Lee, K. A., Ma, W., Zakharov, S., et al. (2021). Cancer symptom checker: evaluation of accuracy, safety, and usability. BMJ Open, 11(6), e045145. https://doi.org/10.1136/bmjopen-2020-045145.

[8] Miah, M. B. A. & Yousuf, M. A. (2015). Detection of lung cancer from CT image using image processing and neural network. In 2015 International Conference on Electrical Engineering and Information Communication Technology (ICEEICT) (pp. 1–6). https://doi.org/10.1109/ICEEICT.2015.7307530.

[9] Yaqoob, A., Verma, N. K. & Aziz, R. M. (2024). Metaheuristic algorithms and their applications in different fields: a comprehensive review. In Metaheuristics for Machine Learning: Algorithms and Applications (pp. 1–35).

[10] Rahane, W., Dalvi, H., Magar, Y., Kalane, A. & Jondhale, S. (2018). Lung cancer detection using image processing and machine learning healthcare. In 2018 International Conference on Current Trends Towards Converging Technologies (ICCTCT) (pp. 1–5). https://doi.org/10.1109/ICCTCT.2018.8551008.

[11] Afreen, S., Bhurjee, A. K. & Aziz, R. M. (2024). Cancer classification using RNA sequencing gene expression data based on Game Shapley local search embedded binary social ski-driver optimization algorithms. Microchem. J., 205, 111280.

[12] Rahman, R. U., Singh, K., Tomar, D. S. & Musheer, R. (2024). Building resilient digital forensic frameworks for NoSQL database: harnessing the blockchain and quantum technology. In Sustainable Security Practices Using Blockchain, Quantum and Post-Quantum Technologies.

[13] Dabade, S., Chaudhari, S., Jadhav, S. & Nichal, A. (2017). A review paper on computer aided system for lung cancer detection. In 2017 International Conference on Big Data, IoT and Data Science (BID) (pp. 97–102). https://doi.org/10.1109/BID.2017.8336580.

[14] Tekade, R. & Rajeswari, K. (2018). Lung cancer detection and classification using deep learning. In 2018 Fourth International Conference on Computing Communication Control and Automation (ICCUBEA) (pp. 1–5). https://doi.org/10.1109/ICCUBEA.2018.8697352.

[15] Chaudhary, A. & Singh, S. S. (2012). Lung cancer detection on CT images by using image processing. In 2012 International Conference on Computing Sciences (pp. 142–146). https://doi.org/10.1109/ICCS.2012.43.

[16] Verma, N. K., Yaqoob, A. & Aziz, R. M. (2023). Applications and techniques of machine learning in cancer classification: a systematic review. Hum.-Cent. Intell. Syst.

[17] Vas, M. & Dessai, A. (2017). Lung cancer detection system using lung CT image processing. In 2017 International Conference on Computing, Communication, Control and Automation (ICCUBEA) (pp. 1–5). https://doi.org/10.1109/ICCUBEA.2017.8463851.

[18] Makrariya, A. & Musheer, R. (2022). Machine learning approach for numerical technique for classifying cysts and malignant tumors in breast.

[19] Aziz, R. M., Joshi, A. A., Kumar, K. & Gaani, A. H. (2023). Hybrid feature selection techniques utilizing soft computing methods for cancer data. In Computational and Analytic Methods in Biological Sciences (pp. 23–39).

[20] Dhaware, B. U. & Pise, A. C. (2016). Lung cancer detection using Bayesian classifier and FCM segmentation. In 2016 IEEE International Conference on Automatic Control and Dynamic Optimization Techniques (ICACDOT) (pp. 170–174).

[21] Yaqoob, A., Verma, N. K. & Aziz, R. M. (2024). Improving breast cancer classification with mRMR+ SS0+ WSVM: a hybrid approach. Multimed. Tools Appl., 1–26.

[22] Bhalerao, R. Y., Jani, H. P., Gaitonde, R. K. & Raut, V. (2019). A novel approach for detection of lung cancer using digital image processing and convolution neural networks. In 2019 5th International Conference on Advanced Computing & Communication Systems (ICACCS) (pp. 577–583). https://doi.org/10.1109/ICACCS.2019.8728348.

[23] Aziz, R. M. (2024). Feature selection using Game Shapley improved grey wolf optimizer for optimizing cancer classification. Knowl. Inf. Syst., 1–32.

[24] Tuncal, K., Sckeroglu, B. & Ozkan, C. (2020). Lung cancer prediction using machine learning algorithms. Turkey.

[25] Kalaivani, S., Chatterjee, P., Juyal, S. & Gupta, R. (2017). Lung cancer detection using digital image processing and artificial neural networks. In 2017 International Conference of Electronics, Communication and Aerospace Technology (ICECA) (pp. 100–103). https://doi.org/10.1109/ICECA.2017.8212773.
[26] Joshi, A. A. & Aziz, R. M. (2024). Soft computing techniques for cancer classification of gene expression microarray data: a three-phase hybrid approach. In Computational Intelligence for Data Analysis (pp. 92–113).
[27] Rahman, R. U., Kumar, P., Mohan, A., Aziz, R. M. & Tomar, D. S. (2025). A novel technique for image captioning based on hierarchical clustering and deep learning. SN Comput. Sci., 6(4), 360.
[28] Karthikeyan, R. D., Raghumahendrakumar G, Vinith V, Ganesh Babu C & Kalaiyarasi M (2021). A review of lung cancer detection using image processing. In 2021 Smart Technologies, Communication and Robotics (STCR) (p. 14). https://doi.org/10.1109/STCR51658.2021.9588835.
[29] Miah, M. B. A. & Yousuf, M. A. (2015). Detection of lung cancer from CT image using image processing and neural network. In 2015 International Conference on Electrical Engineering and Information Communication Technology (ICEEICT) (pp. 1–6). https://doi.org/10.1109/ICEEICT.2015.7307530.
[30] Bhalerao, R. Y., Jani, H. P., Gaitonde, R. K. & Raut, V. (2019). A novel approach for detection of lung cancer using digital image processing and convolution neural networks. In 2019 5th International Conference on Advanced Computing & Communication Systems (ICACCS) (pp. 577–583). https://doi.org/10.1109/ICACCS.2019.8728348.

Abrar Yaqoob, Navneet Kumar Verma, G. V. V. Jagannadha Rao, and Rabia Musheer Aziz

8 Efficient gene selection for breast cancer classification using Brownian Motion Search Algorithm and Support Vector Machine

Abstract: Gene expression datasets provide extensive information about various biological processes, but identifying important genes in high-dimensional data is challenging due to redundancy and irrelevant genes. To overcome this challenge, numerous feature selection (FS) techniques have been developed to identify significant genes amidst complex biological data. This research introduces a novel approach that combines the Brownian Motion Search Algorithm (BMSA) with the Support Vector Machine (SVM) for gene selection in breast cancer classification. Using the breast cancer dataset, our method efficiently identifies relevant gene subsets using BMSA and uses SVM for precise classification. The BMSA navigates the high-dimensional feature space to select relevant genes by simulating random motion, reducing redundancy and irrelevant genes. SVM evaluates these gene subsets for accurate classification. We assess the performance of the algorithm using diverse metrics, including the confusion matrix for accuracy and error distribution, the precision-recall curve for precision-recall balance, and the ROC curve for diagnostic ability. The findings demonstrate the effectiveness of our proposed approach in achieving high classification accuracy. Specifically, the method achieves a best classification accuracy of 99.14 % on 16 genes, along with notable mean and worst-case performances. These results highlight the potential of the BMSA-SVM approach to pro-

---

Data availability statement: The datasets used and/or analyzed during the current study are available from the corresponding author on reasonable request.

Conflict of interest disclosure: The authors confirm that they have no conflicts of interest to disclose.

Funding: No funding has been received.

Authors' contribution: In this study, Abrar Yaqoob made significant contributions by preparing materials, meticulous data collection, and conducting data analysis. Navneet Kumar Verma provided valuable expertise through comprehensive literature reviews, critical insights, and substantial contributions to the manuscript's intellectual content and expertly designing experiments to address key research questions, and supervising the research process to maintain integrity and coherence. This collaborative effort, with each team member leveraging their specific expertise, resulted in a comprehensive and impactful research project.

Abrar Yaqoob, Navneet Kumar Verma, VIT Bhopal University's School of Advanced Science and Language, located at Kothrikalan, Sehore, Bhopal 466114, India, e-mail: abraryaqoob77@gmail.com
G. V. V. Jagannadha Rao, Associate Professor & Head, Department of Mathematics, Kalinga University, Naya Raipur 492001, India
Rabia Musheer Aziz, Researcher Officer (Technical), State Planning Institute (New Division), Planning Department, Lucknow, Utter Pradesh 226001, India

https://doi.org/10.1515/9783111504667-008

vide accurate classifications and valuable insights into breast cancer-associated gene biomarkers, representing a significant advancement in bioinformatics and cancer research.

Keywords: Brownian Motion Search Algorithm, Support Vector Machine, breast cancer, High-Dimensional Data

8.1 Introduction

Breast cancer is a prevalent and potentially life-threatening disease characterized by the abnormal growth of cells in the breast tissue. It is one of the most commonly diagnosed cancers in women worldwide, with a significant impact on both individual health and public health systems. Breast cancer can manifest in various forms, ranging from localized tumors confined to the breast ducts or lobules to invasive cancers that spread to surrounding tissues and organs. Early detection and diagnosis play a crucial role in improving treatment outcomes and patient survival rates. Common diagnostic methods for breast cancer include mammography, breast ultrasound, magnetic resonance imaging (MRI), and biopsy. Treatment options for breast cancer may include surgery, radiation therapy, chemotherapy, hormonal therapy, targeted therapy, or a combination of these approaches, depending on the cancer stage, subtype, and individual patient factors [1]. Advances in research and medical technology have led to significant improvements in the detection, diagnosis, and treatment of breast cancer, offering hope for improved outcomes and quality of life for patients affected by this disease. However, continued efforts in education, screening, early detection, and research are essential to further progress in combating breast cancer and reducing its impact on individuals and society. Gene expression datasets contain vast amounts of information crucial for understanding biological processes. However, the complexity of these datasets poses a significant challenge in identifying important genes amidst redundancy and irrelevant information. Consequently, the development of effective feature selection (FS) techniques has become imperative to sift through this vast biological data and extract meaningful insights. In recent years, researchers have explored various FS methods to improve the efficacy and precision of gene selection [2]. These techniques aim to identify subsets of genes that are most relevant to specific biological phenomena, such as disease classification or treatment response prediction. Among these approaches, the integration of optimization algorithms with machine learning models has shown promise in addressing the challenges of gene selection. The Brownian Motion Search Algorithm (BMSA) is one such optimization technique inspired by the random motion of particles observed in Brownian motion. By simulating the stochastic behavior of particles, BMSA effectively explores solution spaces and identifies optimal solutions. The combination of BMSA with machine learning models, such as the Support Vector Machine (SVM), provides a novel approach to gene selection and classification tasks [3].

In this research, we propose a novel approach that combines BMSA with SVM for gene selection in breast cancer classification. Leveraging the breast cancer dataset, our method aims to efficiently identify relevant gene subsets that contribute to the accurate classification of breast cancer subtypes. By integrating BMSA for feature selection and SVM for classification, we aim to achieve high classification accuracy while providing valuable insights into breast cancer-associated gene biomarkers. In the subsequent sections, we provide a detailed overview of the methods, experimental setup, results, and discussion, to elucidate the effectiveness and implications of our proposed approach for gene selection and breast cancer classification. Figure 8.1 shows various techniques for visualizing breast cancer images.

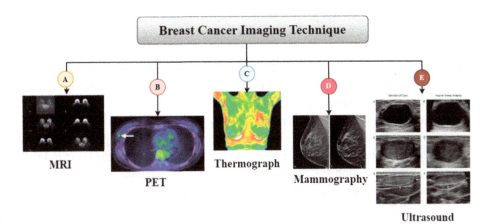

Figure 8.1: Different techniques to visualize breast cancer images.

8.1.1 Objective of the paper

By leveraging diagnostic data and machine learning techniques, our proposed solution aims to address the challenges of cancer classification and contribute to improved patient care and clinical decision making. By developing an accurate and reliable classification system, we strive to empower healthcare professionals with the tools necessary to detect cancerous tumors early and provide timely interventions, ultimately leading to better treatment outcomes and improved patient survival rates.

8.2 Related work

Tehnan I. A. Mohamed et al. propose a CNN model for breast cancer detection using gene expression data from TCGA. The dataset includes 1208 samples with 19,948 genes, comprising 113 normal and 1095 cancerous samples. The Preprocessing involves AAIC for outlier removal and normalization to mitigate bias. Gene reduction is achieved by filtering with a threshold of 0.25. The data are then converted to grayscale images to meet the requirements of the model [4].

Amel Ali Alhussan et al. present a novel framework that integrates metaheuristic optimization with deep learning and feature selection to effectively classify breast cancer from ultrasound images. The methodology consists of five stages: data augmentation to enhance CNN model learning, transfer learning using GoogleNet for feature extraction, feature selection using a hybrid optimization algorithm combining the dipper throated and particle swarm techniques, and classification of selected features using the CNN optimized by the proposed algorithm [5].

Ammar Abdulrahman Ahmed et al. introduce an innovative approach for classifying breast thermography images into normal, benign, or malignant categories. The method incorporates bio-inspired algorithms, namely ant colony optimization (ACO) and particle swarm optimization (PSO), for feature selection. The proposed method consists of four phases: image preprocessing, feature extraction, feature selection, and classification. The evaluation is conducted using a standard thermography dataset and reveals a promising performance of the proposed method [6].

David González-Patiño et al. investigate the application of meta-heuristics to mammographic image segmentation. Contrary to the traditional use for optimization problems, this study focuses on the segmentation of mammograms using the Dunn index as the optimization function and gray levels to represent individuals. The update of grey levels is aimed at maximizing Dunn's index, resulting in improved segmentation quality. The findings demonstrate lower error rates using these meta-heuristics compared to the widely used Otsu method for segmentation [7].

Lingxi Peng et al. blend cutting-edge life science research with artificial intelligence and introduce a semi-supervised learning algorithm to minimize the dependence on labeled data. Using two renowned breast cancer datasets from the UCI machine learning repository, extensive experiments confirm the effectiveness and efficiency of the proposed algorithm. These findings underscore the potential of the algorithm as a promising automated diagnostic method for breast cancer [8].

Ali Al Bataineh et al. introduce a novel application of CSA for training MLP architectures to solve various real-world problems, including breast cancer diagnosis, active sonar target classification, wheat classification, and flower classification. CSA optimizes the weights and biases of MLPs to significantly improve classification accuracy. Comparative analysis against other popular training methods such as GA, ACO, PSO, HHO, MFO, FPA, and BP is conducted using benchmark datasets including Iris Flower, Sonar, Wheat Seeds, Breast Cancer Wisconsin, and Haberman's Survival. The results demonstrate the superior performance of CSA in improving MLP performance across various disciplines, establishing it as a competitive approach for solving real-world applications [9].

Selvakumar Thirumalaisamy et al. propose an advanced breast cancer detection method that combines a synthesized CNN, an optimized optimization algorithm (EACO), and transfer learning. Experimental analysis on MIAS and CBIS-DDSM datasets demonstrates superior accuracy, sensitivity, and specificity compared to conventional methods, highlighting the effectiveness of the proposed EACO–ResNet101 model [10].

Abrar Yaqoob et al. propose a novel gene selection approach named the Sine Cosine and Cuckoo Search Algorithm (SCACSA), which is designed to enhance Support Vector Machine (SVM) classifiers. Using a breast cancer dataset, the performance of the hybrid SCACSA algorithm is rigorously evaluated and compared with other feature selection methods. Initially, the minimum redundancy maximum relevance (mRMR) filtering strategy is employed to improve the quality of the feature set. Subsequently, the SCACSA method is used to optimize the gene selection process. Finally, the dataset is classified using the SVM classifier based on the selected genes. Given the critical role of gene selection in understanding complex biological datasets, SCACSA emerges as a valuable tool for cancer dataset classification to help medical practitioners make informed decisions about cancer diagnosis [11].

8.3 Proposed methodology

In this section, we will explore the use of the Brownian Motion Search Algorithm for feature selection. We will then delve into the role of the Support Vector Machine (SVM) within this hybrid algorithm for classification.

8.3.1 Stage 1: feature selection stage with Brownian Motion Search Algorithm

The Brownian Motion Search Algorithm (BMSA) is a stochastic optimization technique inspired by the random movement of particles observed in Brownian motion. In BMSA, a population of candidate solutions, denoted as particles, is represented by their positions in the search space. Let x_i represent the position of the i-th particle in the d-dimensional search space, where $I = 1, 2, \ldots, N$ and d represents the dimensionality of the problem. The position of each particle is updated iteratively according to the equation (8.1) [12]:

$$x_i^{(t+1)} = x_i^{(t)} + a.\Delta x_i \qquad (8.1)$$

where $x_i^{(t)}$ is the position of the i-th particle at iteration t, a is a step size parameter, and Δx_i represents a random perturbation vector that follows a Gaussian distribution with mean 0 and variance σ^2. This random perturbation allows the particles to explore the search space i in a stochastic manner, similar to the random movement of particles in Brownian motion. The fitness of each particle is evaluated using an objective function $f(x_i)$, which quantifies the quality of the solution associated with the particle's position.

The objective function guides the search process by providing feedback on the performance of candidate solutions. At each iteration, particles update their positions based on the evaluation of their fitness, where $x_i^{(t+1)}$ represents the updated position of the i-th particle at iteration $t+1$. BMSA dynamically balances exploration and exploitation by adjusting the step size α and the variance σ^2 of the random perturbation vector. This allows the algorithm to effectively explore the search space while exploiting promising regions, identified by the fitness evaluations. The iterative optimization process continues until a termination criterion is met, such as reaching a maximum number of iterations or achieving convergence. In summary, the Brownian Motion Search Algorithm provides a powerful framework for stochastic optimization that uses the principles of Brownian motion to efficiently explore solution spaces and find optimal solutions in various optimization problems [13, 14].

In the feature selection stage employing the Brownian Motion Search Algorithm (BMSA), the goal is to identify the most informative subset of features from a high-dimensional dataset. BMSA, inspired by the stochastic movement observed in Brownian motion, offers a novel approach to effectively explore the solution space. Unlike traditional feature selection methods, BMSA exhibits the ability to perform local exploitation and global exploration simultaneously, making it particularly suitable for complex optimization landscapes. At the outset of the feature selection process, BMSA initializes a population of candidate feature subsets within the defined search space. Each candidate solution represents a subset of features from the original dataset. The algorithm then evaluates the fitness of each candidate subset based on a predefined objective function, which typically measures the relevance or discriminative power of the features for the given classification task. During the iterative optimization process, BMSA simulates Brownian motion by introducing random perturbations to the candidate solutions. These perturbations allow the algorithm to stochastically explore the solution space, gradually refining the candidate feature subsets toward more optimal solutions. Throughout the optimization process, BMSA dynamically adjusts the balance between exploration and exploitation, allowing it to escape local optima and discover globally optimal feature subsets. As BMSA iterates, it continuously updates the best feature subset found so far based on the fitness evaluation. This iterative refinement process continues until a termination criterion is met, such as a maximum number of iterations or convergence of the algorithm [15].

In summary, the feature selection stage with the Brownian Motion Search Algorithm offers a robust and efficient approach to identifying the most relevant features for a given classification task. By leveraging the stochastic nature of Brownian motion, BMSA effectively explores the solution space, leading to the discovery of feature subsets that significantly enhance the performance of machine learning models. The pseudocode of the Brownian Motion Search Algorithm is shown in Algorithm 8.1.

Algorithm 8.1: Pseudocode of the Brownian Motion Search Algorithm.

```
Initialize population of gene subsets randomly within
    search space
best_subset = None
best_accuracy = -Infinity
for iteration = 1 to max_iterations:
    for each gene subset:
        Evaluate fitness using SVM classification accuracy
            on training dataset
        if accuracy > best_accuracy:
            Update best_subset
            Update best_accuracy
    for each gene subset:
        Simulate Brownian motion to perturb gene subset
            composition
        Clip gene subset to maintain within search space
            bounds
return best subset
```

8.3.2 Stage 2: classification by using Support Vector Machine

Support Vector Machine (SVM) is a robust classification and regression algorithm, designed to find the optimal hyperplane that separates data points of different classes in high-dimensional space. By maximizing the margin between the decision boundary and the nearest data points (support vectors), SVM improves model generalization. Using kernel functions, SVM transforms data into a higher-dimensional space to create nonlinear decision boundaries. It employs soft margin classification to handle non-linearly separable data, balancing margin maximization and classification error through the regularization parameter (C). SVM is efficient on high-dimensional data and suitable for small to medium-sized datasets. It can manage multi-class problems using one-vs-one or one-vs-all strategies and has applications in text classification, image recognition, bioinformatics, and financial forecasting [16]. In summary, SVM constructs optimal decision boundaries, offers robustness against overfitting, and is effective in various domains, making it a popular choice for diverse machine learning tasks [17].

Parameter settings for the hybrid BMSA-SVM approach

To effectively implement the hybrid Brownian Motion Search Algorithm (BMSA) and Support Vector Machine (SVM) approach for gene selection and classification in breast cancer datasets, the following parameter settings are recommended:

To effectively implement the hybrid Brownian Motion Search Algorithm (BMSA) and Support Vector Machine (SVM) approach for gene selection and classification in breast cancer datasets, specific parameter settings are recommended. For the BMSA, an initial population size of 50 subsets is typically used, with a maximum of 100 iterations. The perturbation rate, which determines how often feature subsets are altered to explore the solution space, usually ranges from 0.1 to 0.3. The fitness function employed is generally based on the classification accuracy provided by the SVM, and the algorithm converges when no significant improvement is observed over the last 20 iterations.

In the SVM component, the Radial Basis Function (RBF) kernel is commonly chosen, although linear, polynomial, and sigmoid kernels are also options. The regularization parameter (C), which balances the tradeoff between low training error and model complexity, is often set between 1 and 10. The kernel coefficient (y), which defines the influence range of a single training example, typically falls between 0.1 and 1 for the RBF kernel. To handle class imbalance, the class weight parameter can be set to 'balanced', which automatically adjusts the weights inversely proportional to the class frequencies. A 10-fold cross-validation is employed to fine-tune the SVM parameters. Performance metrics for evaluating the hybrid algorithm include the confusion matrix, which shows the classification performance, and the precision-recall curve, depicting the trade-off between precision and recall at various thresholds. The ROC curve and the area under the curve (AUC) provide insight into the diagnostic ability and overall performance of the classifier. By carefully setting these parameters, the proposed hybrid BMSA-SVM approach can effectively select relevant gene subsets and achieve high classification accuracy in breast cancer datasets, offering valuable insights into associated gene biomarkers.

8.4 Experimental setup

This study, breast cancer microarray datasets were analyzed to evaluate the effectiveness of a proposed gene selection method. The datasets, which focused on stage II lung cancer, were obtained from https://csse.szu.edu.cn/staff/zhuzx/Datasets.html. Table 8.1 lists their details and characteristics. To ensure robust findings, we employed

Table 8.1: Detailed overview of the used dataset.

Data Set	Classes	Genes	No. of Samples	Short Description
Breast Cancer	2	24481	97	Breast cancer is a type of cancer that originates in the cells of the breast. It can occur in both men and women, but it is far more common in women. The disease typically begins in the milk-producing glands (lobules) or in the ducts that carry milk to the nipple.

the Leave-One-Out Cross-Validation (LOOCV) approach. This method iteratively withholds one data point, trains the model on the remaining data, and assesses performance using the excluded point. This process is repeated for each data point, providing a comprehensive evaluation of the model. Our approach integrates information gain, Harris Hawks Optimization (HHO), and Support Vector Machine (SVM) for gene selection. This hybrid method showed superior performance in selecting relevant genes compared to other techniques. The effectiveness was measured by the classification accuracy of the SVM classifier and the number of genes identified. The classification accuracy of the SVM classifier is determined by the following formula:

$$\text{Classification} = \frac{CC}{N} \times 100$$

where CC denotes correctly classified samples and N represents the total number of samples within a specific class. The experiments were conducted on a desktop with a 64-bit Windows 10 OS, an Intel Core i7-3770 CPU at 3.40 GHz, and 8 GB of RAM, using Python 3.12.0. The fitness function of the proposed approach is based on the classification accuracy of the SVM classifier. If the current fitness score exceeds the previous one, it replaces the previous result; otherwise, the previous solution is retained. The solution with the highest fitness score is selected as the optimal gene subset for prediction.

8.5 Results

Table 8.2 presents the classification accuracy of the proposed hybrid BMSA-SVM method for the breast cancer dataset, evaluating its performance with different numbers of selected genes. The results include the best, average, and worst classification accuracies observed for each subset size. When 12 genes were selected, the proposed method achieved a best classification accuracy of 93.23 %, with a mean accuracy of 85.18 % and a worst case accuracy of 79.34 %. Increasing the number of genes to 14 resulted in an im-

Table 8.2: Classification accuracy of the proposed method for the breast cancer dataset.

No. of genes	Proposed Method		
	Best	Mean	Worst
12	93.23	85.18	79.34
14	95.45	88.89	83.5
16	99.14	92.05	87.81
18	97.09	89.81	84.7
20	96.15	88.73	82.45
24	94.91	86.07	79.33
28	93.37	82.19	74.49

proved best accuracy of 95.45 %, a mean accuracy of 88.89 %, and a worst-case accuracy of 83.5 %. By further increasing the subset to 16 genes, the method reached its highest best accuracy of 99.14 %, with a mean accuracy of 92.05 % and a worst-case accuracy of 87.81 %. However, when 18 genes were selected, the best accuracy decreased slightly to 97.09 %, and the mean and worst-case accuracy also showing slight declines to 89.81 % and 84.7 %, respectively. When Selecting 20 genes resulted in a best accuracy of 96.15 %, a mean accuracy of 88.73 %, and a worst-case accuracy of 82.45 %. For 24 genes, the best accuracy was 94.91 %, with a mean of 86.07 % and a worst-case of 79.33 %. Finally, with 28 genes, the best accuracy dropped to 93.37 %, the mean to 82.19 %, and the worst-case to 74.49 %. These results demonstrate that the proposed method achieves the highest classification accuracy with 16 genes. Beyond this point, adding more genes does not improve the accuracy and may even degrade the performance of the model. This suggests that the proposed BMSA-SVM method is highly effective in selecting a small, yet highly informative subset of genes for accurate breast cancer classification, providing a balance between complexity and performance.

We assess the algorithm's performance using several metrics, including the confusion matrix, which provides a detailed breakdown of true positives, true negatives, false positives, and false negatives, allowing us to evaluate the classifier's accuracy and error distribution. The precision-recall curve is used to measure the balance between precision and recall across different thresholds, providing insight into the trade-offs between false positives and false negatives. Additionally, the ROC curve, along with the area under the curve (AUC), evaluates the diagnostic ability of the classifier, illustrating its performance across various threshold settings and helping to identify the optimal balance between sensitivity and specificity. These metrics collectively offer a comprehensive evaluation of the proposed method's effectiveness in classifying breast cancer data.

8.5.1 Descriptions for each metric based on the provided confusion matrix

1. Accuracy: The model correctly classified 97 samples, resulting in an accuracy of 99.01 %, indicating that the vast majority of predictions were correct.
2. Precision: The precision of the model is 99.01 %, meaning that out of all the samples predicted to be positive (97 total), 42 were actually positive, reflecting a high reliability in positive predictions.
3. Sensitivity (Recall): The sensitivity (or recall) of the model is 100 %, indicating that the model successfully identified all 42 actual positive cases without missing any.
4. F1-Score: The F1-Score is 99.72 %, showing a strong balance between precision (99.01 %) and recall (100 %), making it a robust measure of the model's performance in accurately handling positive predictions.

8.5.2 Confusion matrix

Figure 8.2 illustrates the confusion matrix, a vital evaluation tool for classification models. This matrix compares the model's predictions with actual values in a grid format, divided into four sections: true positives (TP), true negatives (TN), false positives (FP), and false negatives (FN). True positives are correctly identified positive instances, true negatives are accurately identified negative instances, false positives are instances mistakenly classified as positive, and false negatives are instances incorrectly classified as negative.

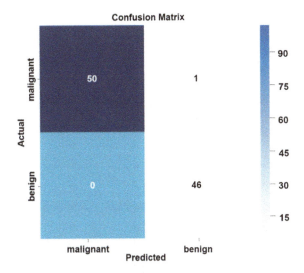

Figure 8.2: Confusion matrix based on the breast cancer dataset.

The confusion matrix provides a clear summary of the model's strengths and weaknesses, helping to understand its predictive capabilities. By examining true positives (TP), true negatives (TN), false positives (FP), and false negatives (FN), performance metrics such as accuracy, precision, recall, and F1-Score can be calculated. These metrics offer a comprehensive evaluation of the model's classification effectiveness. The confusion matrix is essential for refining models and making informed deployment decisions. Calculations for these performance metrics are based on specific equations derived from the confusion matrix values

$$ACC = \frac{TP + TN}{TP + TN + FP + FN} \tag{y}$$

$$P = \frac{TP}{TP + FP} \tag{j}$$

$$Sn = \frac{TP}{TP + FN} \tag{k}$$

$$\text{F-score} = 2 \times \frac{P \times \text{Sn}}{P + \text{Sn}}$$

8.5.3 Precision-recall curve

To enhance its findings, the study uses visual aids such as Figure 8.3, which presents the Precision-Recall (PR) graph. This graph evaluates the proposed approach's performance by illustrating the balance between precision (accuracy of positive predictions) and recall (proportion of actual positives correctly predicted). The PR graph provides deeper insight into the approach's efficacy, contributing to a comprehensive understanding of its predictive capabilities.

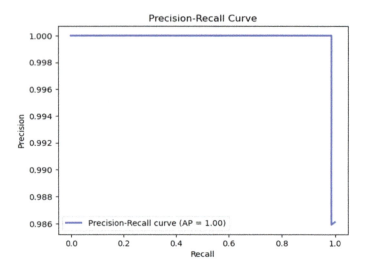

Figure 8.3: Precision-recall curve on the breast cancer dataset.

8.5.4 Area under the curve

A higher area under the curve (AUC) indicates the model's superior performance in distinguishing between positive and negative instances. In the precision-recall (PR) graph, a greater AUC underscores the robustness and efficacy of the proposed method, particularly in accurately identifying positive instances in imbalanced datasets. This detailed assessment highlights the method's reliability and effectiveness, providing valuable insight into its practical applicability in real-world scenarios where precise identification of positive cases is critical.

Figure 8.4 depicts the Receiver Operating Characteristic (ROC) curve, illustrating the balance between the true positive (sensitivity) and false positive (1-specificity) rates. A higher AUC-ROC value indicates the model's superior ability to distinguish between

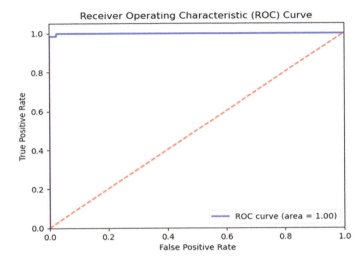

Figure 8.4: ROC curve of the breast cancer dataset.

classes. The ROC curve from the proposed method demonstrates strong discriminatory capability. High AUC values for both the precision-recall (PR) and ROC curves confirm the method's effectiveness and reliability in accurately classifying cancer types. These visual representations provide compelling evidence of the method's proficiency and potential for real-world clinical applications.

Table 8.3 compares the classification accuracy (CA) and standard deviation (STD) of Decision Tree, K-Nearest Neighbors (KNN), and Random Forest (RF) classifiers using the proposed feature selection algorithm for breast cancer classification. The RF classifier consistently achieves the highest accuracy across different gene sets with low variability. For example, with 12 genes, RF achieves a CA of 99.03 %, compared to 97.22 % for Decision Tree and 96.62 % for KNN. As the number of selected genes varies, RF maintains superior performance, highlighting its robustness. In contrast, Decision Tree and KNN show more variability in their performance. These results emphasize the effectiveness

Table 8.3: The comparison between different classifiers with the proposed algorithm for breast cancer classification.

Selected Genes	Decision Tree Mean CA (±STD)	KNN Mean CA (±STD)	RF Mean CA (±STD)
12	97.22 ± 0.04	96.62 ± 2.0	99.03 ± 0.76
14	91.01 ± 1.10	98.23 ± 3.10	96.43 ± 3.15
16	82.30 ± 3.08	99.31 ± 1.01	99.01 ± 1.01
18	90.10 ± 1.24	97.25 ± 2.06	96.54 ± 1.06
20	83.12 ± 2.70	90.13 ± 1.34	99.03 ± 0.11
24	97.53 ± 3.10	93.22 ± 1.98	98.40 ± 0.98

of the proposed feature selection algorithm and the importance of selecting the appropriate classifier for optimal breast cancer classification. Figure 8.5 shows more clearly the comparison of different classifiers used of the same data set.

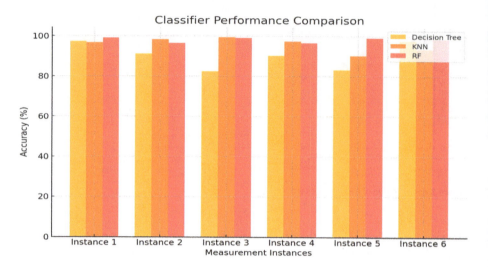

Figure 8.5: Histogram comparison of different classifiers.

Based on the data presented in Table 8.3, Random Forest (RF) consistently outperforms both the Decision Tree and the K-Nearest Neighbors (KNN) classifiers across all listed measurements. The accuracy values for RF are higher than those for the other two classifiers in most cases, which is indicative of RF's robustness and better performance.

To illustrate this, we can create a histogram that visually compares the performance of the three classifiers. In this histogram:
- The x-axis will represent the different measurement instances.
- The y-axis will represent the accuracy percentages.
- Different colors or patterns will distinguish the bars representing Decision Tree, KNN, and RF.

Each group of bars at each measurement instance will show how RF (with the highest bars) performs better than Decision Tree and KNN, emphasizing the superior accuracy of the RF classifier in this context. Figure 8.5 shows a comparison between different classifiers.

The histogram clearly shows that the Random Forest (RF) classifier consistently outperforms both the Decision Tree and K-Nearest Neighbors (KNN) classifiers across all six measurement instances. Each group of bars represents the performance of the three classifiers for a specific instance, with RF (red bars) achieving higher accuracy percentages in most cases. This visual representation highlights the superior performance of RF, demonstrating its robustness and effectiveness compared to Decision Tree and KNN. The consistently higher bars for RF across the instances reinforce the conclusion that RF is the best performing classifier of the three in this particular dataset.

Table 8.4 compares the performance of the proposed BMSA-SVM algorithm with several advanced feature selection and classification methods based on different references. Each method is evaluated on key metrics, including the number of selected genes, classification accuracy, training time, and testing time. The proposed BMSA-SVM method stands out with an impressive classification accuracy of 99.01 % using only 16 genes. It demonstrates efficient performance with a training time of 3.03 seconds and a testing time of 250.9 milliseconds. Reference [24] describes a method that combines mRMR with KNN and CNN, and achieves an accuracy of 98.19 % with 33 genes, a training time of 3.37 seconds, and a testing time of 324.59 milliseconds. Reference [25] presents the SVM-mRMRe approach, which selects 65 genes and achieves an accuracy of 91.17 %, with a training time of 3.88 seconds and a testing time of 248.01 milliseconds. The M-FS method in Reference [26] matches the proposed method's accuracy of 99.01 %, but requires 26 genes and has longer training (4.19 seconds) and testing times (348.89 milliseconds). Reference [27] describes the HER+MLT method, which achieves an accuracy of 82.6 % with 34 genes, with training and testing times of 3.42 seconds and 222.9 milliseconds, respectively. The FR+SE method from Reference [28] achieves the highest accuracy of 99.45 % with only 14 genes, but it has the shortest training time (2.29 seconds) and the longest testing time (352.9 milliseconds). Lastly, the PSO+DT method in Reference [29] achieves an accuracy of 85.48 % using 20 genes, with a training time of 3.72 seconds and a testing time of 243.2 milliseconds. In summary, the proposed BMSA-SVM algorithm excels in balancing high classification accuracy, efficient gene selection, and competitive training and testing times. Compared to other advanced methods, it demonstrates significant efficiency and effectiveness in classifying breast cancer data, highlighting its potential as a robust tool for gene selection and disease classification.

Table 8.4: Comparison of the proposed algorithm with advanced methods.

References	Algorithms	Gene no.	Accuracy	Training Time	Testing Time
Proposed method	BMSA-SVM	16	99.14	3.03 s	250.9 Ms
[18]	mRMR+KNN+CNN	33	98.19	3.37 s	324.59 Ms
[19]	SVM-mRMRe	65	91.17	3.88 s	248.01 Ms
[20]	M-FS	26	99.01	4.19 s	348.89 Ms
[21]	HER+MLT	34	82.6	3.42 s	222.9 Ms
[22]	FR+SE	14	99.45	2.29 s	352.9 Ms
[23]	PSO+DT	20	85.48	3.72 s	1.2 Ms

8.6 Conclusion

In conclusion, the proposed hybrid approach combining the Brownian Motion Search Algorithm (BMSA) and Support Vector Machine (SVM) demonstrates significant efficacy in gene selection and classification for the breast cancer dataset. The results, as shown in the classification accuracy table, indicate that the proposed method achieves the highest classification accuracy of 99.14 % with 16 genes, with a mean accuracy of 92.05 % and a worst-case accuracy of 87.81 %. This method outperforms other feature selection techniques in terms of both accuracy and efficiency. The use of BMSA effectively identifies relevant gene subsets from high-dimensional data, overcoming challenges related to redundancy and irrelevant genes. SVM ensures precise classification of the selected genes, further enhancing the model's performance. The comprehensive assessment of the algorithm using metrics such as the confusion matrix, precision-recall curve, and ROC curve underscores its robustness and reliability. These findings highlight the potential of the proposed BMSA-SVM approach not only to achieve high classification accuracy, but also to provide valuable insights into gene biomarkers associated with breast cancer. This novel method represents a significant advancement in the field of bioinformatics and cancer research, offering a powerful tool for identifying critical genes in complex biological data.

8.7 Future directions

Looking ahead, this research lays a strong foundation for future exploration and advancement in the field of cancer classification and gene expression profiling. Several promising directions emerge from the success of the proposed approach:

Direction 1 (Multi-omics integration). Incorporating data from multiple omics levels, such as genomics, transcriptomics, proteomics, and epigenomics, could yield a comprehensive understanding of cancer mechanisms. The integration of different data sources could potentially improve the precision and reliability of classification models.

Direction 2 (Deep Learning Architectures). Applying deep learning models, such as recurrent neural networks (RNNs) or convolutional neural networks (CNNs), to gene expression data could reveal intricate patterns and relationships, leading to more intricate and precise cancer classifications.

Direction 3 (Interpretable AI). Developing methods that not only achieve a high level of accuracy, but also offer insight into the underlying biological processes responsible for classification decisions is crucial. Enhancing the interpretability of AI models could increase their adoption in clinical settings.

Direction 4 (Personalized Medicine). The use of gene expression profiles for patient-specific treatment recommendations is a promising avenue. Future research could focus on tailoring classification models to individual patients, considering their unique genetic signatures and characteristics.

Direction 5 (Benchmarking and Generalization). Extending the validation and benchmarking of hybrid approaches across different datasets and cancer types can provide a broader understanding of their performance and generalizability.

Bibliography

[1] Rana, N., Shafie, M., Latiff, A., Abdulhamid, M., Chiroma, H. & Rana, N. (2020). Whale optimization algorithm: a systematic review of contemporary applications, modifications and developments. 32(20). Springer London. https://doi.org/10.1007/s00521-020-04849-z.

[2] Poli, R., Kennedy, J. & Blackwell, T. (2007). Particle swarm optimization: an overview. 33–57. https://doi.org/10.1007/s11721-007-0002-0.

[3] Khurma, R. A., Aljarah, I., Sharieh, A., Elaziz, M. A., Damaševičius, R. & Krilavičius, T. (2022). A review of the modification strategies of the Nature Inspired algorithms for Feature Selection problem. Mathematics, 10(3). https://doi.org/10.3390/math10030464.

[4] Mohamed, T. I. A., Ezugwu, A. E., Fonou-Dombeu, J. V., Ikotun, A. M. & Mohammed, M. (2023). A bio-inspired convolution neural network architecture for automatic breast cancer detection and classification using RNA-Seq gene expression data. Sci. Rep., 13(1), 1–19. https://doi.org/10.1038/s41598-023-41731-z.

[5] Alhussan, A. A., Eid, M. M., Towfek, S. K. & Khafaga, D. S. (2023). Breast cancer classification depends on the dynamic dipper throated optimization algorithm. Biomimetics, 8(2), 1–20. https://doi.org/10.3390/biomimetics8020163.

[6] Ahmed, A. A., Ali, M. A. S. & Selim, M. (2019). Bio-inspired based techniques for thermogram breast cancer classification. Int. J. Intell. Eng. Syst., 12(2), 114–124. https://doi.org/10.22266/IJIES2019.0430.12.

[7] González-Patiño, D., Villuendas-Rey, Y., Argüelles-Cruz, A. J. & Karray, F. (2019). A Novel bio-inspired method for early diagnosis of breast cancer through mammographic image analysis. Appl. Sci., 9(21). https://doi.org/10.3390/app9214492.

[8] Peng, L., Chen, W., Zhou, W., Li, F., Yang, J. & Zhang, J. (2016). An immune-inspired semi-supervised algorithm for breast cancer diagnosis. Comput. Methods Programs Biomed., 134(61472092), 259–265. https://doi.org/10.1016/j.cmpb.2016.07.020.

[9] Al Bataineh, A., Kaur, D. & Jalali, S. M. J. (2022). Multi-layer perceptron training optimization using nature inspired computing. IEEE Access, 10, 36963–36977. https://doi.org/10.1109/ACCESS.2022.3164669.

[10] Thirumalaisamy, S., et al. (2023). Breast cancer classification using synthesized deep learning model with metaheuristic optimization algorithm. Diagnostics, 13(18), 1–21. https://doi.org/10.3390/diagnostics13182925.

[11] Yaqoob, A., Kumar, N., Rabia, V. & Aziz, M. (2024). Optimizing gene selection and cancer classification with hybrid Sine Cosine and Cuckoo Search Algorithm. J. Med. Syst. https://doi.org/10.1007/s10916-023-02031-1.

[12] Almufti, S. M. (2019). Historical survey on metaheuristics algorithms. Int. J. Sci. World, 7(1), 1. https://doi.org/10.14419/ijsw.v7i1.29497.

[13] Azizi, M., Talatahari, S. & Gandomi, A. H. (2023). Fire Hawk Optimizer: a novel metaheuristic algorithm. 56(1). Springer Netherlands. https://doi.org/10.1007/s10462-022-10173-w.
[14] Agrawal, P., Abutarboush, H. F., Ganesh, T. & Mohamed, A. W. (2021). Metaheuristic algorithms on feature selection: a survey of one decade of research (2009–2019). IEEE Access, 9, 26766–26791. https://doi.org/10.1109/ACCESS.2021.3056407.
[15] Yang, X. Nature-Inspired Algorithms and Applied Optimization. Studies in Computational Intelligence (Vol. 744).
[16] Mohsen, H., El-Dahshan, E.-S. A., El-Horbaty, E.-S. M. & Salem, A.-B. M. (2018). Classification using deep learning neural networks for brain tumors. Future Comput. Inform. J., 3(1), 68–71. https://doi.org/10.1016/j.fcij.2017.12.001.
[17] Shukla, A. K., Singh, P. & Vardhan, M. (2019). A new hybrid wrapper TLBO and SA with SVM approach for gene expression data. Inf. Sci., 503, 238–254. https://doi.org/10.1016/j.ins.2019.06.063.
[18] Toğaçar, M., Ergen, B. & Cömert, Z. (2020). Detection of lung cancer on chest CT images using minimum redundancy maximum relevance feature selection method with convolutional neural networks. Biocybern. Biomed. Eng., 40(1), 23–39. https://doi.org/10.1016/j.bbe.2019.11.004.
[19] El Kafrawy, P., Fathi, H., Qaraad, M., Kelany, A. K. & Chen, X. (2021). An efficient SVM-based feature selection model for cancer classification using high-dimensional microarray data. IEEE Access, 9, 155353–155369. https://doi.org/10.1109/ACCESS.2021.3123090.
[20] Venkataramana, L., Jacob, S. . & Ramadoss, R. (2020). A Parallel Multilevel Feature Selection algorithm for improved cancer classification. J. Parallel Distrib. Comput., 138, 78–98. https://doi.org/10.1016/j.jpdc.2019.12.015.
[21] Pradeep, K. R. & Naveen, N. C. (2018). Lung cancer survivability prediction based on performance using classification techniques of Support Vector Machines, C4.5 and Naive Bayes Algorithms for healthcare analytics. Proc. Comput. Sci., 132, 412–420. https://doi.org/10.1016/j.procs.2018.05.162.
[22] Kurniawati, P. (2017). Metode Penelitian Kualitatif. Univ. Nusant. PGRI Kediri, 01, 1–7.
[23] Chen, K. H., et al. (2014). Gene selection for cancer identification: a decision tree model empowered by particle swarm optimization algorithm. BMC Bioinform., 15(1), 0–9. https://doi.org/10.1186/1471-2105-15-49.
[24] Yaqoob, A., Verma, N. K., Mir, M. A., Tejani, G. G., Eisa, N. H. B., Mamoun Hussien Osman, H. & Shah, M. A. (2025). SGA-Driven feature selection and random forest classification for enhanced breast cancer diagnosis: a comparative study. Sci. Rep., 15(1), 10944.
[25] Yaqoob, A. & Verma, N. K. (2025). Feature selection in breast cancer gene expression data using KAO and AOA with SVM classification. J. Med. Syst., 49(1), 1–21.
[26] Yaqoob, A. (2024). Combining the mRMR technique with the Northern Goshawk Algorithm (NGHA) to choose genes for cancer classification. Int. J. Inf. Technol., 1–12.
[27] Yaqoob, A., Verma, N. K., Aziz, R. M. & Shah, M. A. (2024). RNA-Seq analysis for breast cancer detection: a study on paired tissue samples using hybrid optimization and deep learning techniques. J. Cancer Res. Clin. Oncol., 150(10), 455.
[28] Yaqoob, A., Verma, N. K., Aziz, R. M. & Shah, M. A. (2024). Optimizing cancer classification: a hybrid RDO-XGBoost approach for feature selection and predictive insights. Cancer Immunol. Immunother., 73(12), 261.
[29] Yaqoob, A., Mir, M. A., Jagannadha Rao, G. V. V. & Tejani, G. G. (2024). Transforming cancer classification: the role of advanced gene selection. Diagnostics, 14(23), 2632.

Abrar Yaqoob, Navneet Kumar Verma, G. V. V. Jagannadha Rao, and Rabia Musheer Aziz

9 A hybrid feature gene selection approach by integrating variance filter, extremely randomized tree, and Cuckoo Search algorithm for cancer classification

Abstract: In biomedical data mining, the challenge of handling high-dimensional gene expression data, where the number of genes often exceeds the number of samples, poses a significant hurdle for accurate classification and analysis. To address this issue, this paper introduces a novel three-stage hybrid gene selection approach that combines a variance filter, an extremely randomized tree, and the Cuckoo Search algorithm. Initially, the variance filter reduces the dimensionality of the gene space by eliminating genes with low variability. Subsequently, the extremely randomized tree method further refines this subset by prioritizing those with strong associations to the target phenotype. Finally, the Cuckoo Search algorithm identifies the optimal feature gene subset from this refined pool. The proposed methodology was evaluated on a breast cancer gene expression dataset using four classifiers: Random Forest, Linear Regression, K-Nearest Neighbors (KNN), and Support Vector Machine (SVM). Experimental results showed that the proposed method consistently outperformed the extremely randomized tree and Variance Filter techniques. For instance, with the Random Forest classifier, the proposed method achieved 100 % accuracy with 11 selected genes, compared to 95.96 % and 83.91 % for the extremely randomized tree and Variance Filter methods, respectively. Similar trends were observed with the other classifiers, where the proposed method achieved the highest accuracies, demonstrating its robustness and effectiveness. These findings underscore the potential of the proposed hybrid approach to significantly improve classification accuracy and reliability in biomedical data mining applications, offering a powerful tool for gene selection and analysis in high-dimensional datasets.

Data availability statement: The data used in this research study are in the public domain.

Conflict of interest disclosure: The authors confirm that they have no conflicts of interest to disclose.

Funding: There is no funding available for this project.

Authors contribution: The authors contributed equally.

Abrar Yaqoob, Navneet Kumar Verma, VIT Bhopal University's School of Advanced Science and Language, located at Kothrikalan, Sehore, Bhopal 466114, India, e-mail: abraryaqoob77@gmail.com
G. V. V. Jagannadha Rao, Associate Professor & Head, Department of Mathematics, Kalinga University, Naya Raipur 492001, India
Rabia Musheer Aziz, Researcher Officer (Technical), State Planning Institute (New Division), Planning Department, Lucknow, Utter Pradesh 226001, India

https://doi.org/10.1515/9783111504667-009

Keywords: Cancer classification, feature selection, Cuckoo Search algorithm, extremely randomized tree, variance filter

9.1 Introduction

Biomedical data encompasses a wide range of information derived from various biological sources, including genomic, proteomic, clinical, and imaging data, among others. Within this landscape, gene microarray data holds special significance as it provides a comprehensive snapshot of gene expression levels across thousands of genes simultaneously. This high-throughput technology enables researchers to gain insight into the molecular mechanisms underlying diseases, including cancer. Cancer, a complex and heterogeneous group of diseases characterized by uncontrolled cell growth and proliferation, poses a major public health challenge worldwide. Among the various types of cancer, breast cancer remains one of the most prevalent and lethal, affecting millions of patients worldwide each year [1]. Gene expression profiling studies in breast cancer have revealed distinct molecular subtypes and identified key biomarkers associated with prognosis and treatment response, facilitating personalized approaches to patient management and therapy selection. The analysis of gene expression profiles has revolutionized biomedical research, offering insight into the molecular basis of disease and guiding the development of targeted therapies. However, the inherent complexity of gene expression data, characterized by a high-dimensional feature space where the number of genes far exceeds the sample size, poses formidable challenges to accurate predictive modeling [2]. In this context, the process of feature selection emerges as a critical step in identifying a subset of genes that are most relevant to the phenotype under investigation, thereby improving model interpretability and generalization. Recognizing the importance of addressing this challenge, our study introduces a comprehensive three-stage hybrid approach to gene selection, that relies on a combination of sophisticated techniques including a variance filter, an extremely randomized tree, and a Cuckoo Search algorithm. High-dimensional gene expression data often suffer from the curse of dimensionality, where the presence of redundant or irrelevant features degrades model performance and interpretability. To mitigate this issue, our approach first applies a variance filter, which serves to reduce the dimensionality of the feature space by eliminating genes with low variance across samples. By focusing on genes with high variability, we aim to retain those that are most likely to capture meaningful biological information and exhibit strong associations with the phenotype of interest [3]. After the initial dimensionality reduction step, we use an extremely randomized tree algorithm to further refine the set of feature genes. Unlike traditional decision trees, which select the best split based on a subset of features, extremely randomized trees introduce an additional layer of randomness by randomly selecting candidate splits at each node. This randomization helps to decorrelate the individual trees in the ensemble, reducing overfitting and improving the robustness of feature selection. By exploiting the inherent diversity of these randomized trees, we aim to identify genes that consistently contribute to predictive accuracy across different subsets of data [4]. In the final stage of our hybrid approach, we employ a Cuckoo Search algorithm to select the optimal subset of feature genes from the refined pool. Inspired by the social behavior of cuckoos, which coordinate their movements to optimize foraging efficiency, the cuckoo algorithm iteratively updates the position of candidate solutions in search of the global optimum. By simulating this process of collective intelligence, we aim to identify the subset of genes that collectively yield the highest predictive performance across multiple evaluation metrics [5]. By integrating these complementary techniques, our hybrid approach offers a systematic and robust framework for gene selection in biomedical data mining. In the following sections of this paper, we provide a detailed overview of each step of our methodology, including the implementation details, experimental setup, and evaluation metrics. Furthermore, we present comprehensive results from our empirical study, comparing the performance of our proposed approach with state-of-the-art gene selection algorithms on a variety of datasets and predictive modeling tasks [6]. By advancing the state-of-the-art in gene selection methods, we aim to facilitate more accurate and interpretable analyses of high-dimensional gene expression data, ultimately contributing to advances in biomedical research and clinical practice.

9.1.1 Problem statement and objectives of the paper

Problem statement

High-dimensional gene expression data pose a significant challenge in biomedical data mining due to the large number of genes compared to the relatively small number of samples. This imbalance can lead to overfitting and reduced classification accuracy, making it difficult to identify the most informative genes relevant to specific phenotypes, such as cancer subtypes. Existing gene selection methods often fail to adequately reduce dimensionality while preserving critical information necessary for accurate classification. Consequently, there is a need for an effective and comprehensive approach that can balance dimensionality reduction and informative gene selection to improve classification performance and provide reliable insights for clinical decision making.

Objectives

- Develop a novel three-stage hybrid feature gene selection approach to address the challenge of high-dimensional gene expression data in biomedical data mining [7].

- Integrate a variance filter, an extremely randomized tree, and the Cuckoo Search algorithm to strategically reduce the dimensionality of the feature gene space while preserving informative genes [8].
- Evaluate the proposed methodology using a breast cancer gene expression profile dataset with three distinct classifiers to assess its effectiveness and robustness [9].
- Compare the performance of the proposed approach with various state-of-the-art feature selection algorithms to highlight its advantages in improving accuracy and reliability [10].
- Demonstrate the efficacy of the proposed method in improving the accuracy and reliability of subsequent analyses in biomedical data mining applications [11].

9.2 Literature review

Hanan et al. present a novel computer-aided diagnosis method for breast cancer classification using a combination of deep neural networks (ResNet 18, ShuffleNet, and Inception-V3Net) and transfer learning. The proposed method provides the best average accuracy for binary classification of benign or malignant cancer cases of 99.7 %, 97.66 %, and 96.94 % for ResNet, InceptionV3Net, and ShuffleNet, respectively. The average accuracies for multi-class classification were 97.81 %, 96.07 %, and 95.79 % for ResNet, Inception-V3Net, and ShuffleNet, respectively [12].

Moloud Abdar et al. proposed two best UQ methods (i. e., DE and EMC) which they applied in two classification phases to analyze two well-known skin cancer datasets to avoid making overconfident decisions in diagnosing the disease. The accuracy and the F1-score of final solution were 88.95 % and 89.00 % for the first dataset, and 90.96 % and 91.00 % for the second dataset. The results suggest that the proposed TWDBDL model can be effectively used in different stages of medical image analysis [13].

Mahmoud Ragab et al. developed an Ensemble Deep-Learning-Enabled Clinical Decision Support System for Breast Cancer Diagnosis and Classification (EDLCDS-BCDC) technique using USIs. The proposed EDLCDS-BCDC technique was designed to identify the presence of breast cancer using USIs. In this technique, USIs initially are first preprocessed through two stages, namely Wiener filtering and contrast enhancement. Furthermore, the Chaotic Krill Herd Algorithm (CKHA) with Kapur's Entropy (KE) is applied for the image segmentation process. In addition, an ensemble of three deep learning models, VGG-16, VGG-19, and SqueezeNet, is used for feature extraction. Finally, Cat Swarm Optimization (CSO) with the Multilayer Perceptron (MLP) model is used to classify the images based on the presence or absence of breast cancer. A wide range of simulations have been performed on benchmark databases and the extensive results highlight the better outcomes of the proposed EDLCDS-BCDC technique over recent methods [14].

Ruxandra Stoean introduces a novel modality to efficiently tune the convolutional layers of a deep neural network (CNN) and an approach to rank the importance of the hyperparameters involved. Three models have been used and evaluated as surrogates: random forests (RF), support vector machines (SVM), and Kriging. Sample convolutional configurations are generated by Latin hypercube sampling and are accompanied by computed accuracy outcomes from real CNN runs. For the hyperparameter estimation task, the fitness of an individual from the EA associated with a surrogate model is subsequently derived from the CNN accuracy estimation on these variable values. For the ranking and variable selection task, RF includes implicit variable selection, the SVM can be easily supported by a second EA, and Kriging offers a ranking based on the corresponding h-values. The estimated accuracy of the found hyperparameter values is compared to the true validation accuracy, and is then used for the prediction on the test cases. The ranking of the variables for each of the three surrogate models is compared, and their influence is also revealed by response surface methodology. The experimental testing of the proposed EA surrogate approaches is conducted on a real-world scenario of histopathological image interpretation in colorectal cancer diagnosis [15].

Shallu Sharma et al. proposed two machine learning approaches which were thoroughly investigated and compared for the task of automatic magnification-dependent multi-classification on a balanced BreakHis dataset for the breast cancer detection. The first approach is based on handcrafted features which are extracted using Hu moment, color histogram, and Haralick textures. The extracted features are then used to train the conventional classifiers, while the second approach is based on transfer learning where the pre-existing networks (VGG16, VGG19, and ResNet50) are used as a feature extractor and as a baseline model. The results show that the use of pre-trained networks as feature extractors showed superior performance compared to the baseline and hand-crafted approaches for all the magnifications. Moreover, it has been observed that the augmentation plays a pivotal role in further improving the classification accuracy. In this context, the VGG16 network with linear SVM provides the highest accuracy that is computed in two forms, (a) patch-based accuracies (93.97 % for 40×, 92.92 % for 100×, 91.23 % for 200×, and 91.79 % for 400×); (b) patient-based accuracies (93.25 % for 40×, 91.87 % for 100×, 91.5 % for 200×, and 92.31 % for 400×) for the classification of magnification-dependent histopathologic images. Additionally, the "fibroadenoma" (benign) and "mucous carcinoma" (malignant) classes were found to be the most complex classes for all magnification factors [16].

Devakishan Adla et al. proposed an automated deep learning with class attention layer-based CAD model for skin lesion detection and classification, known as DLCAL-SLDC. The goal of the DLCAL-SLDC model is to detect and classify the different types of skin cancer using dermoscopic images. During image preprocessing, hair removal based on the Dull razor approach and noise removal based on average median filtering are performed. Tsallis entropy-based segmentation technique is applied to detect the affected lesion areas in the dermoscopic images. Also, a DLCAL-based feature extractor is used to extract the features from the segmented lesions using Capsule Network (CapsNet) along with CAL and Adagrad optimizer. The CAL layer incorporated in the CapsNet is intended to capture the discriminative class-specific features to cover the class dependencies and effectively bridge the CapsNet for further processing. Finally, the classification is performed by the Swallow Swarm Optimization (SSO) algorithm based Convolutional Sparse Autoencoder (CSAE) known as SSO-CSAE model. The proposed DLCAL-SLDC technique is validated using a benchmark ISIC dataset. The proposed framework has achieved promising results with 98.50 % accuracy, 94.5 % sensitivity and 99.1 % specificity over the other methods in terms of different measures [17].

Maad M. Mijwil proposed a deep learning network which was selected and trained for the analysis of more than 24,000 skin cancer images by applying convolutional neural network (ConvNet) model with three architectures (InceptionV3, ResNet, and VGG19) with many parameters to identify the best architectures in the classification of these images and get very satisfactory results, and classify the cancer type as benign or malignant with high accuracy. The dataset contains high-resolution images obtained from the ISIC archive between 2019 and 2020. After all the tests were done, the best architecture is InceptionV3. This architecture has achieved a diagnostic accuracy of approximately 86.90 %, precision of 87.47 %, sensitivity of 86.14 %, and the specificity of 87.66 % [18].

Nonita Sharma et al. propose the implementation of the snapshot assembling technique to create an efficient model that could potentially assist medical professionals in diagnosing disease. Employing t-SNE enables the generation of improved scatter plots in addition to cost optimization. Furthermore, the current manuscript also uses a snapshot ensemble deep learning framework that integrates the predictions from various base models, leading to an improvement in accuracy. The proposed model is implemented on the Wisconsin Breast Cancer Dataset (WBCD), which is openly available at the UCI Machine Repository. During the experimental evaluation, the proposed model yields an accuracy of 86.6 %, which is higher than the state-of-art models such as averaging, weighted averaging, stacked ensemble, and Polyak Rupert, that yield an accuracy of 81 %, 81.7 %, 84.7 %, and 82.2 %, respectively, and hence establishes the competence of proposed model [19]. Lei Cui et al. proposed a survival analysis system that takes advantage of recently emerging deep learning techniques. The proposed system consists of three main components. 1) The first component is an end-to-end cellular feature learning module using a deep neural network with global average pooling. The learned cellular representations encode high-level biologically relevant information without requiring individual cell segmentation, which is aggregated into patient-level feature vectors by using a locality-constrained linear coding (LLC)-based bag of words (BoW) encoding algorithm. 2) The second component is a Cox proportional hazards model with an elastic net penalty for robust feature selection and survival analysis. 3) The third component is a biomarker interpretation module that can help localize the image regions that contribute to the survival model decision. Extensive experiments show that the proposed survival model has excellent predictive power for a public (i. e., The Cancer Genome Atlas) lung cancer dataset in terms of two commonly used metrics: the log-rank test (p-value) of the Kaplan-Meier estimate and the concordance index (c-index) [20].

9.3 Methods

9.3.1 Variance filter (VF)

In the field of biomedical data mining, where the gene dimension often exceeds the sample size, managing high dimensionality is crucial. A key strategy to address this challenge is the use of a variance filter, a fundamental technique designed to streamline the feature gene space while preserving essential genes. The variance filter operates on the principle that genes with limited variability across samples offer less predictive value. Thus, by prioritizing genes with higher variance – indicative of greater diversity in expression levels across various biological conditions – this method effectively concentrates on genes with greater potential for meaningful insight [21]. The variance filter starts by computing the variance of each gene across the samples in the dataset. Genes with low variance, indicating minimal variation in expression levels, are subsequently excluded, thereby reducing the overall dimensionality of the feature gene space. This process serves to counteract the curse of dimensionality by eliminating redundant or uninformative genes that are less likely to capture meaningful biological patterns [22]. Furthermore, by favoring genes with higher variance, the variance filter highlights those that are more likely to be associated with the phenotype of interest, thereby enhancing the significance and interpretability of subsequent analyses. Despite its simplicity, the variance filter plays a critical role as an initial preprocessing step within feature selection methods, laying the groundwork for subsequent, more intricate techniques. By efficiently reducing the dimensionality of the feature gene space, the variance filter not only improves computational efficiency, but also mitigates the risk of overfitting in predictive modeling endeavors. Additionally, its straightforward implementation makes it adaptable to various biomedical datasets, providing researchers with a valuable tool for data preprocessing and dimensionality reduction [23].

In summary, the variance filter plays a pivotal role in biomedical data mining by facilitating the initial dimensionality reduction of gene expression datasets. By prioritizing genes with greater variability across samples, this technique effectively retains the most informative features while discarding redundant or less informative ones. As an integral component of comprehensive feature selection pipelines, the variance filter contributes to more efficient and effective analyses, ultimately advancing our understanding of complex biological processes and aiding clinical decision making [24].

9.3.2 Extremely randomized tree (ERT)

Within the biomedical data mining landscape, the management of high-dimensional gene expression datasets requires innovative approaches, including the use of sophisticated techniques such as the extremely randomized tree (ERT) algorithm. The ERT algorithm represents a powerful feature selection tool, particularly in scenarios where traditional decision tree-based methods may struggle to effectively handle large volumes of features [25]. Unlike conventional decision trees, which select splits based on the optimal criteria within a subset of features, ERT introduces an additional layer of randomness by selecting candidate splits at each node without any regard for optimal criteria. This unique approach effectively decorrelates individual trees within the ensemble, mitigating the risk of overfitting and enhancing the robustness of feature selection [26]. By aggregating the predictions from multiple randomly constructed trees, ERT provides a more stable and reliable estimate of feature importance, allowing the identification of genes with stronger correlations to the phenotype of interest. Furthermore, the inherent diversity of ERT's ensemble of trees allows it to capture complex nonlinear relationships and interactions within high-dimensional gene expression data, thus facilitating more accurate and interpretable predictive modeling. The versatility and effectiveness of ERT make it a valuable asset in biomedical data mining, empowering researchers to extract meaningful insights from complex genomic datasets and advance our understanding of the biological mechanisms underlying diseases such as cancer [27].

9.3.3 Cuckoo Search algorithm (CSA)

The optimization method used in computer science is inspired by the reproductive behavior of the cuckoo bird. This nature-inspired strategy employs a technique known as Lévy flying, rather than relying on random movements characterized by wide-ranging and unpredictable patterns [28]. Lévy flying involves making subtle adjustments to the existing position rather than large shifts, similar to the nuanced adjustments made by the cuckoo bird. In nature, the cuckoo ensures the survival of its offspring by laying its eggs in the nests of other birds, tricking the host birds into raising the cuckoo chicks as their own [29]. Similarly, in the optimization method, the concept of laying eggs corresponds to the generation of new candidate solutions, while the process of host birds raising the cuckoo chicks reflects the evaluation and potential improvement of these solutions. This biomimetic approach exploits the efficiency and effectiveness observed in natural systems, and offers a novel and adaptive optimization strategy in computer science [30].

Brood parasitism: It uses another bird's nest as its own, hides its eggs inside, and then depends on the host bird to care for the offspring [31].

Host bird: The owner of the host nest is tasked with nurturing and providing sustenance for the cuckoo chicks [32].

Parasite bird: Birds that lay their eggs in another bird's nest [33].

Lévy Flight: A Lévy flight is a natural occurrence where the duration of each phase follows a probability distribution characterized by a distinct tail, referred to as the Lévy distribution. This distribution governs the probability of transitions during Lévy flights as outlined below [34]:

For $1 < \lambda \leq 3$

We have $\quad Lévy(\lambda) \approx g^{-\lambda}$. (9.1)

From an implementation standpoint, the use of Lévy flights to generate random numbers involves two distinct components
1. Random selection of the direction based on a uniform distribution [35].
2. Making decisions according to with the chosen Lévy distribution [36].

Random Walk: A stochastic process that delineates a trajectory consisting of a series of discrete steps of constant length in random directions within a mathematical space (e. g., 1D, 2D, or nD), such as integers [37].
Random Walk Equation:

$$S_i^{t+1} = E_i^t + a \odot L(\lambda).$$ (9.2)

Where S_i^{t+1} = new solution, E_i^t = existing solution, a = *length of walk*, $\odot$ = entry considering multiplication $L(\lambda)$ = Lévy expositor.
Implementation rules:
- Typically, each cuckoo lays only one egg at a time into a randomly chosen nest.

Mathematical representation: Since a cuckoo can only lay one egg at a time, each egg found in the nest represents a potential solution [38].
- In subsequent generations, even the most exceptional nests and the highest quality eggs can be surpassed [39].

Mathematical representation: Eggs that are very similar have the potential to develop. The host bird faces a choice: either abandon the current nest and establish a new one elsewhere, where the number of potential host nests is reduced and there is a probability (Pa) ranging between 0 and 1 [40].
Mathematical representation: The current number of nesting hosts remains stable as a population. If the host bird detects a cuckoo hatch, it represents the worst solution, far from the optimal one. The fundamental Cuckoo Search algorithm is outlined in pseudocode based on these criteria. Maintaining control while searching for new solutions is crucial. Lévy flights, which involve random walks, help prevent large movements that could lead to escaping the search area. The step size is determined by the size of the problem, which should be adjusted accordingly to maintain interest. Exploring the optimal use of Lévy flights for optimization is an intriguing area for further investigation. To simplify the process, a common step size factor of 0.01 is employed. Figure 9.1 shows the schematic view of the proposed method and Algorithm 9.1 shows the hybrid code of the proposed method [41].

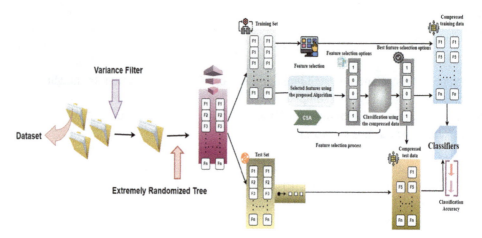

Figure 9.1: Graphical view of the proposed method.

Algorithm 9.1: Pseudocode for the proposed hybrid algorithm.

```
import numPy as np
from sklearn. feature_ selection import Variance Threshold
from sklearn. ensemble import Extra Trees Classifier
from sklearn. Model _ selection import cross_ val_ score
from sklearn. metrics import accuracy_ score
from cuckoo_ search import Cuckoo Search # Assuming
    implementation of Cuckoo Search Algorithm
# Step 1: Variance Filter
def apply_ variance_ filter (X, threshold):
    selector = Variance Threshold (threshold=threshold)
    X_ filtered = selector. Fit _ transform(X)
    return X_ filtered
# Step 2: Extremely Randomized Tree
def apply_ extra_ trees (X, y, n_ estimators):
    clf = Extra Trees Classifier (n_ estimators=n_
        estimators, random_ state=42)
    clf. fit (X, y)
    feature_ importances = clf. feature _ importances_
    return feature_ importances
# Step 3: Cuckoo Search Algorithm
def apply_ cuckoo_ search (X, y, num_ agents, max_ iter):
    cuckoo_ search = Cuckoo Search (n_ agents=num_ agents,
        max_ iter= max_iter)
    selected_ features = cuckoo_ search. fit (X, y)
    return selected_ features
```

```
# Evaluation
def evaluate_ method (X, y, selected_ features):
    X_ selected = X [: selected_ features]
    # Perform classification using selected features
    # Assuming classifiers are imported and defined
        elsewhere
    # classifier. fit (X _selected, y)
    # y_ pred = classifier. predict (X_ selected)
    # accuracy = accuracy_ score (y, y_ pred)
    # return accuracy
# Main
if _name_ == "_main_":
    # Load breast cancer dataset (X, y)
    # Assuming X contains gene expression features and y
        contains target labels
    # Step 1: Variance Filter
    X_ filtered = apply_ variance_ filter (X, threshold=0.1)
    # Step 2: Extremely Randomized Tree
    feature_ importances = apply_ extra_ trees (X_ filtered,
        y, n_ estimators=100)
    selected_ features = np. arg sort (feature_ importances)
        [:-1][:50]  # Select top 50 features
    # Step 3: Cuckoo Search Algorithm
    selected_ features = apply_ cuckoo_ search (X_ filtered,
        y, num_ agents=10, max_ iter=100)
    # Evaluation
    accuracy = evaluate_ method (X_ filtered, y, selected_
        features)
print ("Accuracy:", accuracy)
```

Table 9.1: Parameter setting for the proposed method.

Step	Parameter	Setting
Variance Filter	Threshold	0.1
Extremely randomized tree	Number of Estimators	100
Cuckoo Search algorithm	Number of Agents	10
Maximum iterations	100	100

Table 9.1 shows the parameter setting which we have used during the implementation of the model.

9.4 Experimental setup

In our research, we harnessed the computational capabilities of the Ubuntu 20.04.5 LTS operating system, and used the Windows Subsystem for Linux (WSL) to seamlessly integrate our work environment. We relied on the Visual Studio Code (VS Code) integrated development environment (IDE) to facilitate our coding efforts, as it offers a robust platform that integrates well with the Python programming language. To ensure the reliability and robustness of our findings, we employed the Leave-One-Out Cross-Validation (LOOCV) technique, a powerful method for evaluating model performance. LOOCV systematically omits one data point from the dataset at each iteration, trains the model on the remaining data, and evaluates its performance on the excluded data point. This iterative process provides a comprehensive assessment of the model's effectiveness across the entire dataset. Our experiments were conducted on a high-performance computing system equipped with an Intel(R) Core™ i9-12900k processor with a clock speed of 5.20 GHz, and 64 GB of RAM, which provides ample memory for processing complex algorithms and datasets. Additionally, we used an Nvidia RTX Quadro A5000 Graphics Processing Unit (GPU) to improve parallelization and accelerate tasks that benefit from GPU acceleration. The dataset under analysis, detailed in Table 9.3, served as the basis for our investigation. Our meticulous attention to the details of the dataset emphasizes the transparency and reproducibility of our methodology, setting the stage for thorough analysis and informed conclusions. Table 9.2 shows the details based on the dataset used in the proposed model.

Table 9.2: Comprehensive details regarding a dataset focused on gene expression.

Data set	Short Description	samples	Categories	Genes
Breast Cancer [42]	Breast cancer originates in the cells of the breast tissue and ranks as one of the prevalent cancer types affecting women.	97	2	24481

9.5 Results and discussion

Tables 9.3, 9.4, 9.5, and 9.6 depict the classification accuracies achieved using the proposed methods on the breast cancer dataset. These tables provide a comprehensive analysis of the accuracy performance of the proposed method, extremely randomized tree, and variance filter algorithms under various conditions and gene subsets. The results clearly demonstrate that the proposed method outperforms the other two algorithms in terms of accuracy, indicating its effectiveness in gene selection. To further visualize and compare the performance of these algorithms, additional graphical representations such as AUC curves, precision-recall curves, and confusion matrix are provided. These

Table 9.3: Using the random forest classifier, the classification accuracy of the breast cancer dataset was tested for the proposed method, extremely randomized tree and variance filter.

Selected Genes	Accuracy								
	Proposed Method			Extremely Randomized Tree			Variance filter		
	Best	Average	Worst	Best	Average	Worst	Best	Average	Worst
3	95.57	87.45	81.61	87.72	81.75	77.08	85.08	71.75	75.08
7	97.72	91.16	85.77	89.62	83.86	81.87	90.87	73.86	80.87
11	**100**	**94.32**	**90.08**	95.96	85.94	85.91	83.91	85.94	73.91
15	99.36	92.08	86.97	**98.52**	**93.86**	**88.94**	**86.94**	**93.86**	76.94
19	98.42	90.97	84.72	95.64	90.12	86.94	84.94	80.12	**82.94**
23	97.18	88.34	81.57	93.99	87.53	84.07	81.07	85.53	80.07
27	95.64	84.46	76.76	92.07	84.09	81.19	83.19	84.09	81.19

figures, accompanied by legends, offer a visual summary of the classification accuracies achieved by the proposed method, complementing the numerical results presented in the tables. The integration of tabular data and visualizations facilitates a comprehensive evaluation of the suggested technique's performance on different datasets, underscoring the superiority of the proposed algorithm in optimizing gene selection for cancer classification. The robustness and effectiveness of the proposed approach across various datasets are evident from the distinct trends and consistent improvements observed in both tables and visual representations.

Figure 9.4 presents the area under the curve (AUC) values, which assess the ability of the model to distinguish between positive and negative classes based on the selected genes. Higher AUC values, which are commonly used in binary classification problems, indicate better performance. Presumably, the multiple subplots or data points in the figure represent the performance of the three binary adaptations across various gene subsets in the breast cancer dataset. Similarly, Figures 9.2 and 9.3 display the precision recall and confusion matrix with values for the three binary adaptations across selected genes in the same dataset, providing additional context and validating the efficacy of the models across different gene sets. It is crucial to compare the proposed method, the extremely randomized tree, and the variance filter in all figures to determine which adaptation performs better under different scenarios and gene selections. Examining trends, patterns, and variances in AUC scores across datasets and gene sets helps better understand the strengths and weaknesses of the models.

Table 9.3 presents the classification accuracy results of the breast cancer dataset using the Random Forest classifier for different approaches: the proposed method, the extremely randomized tree, and the variance filter. The accuracy metrics are provided for various numbers of selected genes, ranging from 3 to 27. Each cell in the table displays the accuracy values corresponding to the best, average, and worst performance achieved by each approach. The analysis shows that the proposed method consistently outperforms both the extremely randomized tree and the variance filter over all configurations of selected genes. For instance, when only three genes are selected, the proposed method achieves the best accuracy of 95.57 %, significantly higher than the best accuracy of 87.72 % achieved by the extremely randomized tree and 85.08 % achieved by the variance filter. This trend persists over different numbers of selected genes, with the proposed method consistently yielding higher accuracy values compared to the other approaches. Furthermore, as the number of selected genes increases, there is a noticeable improvement in accuracy for all methods. However, the proposed method consistently maintains the highest accuracy values, reaching 100 % accuracy with 11 selected genes. In contrast, the extremely randomized tree and the variance filter achieve lower accuracy values, with the proposed method consistently outperforming them. Overall, Table 9.3 highlights the superiority of the proposed method in terms of classification accuracy on the breast cancer dataset. These results underscore the effectiveness of the proposed approach in selecting informative genes for cancer classification, thereby contributing to improved diagnostic accuracy and potentially better patient outcomes.

Table 9.4 displays the classification accuracy results of the breast cancer dataset using linear regression across different methodologies: the proposed method, the extremely randomized tree, and the variance filter. Similar to Table 9.3, the accuracy metrics are provided for varying numbers of selected genes, ranging from 2 to 26, and each cell in the table represents the best, average, and worst accuracy values achieved by each approach. Upon analysis of the table, it is apparent that the proposed method generally performs competitively with the other approaches, demonstrating consistent accuracy across different configurations of selected genes. Notably, the proposed method achieves high accuracy values, especially when a larger number of genes are selected. For instance, with 8 selected genes, the proposed method achieves 100 % accuracy at its best, outperforming both the extremely randomized tree and the variance filter. Moreover, as the number of selected genes increases, there is a tendency for accuracy to improve

Table 9.4: Using linear regression, the classification accuracy of the breast cancer dataset was tested for the proposed method, the extremely randomized tree, and the variance filter.

Selected Genes	Proposed Method Best	Proposed Method Average	Proposed Method Worst	Extremely Randomized Tree Best	Extremely Randomized Tree Average	Extremely Randomized Tree Worst	Variance filter Best	Variance filter Average	Variance filter Worst
2	92.72	83.04	79.22	91.37	82.01	76.52	83.04	79.22	73.52
5	96.02	88.07	82.03	93.27	85.55	78.22	88.07	82.03	76.22
8	**100**	**97.25**	**91.15**	94.53	88.17	85.89	97.25	91.15	81.89
11	98.28	95.85	89.35	**100**	**95.12**	**89.66**	95.85	89.35	**89.66**
14	97.06	92.76	83.54	97.52	91.52	85.46	92.76	83.54	86.46
17	94.67	88.75	81.16	93.64	88.51	81.06	88.75	81.16	82.06
20	90.46	84.72	77.08	91.81	83.57	76.31	84.72	77.08	78.31
23	88.78	82.36	75.23	88.23	81.48	79.22	82.36	75.23	73.22
26	86.72	80.84	73.39	83.43	78.66	77.12	80.84	73.39	71.12

for all methods, highlighting the importance of gene selection in enhancing classification performance. However, it's worth noting that once the number of selected genes exceeds a certain threshold, the accuracy of all approaches tends to plateau or slightly decrease, indicating diminishing returns in terms of additional gene selection. Overall, Table 9.4 underscores the effectiveness of the proposed method in achieving competitive classification accuracy using linear regression on the breast cancer dataset. While there may be fluctuations in performance with different numbers of selected genes, the proposed method consistently demonstrates robust performance, making it a promising approach for gene selection in cancer classification tasks.

Table 9.5 provides an overview of the classification accuracy results obtained from the breast cancer dataset using the K-Nearest Neighbors algorithm, focusing on three different methods: the proposed method, the extremely randomized tree, and the variance filter. The table presents accuracy metrics for various numbers of selected genes, ranging from 3 to 47, with each cell showing the best, average, and worst accuracy values achieved by each approach. Several observations can be made by examining the table. Firstly, it is evident that the proposed method consistently outperforms both the extremely randomized tree and the variance filter over different configurations of selected genes. Notably, the proposed method demonstrates higher accuracy values, particularly as the number of selected genes increases. For instance, with 11 selected genes, the proposed method achieves an accuracy of 99.01 % at its best, surpassing the accuracy achieved by the other approaches. This trend persists over different numbers of selected genes, highlighting the effectiveness of the proposed method in enhancing classification accuracy with K-Nearest Neighbors. Furthermore, as the number of selected genes increases, there is generally an improvement in accuracy for all methods, although dimin-

Table 9.5: Using the K-Nearest Neighbors, the classification accuracy of the breast cancer dataset was tested for the proposed method, extremely randomized tree and variance filter.

Selected Genes	Proposed Method			Extremely Randomized Tree			Variance filter		
	Best	Average	Worst	Best	Average	Worst	Best	Average	Worst
3	89.27	81.94	75.98	83.56	75.21	69.67	81.94	75.98	65.66
7	96.63	87.86	77.89	88.35	78.65	68.76	87.86	77.89	67.76
11	99.01	91.26	82.93	93.44	82.54	71.44	91.26	82.93	70.44
15	96.87	89.66	81.53	92.30	91.04	81.44	89.66	81.53	80.44
19	96.54	88.08	80.98	97.34	88.65	79.77	88.08	80.98	78.77
23	94.68	84.94	77.97	95.45	85.23	77.81	84.94	77.97	73.81
27	93.16	83.78	76.23	93.57	83.08	75.39	83.78	76.23	71.39
31	92.84	82.58	74.35	91.29	81.35	71.21	82.58	74.35	70.21
35	90.77	80.38	73.36	88.76	79.22	69.48	80.38	73.36	68.48
39	88.96	78.97	71.17	87.06	77.02	67.78	78.97	71.17	65.78
43	87.15	76.99	69.31	84.35	74.37	64.12	76.99	69.31	63.2
47	86.29	75.12	67.76	83.65	73.58	65.31	75.12	67.76	62.31

ishing returns are observed beyond a certain threshold. This suggests the importance of selecting an optimal number of genes to achieve the best classification performance. Additionally, it's worth noting that while the accuracy values may fluctuate with different numbers of selected genes, the proposed method consistently maintains superior performance compared to the other approaches. In summary, Table 9.5 underscores the efficacy of the proposed method in achieving higher classification accuracy with the K-Nearest Neighbors algorithm on the breast cancer dataset. These results highlight the potential of the proposed method to improve cancer classification results by selecting informative gene subsets, thereby contributing to advances in diagnostic accuracy and patient care.

Table 9.6 outlines the classification accuracy results of the breast cancer dataset using the Support Vector Machine (SVM) classifier across different methods: the proposed method, the extremely randomized tree, and the variance filter. The table presents accuracy metrics for different numbers of selected genes, ranging from 2 to 23, with each cell indicating the best, average, and worst accuracy values achieved by each approach. Upon analysis of the table, several insights emerge. Firstly, it is apparent that the proposed method generally exhibits competitive performance compared to the extremely randomized tree and the variance filter over different configurations of selected genes. Particularly noteworthy is the consistency of the proposed method in maintaining higher accuracy values, especially as the number of selected genes increases. For example, with 8 selected genes, the proposed method achieves an accuracy of 98.21 % at its best, outperforming the other methods. This trend persists over various numbers of selected genes, underscoring the effectiveness of the proposed method in improving the classification accuracy of the SVM classifier. Furthermore, as the number of selected genes increases, there is typically an improvement in accuracy for all methods, although with diminishing returns observed beyond a certain threshold. This emphasizes the importance of selecting an optimal number of genes to achieve the best classification per-

Table 9.6: Using the support vector machine classifier, the classification accuracy of the breast cancer dataset was tested for the proposed method, extremely randomized tree and variance filter.

Selected Genes	Proposed Method			Extremely Randomized Tree			Variance filter		
	Best	Average	Worst	Best	Average	Worst	Best	Average	Worst
2	92.83	86.14	78.25	89.95	81.85	75.56	86.14	78.25	72.56
5	94.12	87.92	80.52	93.12	86.68	80.05	87.92	80.52	79.05
8	**98.21**	**91.71**	**84.72**	97.42	90.11	81.61	91.71	84.72	81.61
11	95.16	89.69	83.03	91.28	86.29	82.11	89.69	83.03	80.1
14	91.43	86.78	80.94	89.71	83.87	77.85	86.78	80.94	76.84
17	89.57	84.15	77.53	87.56	81.89	76.03	84.15	77.53	75.02
20	88.65	82.4	74.95	86.13	80.41	74.15	82.4	74.95	73.5
23	87.45	80.7	72.75	83.73	79.05	74.18	80.7	72.75	73.17

formance. Additionally, while there may be fluctuations in accuracy values for different numbers of genes selected, the proposed method consistently demonstrates robust performance compared to the other approaches. In summary, Table 9.6 highlights the efficacy of the proposed method in achieving competitive classification accuracy with the SVM classifier on the breast cancer dataset. These results underscore the potential of the proposed method to improve cancer classification outcomes by selecting informative gene subsets, thus contributing to advances in diagnostic accuracy and patient care.

9.5.1 Confusion matrix

Figure 9.2 illustrates a significant evaluation metric for classification models called the confusion matrix. This matrix provides a comprehensive breakdown of the model's performance by presenting its predictions compared to the actual ground truth values in a grid format. It comprises four sections: true positives (TP), true negatives (TN), false positives (FP), and false negatives (FN). True positives represent correctly identified positive instances, while true negatives indicate correctly identified negative instances. False positives represent instances misclassified as positive, and false negatives denote instances misclassified as negative.

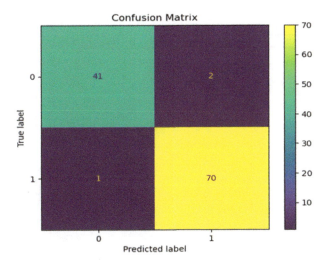

Figure 9.2: Confusion matrix based on the breast cancer dataset by using proposed method.

The matrix offers a concise and transparent summary of the model's strengths and limitations, facilitating a deeper insight into its predictive capabilities. Through a detailed examination of these elements, metrics such as accuracy, precision, recall, and F1-score can be calculated, providing a thorough evaluation of the model's effectiveness in making precise classifications. The use of the confusion matrix allows for the refinement of models and the making of informed decisions regarding their practical deployment. Equations (a) through (d) determine the computation of these performance metrics based on the values within the confusion matrix.

$$ACC = \frac{TP + TN}{TP + TN + FP + FN} \qquad (a)$$

$$P = \frac{TP}{TP + FP} \qquad (b)$$

$$Sn = \frac{TP}{TP + FN} \qquad (c)$$

$$F\text{-score} = 2 \times \frac{P \times Sn}{P + Sn} \qquad (d)$$

9.5.2 Precesion recall curve

The research also uses crucial visual aids to support its conclusions. Figure 9.3 presents the precision-recall (PR) curve, which provides a detailed evaluation of the proposed method' performance. This graph illustrates the balance between precision, which represents the accuracy of positive predictions, and recall, which indicates the proportion of actual positives that are correctly identified.

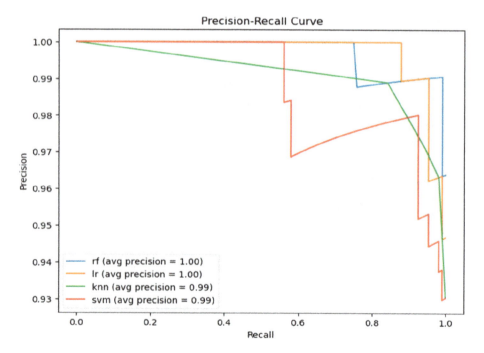

Figure 9.3: Precision-recall curves.

9.5.3 Area under the curve

A higher area under the curve (AUC) in ROC curves indicates superior model performance. These curves demonstrate the trade-off between the true positive rate (sensitivity) and the false positive rate (1 – specificity), offering insight into the classification accuracy of the model at different thresholds. Similarly, the ROC curves show the robustness and effectiveness of the proposed method in accurately distinguishing between positive and negative instances, which is particularly important in scenarios with unbalanced class distributions.

Similarly, Figure 9.4 presents the Receiver Operating Characteristic (ROC) curve, a vital measure for evaluating classifiers. This curve visually illustrates the trade-off between the true positive rate (sensitivity) and the false positive rate (1-specificity), offering insight into the model's ability to discriminate. A higher AUC-ROC value indicates a greater proficiency of the model to discriminate between classes. The ROC curve generated by the proposed method highlights its impressive discriminative power. The substantial AUC values observed in both the PR and ROC curves confirm the effectiveness and reliability of the combined approach in accurately classifying cancer types. These visual representations provide compelling evidence for the efficacy of the method and hold great promise for its use in real-world clinical settings.

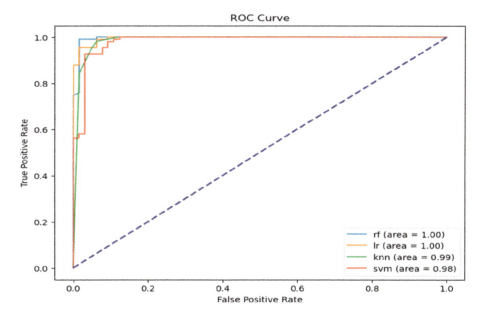

Figure 9.4: ROC curves.

9.6 Conclusion

In conclusion, this research paper introduces a novel three-stage hybrid feature gene selection approach to address the prevalent challenge of dealing with high-dimensional gene data in biomedical data mining. By integrating a variance filter, an extremely randomized tree, and the Cuckoo Search algorithm, this method effectively narrows down the pool of potential genes and selects an optimal feature gene subset. The experimental evaluation conducted on a breast cancer gene expression dataset, employing four distinct classifiers and compared with various state-of-the-art feature selection algorithms, demonstrates the notable advantages of the proposed method. The results highlight its efficacy in improving accuracy and reliability across multiple evaluation metrics. Overall, the comprehensive methodology presented in this study holds promise for improving subsequent analyses in biomedical data mining applications, contributing to advances in the understanding and diagnosis of complex diseases.

Future directions

Based on the promising results of the three-stage hybrid gene selection approach, several future research directions can be considered to further improve its performance and applicability in biomedical data mining:

1. Exploration of alternative filtering techniques:
   - Investigate the use of alternative dimensionality reduction techniques, such as Principal Component Analysis (PCA) or Mutual Information (MI), instead of or in combination with the variance filter. This could reveal more nuanced relationships between genes and phenotypes, potentially leading to improved initial gene selection.
2. Integration with deep learning-based feature selection:
   - Explore the integration of deep learning models, such as autoencoders or convolutional neural networks (CNNs), for feature extraction and selection in the initial stages. These models can capture complex, non-linear relationships in high-dimensional gene expression data, potentially improving the selection of informative genes.
3. Application to multi-omics and multi-modal data:
   - Extend the proposed methodology to incorporate multi-omics data (e. g., proteomics, metabolomics) or integrate different data types (e. g., imaging and clinical data). This holistic approach could provide a more comprehensive understanding of disease mechanisms and improve classification performance.

4. Dynamic parameter optimization in Cuckoo Search:
   – Develop adaptive mechanisms to dynamically tune the parameters of the Cuckoo Search algorithm based on dataset characteristics. This could improve the efficiency and effectiveness of the optimization process, leading to more precise selection of feature genes.
5. Handling class imbalance and rare phenotypes:
   – Investigate methods to handle class imbalance, such as Synthetic Minority Over-sampling Technique (SMOTE) or ensemble techniques, to ensure that the proposed method performs well even with imbalanced datasets or rare phenotypes. This is especially important for diseases with low prevalence or subtypes.
6. Development of a real-time gene selection tool:
   – Create a user-friendly software or web application that implements the three-stage hybrid gene selection approach for real-time gene analysis and classification. This tool could be valuable for clinicians and researchers to quickly identify key genes associated with to various diseases.
7. Investigation of gene-gene interaction networks:
   – Extend the approach to include gene-gene interaction networks using graph-based methods or network analysis. This could help identify sets of genes that work synergistically and contribute more effectively to the classification task.
8. Validation on larger and more diverse datasets:
   – Validate the proposed methodology on larger and more diverse gene expression datasets, including different cancer types and non-cancerous diseases. This would demonstrate the generalizability and robustness of the approach in different biomedical contexts.
9. Combination with ensemble learning techniques:
   – Explore combining the proposed method with ensemble learning techniques, such as random forest or gradient boosting, to further improve classification accuracy. This could help mitigate overfitting and improve generalization to new datasets.
10. Prognostic and predictive modeling:
    – Extend the application of the proposed method to prognostic and predictive modeling, such as survival analysis or treatment response prediction. This could provide valuable insights for personalized medicine and targeted therapeutic interventions.

By pursuing these future directions, the three-stage hybrid gene selection approach can be further refined and adapted to address more complex challenges in biomedical data mining, ultimately contributing to more accurate and reliable disease diagnosis and prognosis.

Bibliography

[1] Zhou, X., Liu, K. Y. & Wong, S. T. C. (2004). Cancer classification and prediction using logistic regression with Bayesian gene selection. J. Biomed. Inform., 37(4), 249–259. https://doi.org/10.1016/j.jbi.2004.07.009.

[2] Mrózek, K., Heerema, N. A. & Bloomfield, C. D. (2004). Cytogenetics in acute leukemia. Blood Rev., 18(2), 115–136. https://doi.org/10.1016/S0268-960X(03)00040-7.

[3] Mohammad, L. & Abualigah, Q. (2018). Feature Selection and Enhanced Krill.

[4] Gaur, H., Vashishtha, S., Singh, V. K. & Hemanth, D. J. (2023). A fuzzy rule-based system with decision tree for breast cancer. February, 1–14. https://doi.org/10.1049/ipr2.12774.

[5] Askarzadeh, A. (2016). A novel metaheuristic method for solving constrained engineering optimization problems: crow search algorithm. Comput. Struct., 169, 1–12. https://doi.org/10.1016/j.compstruc.2016.03.001.

[6] Akkur, E., Türk, F. & Eroğul, O. (2023). Breast cancer classification using a novel hybrid feature selection approach. Neural Netw. World, 33(2), 67–83. https://doi.org/10.14311/NNW.2023.33.005.

[7] Al-Betar, M. A., Alomari, O. A. & Abu-Romman, S. M. (2020). A TRIZ-inspired bat algorithm for gene selection in cancer classification. Genomics, 112(1), 114–126. https://doi.org/10.1016/j.ygeno.2019.09.015.

[8] Aziz, R., Verma, C. K. & Srivastava, N. (2017). Dimension reduction methods for microarray data: a review. AIMS Bioeng., 4(1), 179–197. https://doi.org/10.3934/bioeng.2017.1.179.

[9] Wang, X., Bo, D., Shi, C., Fan, S., Ye, Y. & Yu, P. S. (2022). A survey on heterogeneous graph embedding: methods, techniques, applications and sources. IEEE Trans. Big Data, 1–23. https://doi.org/10.1109/TBDATA.2022.3177455.

[10] Nakariyakul, S. (2019). A hybrid gene selection algorithm based on interaction information for microarray-based cancer classification. PLoS ONE, 14(2), 1–17. https://doi.org/10.1371/journal.pone.0212333.

[11] Shrivastava, P., Shukla, A., Vepakomma, P., Bhansali, N. & Verma, K. (2017). A survey of nature-inspired algorithms for feature selection to identify Parkinson's disease. Comput. Methods Programs Biomed., 139, 171–179. https://doi.org/10.1016/j.cmpb.2016.07.029.

[12] Aljuaid, H., Alturki, N., Alsubaie, N., Cavallaro, L. & Liotta, A. (2022). Computer-aided diagnosis for breast cancer classification using deep neural networks and transfer learning. Comput. Methods Programs Biomed., 223, 106951. https://doi.org/10.1016/j.cmpb.2022.106951.

[13] Abdar, M., et al. (2021). Uncertainty quantification in skin cancer classification using three-way decision-based Bayesian deep learning. Comput. Biol. Med., 135(January), 104418. https://doi.org/10.1016/j.compbiomed.2021.104418.

[14] Ragab, M., Albukhari, A., Alyami, J. & Mansour, R. F. (2022). Ensemble deep-learning-enabled clinical decision support ultrasound images. Biology (Basel), 11, 439.

[15] Stoean, R. (2020). Analysis on the potential of an EA–surrogate modelling tandem for deep learning parametrization: an example for cancer classification from medical images. Neural Comput. Appl., 32(2), 313–322. https://doi.org/10.1007/s00521-018-3709-5.

[16] Sharma, S. & Mehra, R. (2020). Conventional machine learning and deep learning approach for multi-classification of breast cancer histopathology images—a comparative insight. J. Digit. Imag., 33(3), 632–654. https://doi.org/10.1007/s10278-019-00307-y.

[17] Adla, D., Reddy, G. V. R., Nayak, P. & Karuna, G. (2022). Deep learning-based computer aided diagnosis model for skin cancer detection and classification. Distrib. Parallel Databases, 40(4), 717–736. https://doi.org/10.1007/s10619-021-07360-z.

[18] Mijwil, M. M. (2021). Skin cancer disease images classification using deep learning solutions. Multimed. Tools Appl., 80(17), 26255–26271. https://doi.org/10.1007/s11042-021-10952-7.

[19] Sharma, N., Sharma, K. P., Mangla, M. & Rani, R. (2023). Breast cancer classification using snapshot ensemble deep learning model and t-distributed stochastic neighbor embedding. Multimed. Tools Appl., 82(3), 4011–4029. https://doi.org/10.1007/s11042-022-13419-5.
[20] Cui, L., et al. (2020). A deep learning-based framework for lung cancer survival analysis with biomarker interpretation. BMC Bioinform., 21(1), 1–14. https://doi.org/10.1186/s12859-020-3431-z.
[21] Lee, A. & Whiteley, N. (2018). Variance estimation in the particle filter. Biometrika, 105(3), 609–625. https://doi.org/10.1093/biomet/asy028.
[22] Fabijańska, A. (2011). Variance filter for edge detection and edge-based image segmentation. In 2011 Proc. 7th Int. Conf. Perspect. Technol. Methods MEMS Des. MEMSTECH 2011, no. May (pp. 151–154).
[23] Reiss, J. D. & McPherson, A. (2020). Filter design. Audio Eff., 49(11), 74–103. https://doi.org/10.1201/b17593-6.
[24] Schlangen, I., Delande, E. D., Houssineau, J. & Clark, D. E. (2018). A second-order PHD filter with mean and variance in target number. IEEE Trans. Signal Process., 66(1), 48–63. https://doi.org/10.1109/TSP.2017.2757905.
[25] Gotz, M., Weber, C., Blocher, J., Stieltjes, B., Meinzer, H. & Maier-Hein, K. (2014). Extremely randomized trees based brain tumor segmentation. In Proceedings of BRATS Challenge – MICCAI. 2014, Researchgate.Net, no. March 2015 (pp. 1–6). [Online]. Available, http://people.csail.mit.edu/menze/papers/proceedings_miccai_brats_2014.pdf.
[26] Saeed, U., Jan, S. U., Lee, Y. D. & Koo, I. (2021). Fault diagnosis based on extremely randomized trees in wireless sensor networks. Reliab. Eng. Syst. Saf., 205, May 2020. https://doi.org/10.1016/j.ress.2020.107284.
[27] Geurts, P., Ernst, D. & Wehenkel, L. (2006). Extremely randomized trees. Mach. Learn., 63(1), 3–42. https://doi.org/10.1007/s10994-006-6226-1.
[28] Zheng, Y., et al. (2019). A novel hybrid algorithm for feature selection based on whale optimization algorithm. IEEE Access, 7, 14908–14923. https://doi.org/10.1109/ACCESS.2018.2879848.
[29] Bandaru, S. & Deb, K. Metaheuristic techniques (pp. 1–49).
[30] Fister, I., Yang, X. S., Fister, D. & Fister, I. (2014). Cuckoo search: a brief literature review. https://doi.org/10.1007/978-3-319-02141-6_3.
[31] Mirjalili, S. (2015). Knowledge-based systems Moth-flame optimization algorithm: a novel nature-inspired heuristic paradigm. Knowl.-Based Syst., 89, 228–249. https://doi.org/10.1016/j.knosys.2015.07.006.
[32] Singh, N., Singh, S. B. & Houssein, E. H. (2022). Hybridizing salp swarm algorithm with particle swarm optimization algorithm for recent optimization functions. 15(1). Springer Berlin Heidelberg. https://doi.org/10.1007/s12065-020-00486-6.
[33] Azizi, M., Talatahari, S. & Gandomi, A. H. (2023). Fire Hawk Optimizer: a novel metaheuristic algorithm. 56(1). Springer Netherlands. https://doi.org/10.1007/s10462-022-10173-w.
[34] Guo, Z., Yang, H., Wang, S., Zhou, C. & Liu, X. (2018). Adaptive harmony search with best-based search strategy. Soft Comput., 22(4), 1335–1349. https://doi.org/10.1007/s00500-016-2424-3.
[35] Yang, X. (2020). Nature-inspired optimization algorithms: challenges and open problems. J. Comput. Sci., 46, 101104. https://doi.org/10.1016/j.jocs.2020.101104.
[36] Sharma, M. & Kaur, P. (2021). A comprehensive analysis of nature – inspired meta – heuristic techniques for feature selection problem. Arch. Comput. Methods Eng., 28(3), 1103–1127. https://doi.org/10.1007/s11831-020-09412-6.
[37] Ayyad, S. M., Saleh, A. I. & Labib, L. M. (2019). Gene expression cancer classification using modified K-Nearest Neighbors technique. Biosystems, 176(January), 41–51. https://doi.org/10.1016/j.biosystems.2018.12.009.
[38] Yaqoob, A., Aziz, R. M. & Verma, N. K. (2023). Applications and techniques of machine learning in cancer classification: a systematic review. Hum.-Cent. Intell. Syst. https://doi.org/10.1007/s44230-023-00041-3.

[39] Yaqoob, A., Kumar, N., Rabia, V. & Aziz, M. (2024). Optimizing gene selection and cancer classification with hybrid Sine Cosine and Cuckoo Search algorithm. J. Med. Syst. https://doi.org/10.1007/s10916-023-02031-1.

[40] Yaqoob, A., Aziz, R. M., Verma, N. K., Lalwani, P. & Makrariya, A. (2023). A review on nature-inspired algorithms for cancer disease prediction and classification.

[41] Jawad, K., Mahto, R., Das, A., Ahmed, S. U., Aziz, R. M. & Kumar, P. (2023). Applied sciences novel Cuckoo Search-based metaheuristic approach for deep learning prediction of depression.

[42] Van't Veer, L. J., et al. (2002). Gene expression profiling predicts clinical outcome of breast cancer. Nature, 415(6871), 530–536. https://doi.org/10.1038/415530a.

Kingshuk Kirtania, Anogh Dalal, and Pawan Kumar Singh

10 HySleep_Net: a hybrid deep learning model for automatic sleep stage detection from polysomnographic signals

Abstract: Sleep stage identification is crucial as a first step in the analysis and diagnosis of subjects with sleep disorders. However, the standard sleep staging procedures are cumbersome and time-consuming, accurately determining the stages of wakefulness prior to NREM or REM periods through extensive but manual analysis carried of polysomnographic (PSG) data. In the following study, we propose a new hybrid architecture using deep learning (DL) to study PSG sleep recording data in order to detect the sleep stages. We propose an approach to automatically detect sleep stages from PSG data using a model that uses convolutional neural networks (CNN), long short-term memory (LSTM), and gated recurrent units (GRU), called HySleep_Net. HySleep_Net is essentially a hybrid model, and this hybrid nature provides it with the ability to automatically perform data-driven feature selection that has not been possible with existing best-performing methods. HySleep_Net focuses on spatial and temporal dependencies of the PSG data that are important for appropriate sleep stage classification. The functionality of the model has been assessed on 4 public datasets, including Sleep-EDF, Sleep-EDF 78, Sleep Heart Health Study (SHHS) and ISRUC. The experimental results have concluded that our HySleep_Net method performs well with accuracies of 94 %, 89 %, 89 % and 90 % on the above datasets, respectively. These results suggest that HySleep_Net is not only superior to the traditional methods, but also becomes a new state-of-the-art model for automatic sleep stage detection – enabling the use of an efficient tool in the practice of clinical and research-based studies related to prospective applications regarding sleep medicine.

Keywords: Sleep stage detection, HySleep_Net, convolutional neural network, long short-term memory, gated recurrent unit, Sleep-EDF, CNN, GRU, Sleep-EDF 78, SHHS, ISRUC

10.1 Introduction

Sleep is essential for mental and physical well-being, allowing the human body to repair tissues, strengthen the immune system, and consolidate memories for optimal brain

---

Kingshuk Kirtania, Anogh Dalal, Pawan Kumar Singh, Department of Information Technology, Jadavpur University, Jadavpur University Second Campus, Plot No. 8, Salt Lake Bypass, LB Block, Sector III, Salt Lake City, Kolkata, 700106, West Bengal, India, e-mails: bttb.kingshukk@gmail.com, anogh25@gmail.com, pawansingh.ju@gmail.com, https://orcid.org/0000-0002-9598-7981

function. Without sufficient sleep, one can experience decreased energy, difficulty concentrating, and even an increased risk of chronic disease. Short-term (acute) sleep deprivation can impair cognitive function, mood regulation, and immune response. An increased risk of chronic diseases such as obesity, diabetes, and even some cancers has been associated with long-term sleep deprivation [1, 2]. Figure 10.1 illustrates the different forms of sleep [3], which are as follows:

1. *Non-rapid eye movement (NREM):* Breathing and heart rate slow down, muscles relax, and brain waves slow down during this deeper, more restorative stage of sleep. Three stages are further classifications of NREM sleep:
   - *Stage 1:* The transition from wakefulness to sleep. It's rapid and easily interrupted.
   - *Stage 2:* During light sleep, the body gets ready for deeper sleep. Approximately 50 % of the sleep cycle is spent in this phase.
   - *Stage 3:* Deep sleep, where the body repairs and restores itself. This stage is crucial for feeling refreshed in the morning.
2. *Rapid eye movement (REM) sleep:* The lightest stage of sleep, characterized by vivid dreams, rapid eye movements, and greater brain activity. Learning, processing emotions, and retaining memories all depend on getting enough REM sleep.

We cycle through these stages of sleep throughout the night, typically 4–5 times. Each of these cycles last approximately 1.5 hours. While adults go through NREM more frequently, particularly stage 3, newborns spend the majority of their sleep in REM.

Sleep stages are assessed by analyzing the EEG, EOG, and EMG during sleep [4]. Trained technicians visually inspect these signals, dividing sleep into 30-second "epochs". They assign a stage (awake, REM, or NREM 1–3) to specific epochs based on specific criteria such as wave patterns and frequency. While this process is critical for diagnosing sleep disorders, it is time-consuming and prone to subjectivity, prompting the development of automated scoring methods using machine learning.

In this study, we concentrated the evaluation process on DL approaches because, based on our experience in the field, DL is the most appropriate for sleep stage detec-

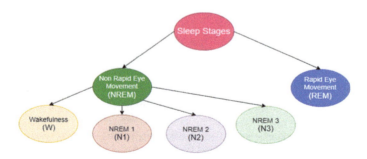

Figure 10.1: Different Sleep Stages.

tion. In this paper we discuss our sophisticated DL model which can be used in sleep stage classification. Our goal is to provide specialists in the field with deep, coherent information so that they can expand and enhance their expertise.

Currently, sleep staging is largely conducted manually, which is not only very time-consuming, but it can also introduce human errors. Automated sleep staging is very beneficial for reducing the workload of medical practitioners. The framework can work on a large amount of patient data and evaluate their sleep stages quickly and accurately, thus using the results to serve the needs of the millions [5] who suffer from sleep disorders.

The contributions made by the proposed work are listed below:
- Our proposed HySleep_Net architecture is based on a hybrid DL approach involving CNN, LSTM networks and GRU networks for the automatic detection of sleep stages. This novelty of using a hybrid DL structure allows our model to extract and analyze both the spatial and temporal dependencies present in the data.
- HySleep_Net is tested on four prominent datasets, namely Sleep-EDF [6], Sleep-EDF Exp. [6], SHHS [7] and ISRUC [8]. It achieves outstanding classification accuracies of 94 %, 89 %, 89 % and 90 % on the aforementioned datasets, respectively, setting a new benchmark for these datasets. Thus, it not only demonstrates the robustness of our model, but also shows the cross-dataset applicability of our model.
- This paper includes a concise report on why automatic sleep staging is needed in modern society, why HySleep_Net should be used and the future prospects of HySleep_Net in a neat and precise way.

10.2 Related study

Recently, artificial intelligence (AI), especially machine learning (ML) and deep learning (DL) have seen a significant increase in research. This has led to the contribution to various domains and intricate research tasks, such as emotion recognition [9], activity recognition [10, 11], cancer analysis [12], speech identification [13], feature selection [14], biomedical image classification [15], etc. Automatic sleep stage detection from physiological signals is no exception. DL techniques can easily learn features using EEG signals. Table 10.1 shows us the dataset name and how frequently it has been applied to categorize sleep stages. The Sleep-EDF and Sleep-EDF 78 datasets are the most frequently used for sleep stage classification, with a rate of 15.32 % and 8.17 %, respectively. We have also tested our HySleep_Net model on the SHHS and ISRUC datasets, as the usage rates of these two datasets are relatively low while still being a prominent dataset in their respective fields of research.

Zhu et al. [16] propose a model that mimics this process and offers a clearer understanding of its decisions. The model combines a CNN to detect local signals with an attention-based architecture to identify features within the sleep stages. Qureshi

Table 10.1: Datasets and their Usage.

Dataset	Used (%)
SLEEP-EDF	15.32
SLEEP-EDF 78	8.17
MASS	6.13
PRIVATE DATASET	4.8
SHHS	5.11
MIT-BIH	4.9
UCD	3.6
ISRUC	2.4

et al. [17] introduce a CNN based method for categorizing sleep stages sleep from an EEG channel. It achieved overall accuracy rates and kappa statistics of 92.51 % and 0.90 in the case of the Sleep-EDF dataset. The method automatically learns features for sleep stage classification without the need for manual feature extraction. Hsu et al. [18] introduce a recurrent neural classifier designed for automatic classification of sleep stages. The proposed method was validated using 8 recordings from the Sleep-EDF dataset. The results indicate that the recurrent neural classifier achieved a superior classification rate of 87.2 %, outperforming both the FNN (81.1 %) and PNN (81.8 %) classifiers.

Michielli et al. [19] introduce a cascaded recurrent neural network in their study. The architecture consists of two LSTM RNNs (i. e., the first network) is used for 4-class classification, mixing stages N1 and REM into a one stage and classifying the respective phases, achieving an accuracy rate = 90.8 %, while the second network pairs with recognition performance = 83.6 % intended to discriminate between phasic categories (N1 vs. REM). The combined performance for all five sleep stages yields an overall classification rate of 86.7 %. Mousavi et al. [20] refer to a single-channel EEG signal based method for automatic sleep stage annotation. Moreover, to address the class imbalance problem with current sleep datasets, their loss functions are designed so that each of these misclassified errors is penalized equally during network training. The authors test the effectiveness of such a method on multiple single-EEG channels from the Sleep-EDF database. The evaluation results show that the proposed method achieves an overall accuracy of 84.26 %. Seo et al. [21] propose a DL model to capture intra- and inter-epoch temporal context information of raw single-channel EEG. The performance of IITNet was tested on three different datasets. The highest accuracies were obtained in 83.9 % for Sleep-EDF, 86.5 % for MASS, and finally with SHHS, the overall accuracy reaching up to 86.7 %.

Zhang et al. [22] develop an automated framework using a DL model was introduced for sleep stage detection based on the PSG data. The network managed to reach an accuracy of 0.8181. Supratak et al. [23] introduce a system for automatic analysis of sleep stages using raw EEG data. It uses two types of DL models: CNNs to identify unchanging patterns and LSTMs to understand the flow between sleep stages. The researchers trained DeepSleepNet on publicly available EEG recordings with different data formats and sleep scoring rules. Phan et al. [24] present a new, efficient way to automatically classify sleep stages. It uses a CNN that's simpler than other methods, but with a twist. It uses a unique pooling method to better handle the way EEG signals change over time. To further improve accuracy, the researchers developed a method to preprocess the data using a filter bank trained with another DL model.

Xu et al. [25] introduce a powerful but efficient DL method for automatic classification of sleep stages. It combines signals from multiple channels and includes a technique to automatically identify and remove corrupted data. The design of the neural network itself is streamlined, using special techniques to significantly reduce the number of parameters required. Tsinalis et al. [26] explore the use of CNNs to automatically analyze sleep stages from EEG recordings. The model is able to learn the patterns needed to classify sleep stages without needing any preprogrammed knowledge of sleep analysis. The researchers tested their method on publicly available data from healthy young adults and used a rigorous evaluation technique. To ensure a fair evaluation, they balanced the data and used a special training method. This suggests that CNNs can be a powerful tool for automatic sleep analysis, achieving performance comparable to existing methods that rely on expert knowledge.

Sokolovsky et al. [27] introduce a CNN-based model. The study reveals that the improved performance comes from the depth of the network, not necessarily from the use of multiple signal channels. By analyzing the internal activity of this model, the researchers observe that it naturally learns to identify features such as sleep spindles and slow waves. Sors et al. [28] use a CNN trained directly on raw EEG samples to predict the five different sleep stages. This approach eliminates the need for any preprocessing or feature extraction steps before feeding the data into the CNN. The researchers trained and tested their system on a large dataset from a multi-center sleep study with expert-rated sleep recordings. Finally, they developed a method to visualize the sleep stage patterns learned by the network.

Fernández-Varela et al. [29] use a DL model, specifically an ensemble of five CNNs, to automatically learn the important features from the data without needing human intervention. Their model achieved a kappa index of 0.83, demonstrating strong performance in classifying sleep stages from a dataset of 500 sleep recordings. L. Zhang et al. [30] trained a DL system to analyze PSG data from a large sleep study. The best performing model used spectrograms as input, processed them through CNN layers, and then used an LSTM layer. Evidently, DL has the potential to become a powerful tool for automatically scoring sleep stages, potentially reducing the workload and improving the consistency of PSG analysis.

Li et al. [31] extracted several features from the ECG signal, including breathing patterns, heart rate variability, and a measure of interaction between these two signals. They then use a deep CNN to analyze these features and categorize sleep stages. Chen et al. [32] introduce MVF-SleepNet. Their model combines the VGG-16 and GRU networks. It achieves an accuracy of 0.841 and an F1-score of 0.828. Li et al. [33] use a random forest algorithm to identify the five sleep stages. Their method achieves results of over 80 % accuracy using only two types of signals (EOG and EMG) with less data (114 features) compared to the traditional method using three signals (EEG, EOG, and EMG) and more data (438 features).

Ji et al. [34] introduce a multi-channel-based 3D-CNN. They conduct classification experiments on ISRUC dataset. Their results on the ISRUC dataset demonstrated an overall accuracy of 0.832 and an F1-score of 0.814. Giannakeas et al. [35] present a methodology for sleep staging that relies exclusively on EEG signals from PSG recordings. Using EEG data from the ISRUC dataset, their goal is to automatically classify the five sleep stages. Their Random Forest classifier achieves an accuracy of 75.29 %. Xiaopeng et al. [36] propose a multi-channel biosignal-based model, that integrates the 3D convolution operations and graph convolution operations. Time-domain-based and frequency-domain-based features are extracted from EEG, EMG, EOG and ECG signals. These features are then fed into the 3D and graph convolution branches. Which has an accuracy = 0.830, and F1-score = 0.821 on ISRUC.

10.2.1 Motivation of our proposed work

This work is primarily motivated by the constraints discovered in previous studies for automatic sleep stage detection. Our examination of the previous works shed light on our focus in conventional machine learning models, which often require manual feature extraction, and this approach is highly dataset dependent. Moreover, to make matters worse, each feature set could be finely configured as required for a very specific dataset, but at the same time not have good generalization across many other types of datasets.

The recent emergence of DL models has the ability to automate feature extraction and learn inherent intrinsic patterns more robustly. However, most of these DL models have been trained and tested on single datasets resulting in very limited generalizability. Models may perform well on the given dataset, but fail to perform decently when subjected to other similar datasets, indicating a significant gap in the development of robust, stand-alone models that can perform consistently across multiple datasets, and this need for development is inculcated by the dire need to develop highly accurate and efficient diagnostic tools due to the increasing prevalence of sleep disorders.

Therefore, the focus of our work is to create a robust DL model capable of accurate sleep stage detection across multiple standard datasets.

In this project, we have tested HySleep_Net on four publicly available and widely recognized datasets: Sleep-EDF, Sleep-EDF 78, SHHS, and ISRUC. Our results show that HySleep_Net performs well compared to other contemporary works, achieving high accuracy and robustness. The validation on a range of datasets demonstrates the possibility to advance toward an independent model with broader applicability, reducing the need for dataset-specific feature engineering and improving the generalizability of automatic sleep stage detection systems that could be applied in real clinical practice.

10.3 Dataset description

10.3.1 Sleep-EDF

The Sleep-EDF Database, contributed to PhysioNet [37] by Bob Kemp et al., is a compilation of PSG [38] recordings from healthy subjects. These recordings, which monitor various physiological parameters during sleep, are stored in the European Data Format (EDF) [39]. Researchers and clinicians use databases such as Sleep-EDF to explore sleep patterns and disorders, contributing to advances in sleep research and our understanding of related conditions. 42,308 samples were taken from the dataset for both training and testing, and an oversampling technique i. e. SMOTE [40], was used to create synthetic examples for the underrepresented classes. The total number of samples is 88,995. We show the class-wise samples taken (before and after oversampling) from the Sleep-EDF dataset in Figure 10.2(a) and 10.2(b).

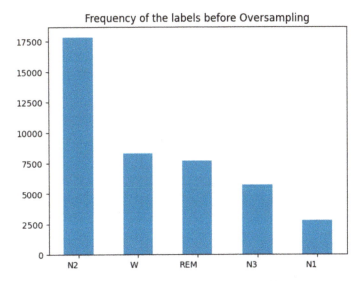

Figure 10.2(a): Class-wise samples for the *Sleep-EDF* dataset before oversampling.

10.3.2 Sleep-EDF 78

The Sleep-EDF dataset has been expanded by Kemp et al. to encompass a total of 197 complete PSG sleep recordings that span entire nights. The *PSG.edf files comprise comprehensive PSG sleep recordings that extend throughout the entire night. These patterns, known as hypnograms, include sleep stages W (Wake), R (REM) and ? (not determined). We collected 116,418 samples from the dataset for both training and testing and employed SMOTE to generate additional synthetic examples for the underrepresented

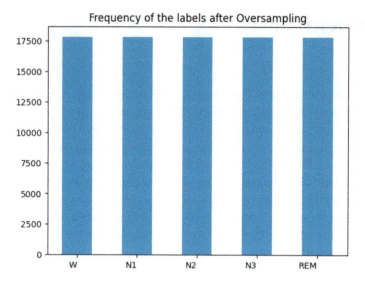

Figure 10.2(b): Class-wise samples for the *Sleep-EDF* dataset after oversampling.

classes. In total, we now have 225,080 samples in our dataset. Figures 10.3(a) and 10.3(b) illustrate the number of samples in each class before and after oversampling.

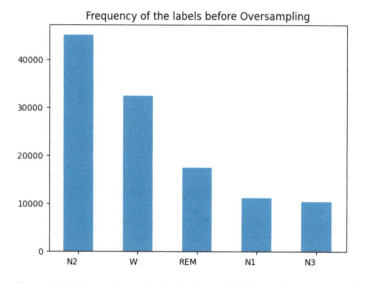

Figure 10.3(a): Class-wise samples for the *Sleep-EDF 78* dataset before oversampling.

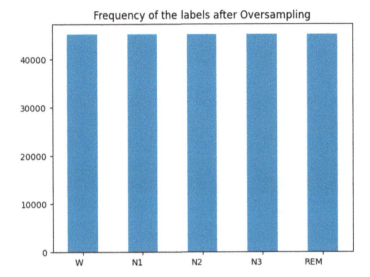

Figure 10.3(b): Class-wise samples for the *Sleep-EDF 78* dataset after oversampling.

10.3.3 SHHS dataset

SHHS is a comprehensive study conducted by the National Heart-Lung-Blood Institute. This dataset contains PSG data, which provides additional data to further analyze and understand sleep-related breathing and its potential cardiovascular implications. We obtained 246,290 samples for from the dataset and applied ADASYN [41] oversampling to balance out the dataset. The total number of available samples is now 493,404. Figure 10.4(a) and 10.4(b) illustrate the sample distribution for each class both before and after applying oversampling techniques to the SHHS dataset.

10.3.4 ISRUC

The ISRUC dataset, a comprehensive PSG collection, was created to assist sleep researchers in their studies. This dataset contains data from adults, including both healthy individuals and individuals with sleep disorders.

Each PSG recording was visually graded by 2 professionals and includes electrophysiological signals, pneumological signals, and other contextual information about the subjects. We used subgroup 3 in our model evaluation.

We obtained 8589 samples and applied SMOTE to address class imbalance. This increased the total number of samples in our dataset to 13080. Figures 10.5(a) and 10.5(b) depict the sample distribution for each class before and after applying the oversampling techniques to the ISRUC dataset.

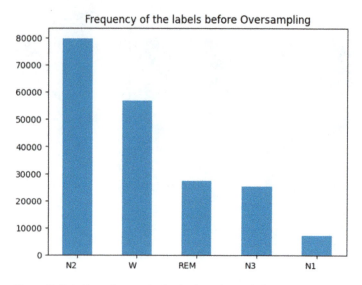

Figure 10.4(a): Class-wise samples for the *SHHS* dataset before oversampling.

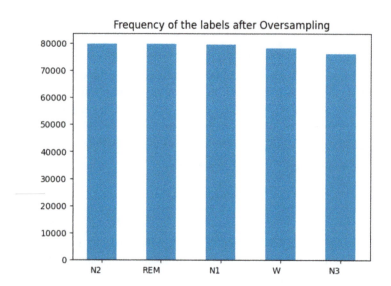

Figure 10.4(b): Class-wise samples for the *SHHS* dataset after oversampling.

10.4 Proposed methodology

10.4.1 Data procurement

We acquired preprocessed versions of the Sleep-EDF and the Sleep-EDF 78 datasets from the DR-NTU website. The PSG recordings and the annotations for the SHHS dataset were

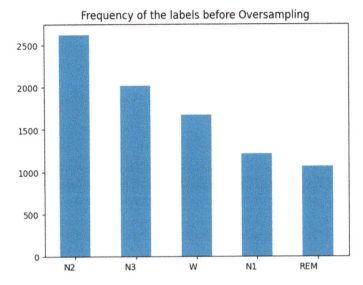

Figure 10.5(a): Class-wise samples for the *ISRUC* dataset before oversampling.

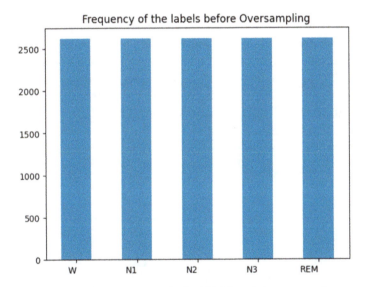

Figure 10.5(b): Class-wise samples for the *ISRUC* dataset after oversampling.

downloaded from the sleepdata website. For the ISRUC dataset, the data of the subgroup 3 was obtained from the sleeptight website.

10.4.2 Data loading

After obtaining the preprocessed data, the data were loaded into specific data frames using the "glob" package in the case of the Sleep-EDF and the Sleep-EDF 78 datasets and using the "pickle" package for the SHHS and the ISRUC datasets.

10.4.3 Data splitting

The 'train test split' function from the scikit-learn library splits each data frame into training and test sets using a 70–30 split ratio. This ensures that the model can be trained on a significant amount of the data and then tested on a different set to see how well it performs in terms of generalization. Using the 'train test split' function ensures that there are no overlapping sequences between the training and testing datasets.

10.4.4 GRU

GRU [42] is a simplified variant of LSTM networks, designed for sequential data processing. GRUs selectively remember or forget information over time using two gates: update and reset. The reset gate determines the impact of past hidden states, and the update gate regulates which part of the candidate activation vector should be added to the new hidden state. It is able to handle long-term dependencies over sequential data with comparable performance as LSTMs, but requires fewer parameters and is more computationally efficient. Figure 10.6 shows the inner workings of a GRU.

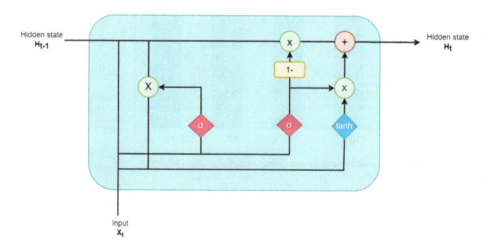

Figure 10.6: Illustration of the internal architecture of the GRU neuron.

Using the previous concealed state H_{t-1} and the current input I, the reset gate Z and the update gate U are calculated, where the weight matrices are W_z and W_u.

$$Z_t = \sigma(W_z \times [H_{t-1}, I_t]) \tag{10.1}$$
$$U_t = \sigma(W_u \times [H_{t-1}, I_t]) \tag{10.2}$$

The candidate activation vector $\tilde{C}_t$ is generated by using a reset-modified version of the previous hidden state and the current input I, where the reset gate determines the modification, where W_h is the weight matrix.

$$\tilde{C}_t = \tanh(W_h \times [Z_t \cdot H_{t-1}, I_t]) \tag{10.3}$$

The new hidden state H_t is derived by integrating the candidate activation vector and the previous hidden state, with the update gate providing the weights for this combination.

$$H_t = (1 - U_t) \times H_{t-1} + U_t \cdot \tilde{C}_t \tag{10.4}$$

10.4.5 LSTM networks

LSTM [43] networks are a type of RNN with the ability to recognize long-term relationships and inherent temporal sequences. Unlike conventional RNNs, LSTMs incorporate memory cells that retain information over extended periods of time, addressing the issue of vanishing gradients. Figure 10.7 shows the key components of LSTM which include:
1. *Input Gate*: Regulates the rate at which new data enters the memory cell.
2. *Forget Gate*: Controls the amount of memory to be discarded from the cell.
3. *Output Gate*: Controls the output flow from the cell.

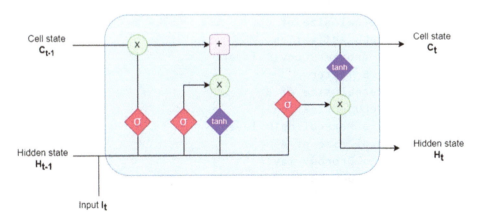

Figure 10.7: Illustration of internal architecture of LSTM neuron.

Together, these gates decide how much information from the input should be stored, forgotten, and output, thereby helping LSTMs handle both short-term and long-term dependencies in data processed by recurrent models. This architecture is well suited for various purposes such as speech recognition, language modeling and handwriting recognition.

10.4.6 Proposed HySleep_Net Model

The construction of the sleep stage detection model involves of a combination of CNN, LSTM layers and GRU layers as shown in Figure 10.8 to efficiently extract and assimilate temporal and hierarchical information from the sleep data. Algorithm 10.1 shows the pseudocode of our HySleep_Net model.

Algorithm 10.1: Pseudo code of Proposed HySleep_Net model.

```
START
Step 1:  CREATE an instance of a Sequential model.
Step 2:  ADD a Conv1D layer:
         - 64 filters
         - kernel size of 8
         - ReLU activation
Step 3:  ADD a MaxPooling1D layer:
         - pool size of 8
Step 4:  ADD a Conv1D layer:
         - 128 filters
         - kernel size of 8
         - ReLU activation
Step 5:  ADD another Conv1D layer:
         - 128 filters
         - kernel size of 8
         - ReLU activation
Step 6:  ADD another Conv1D layer:
         - 128 filters
         - kernel size of 8
         - ReLU activation
Step 7:  ADD a MaxPooling1D layer:
         - pool size of 4
Step 8:  ADD a Dropout layer:
         - dropout rate of 0.3
Step 9:  ADD a Conv1D layer:
         - 32 filters
         - kernel size of 400
```

```
               - ReLU activation
Step 10: ADD a MaxPooling1D layer:
               - pool size of 4
Step 11: ADD a Conv1D layer:
               - 128 filters
               - kernel size of 6
               - ReLU activation
Step 12: ADD another Conv1D layer:
               - 128 filters
               - kernel size of 6
               - ReLU activation
Step 13: ADD another Conv1D layer:
               - 128 filters
               - kernel size of 6
               - ReLU activation
Step 14: ADD a MaxPooling1D layer:
               - pool size of 2
Step 15: ADD a Dropout layer:
               - dropout rate of 0.3
Step 16: ADD a Dense layer:
               - 256 units
               - ReLU activation
Step 17: ADD a Dropout layer:
               - dropout rate of 0.35
Step 18: ADD an LSTM layer:
               - 256 units
               - return sequences set to True
Step 19: ADD a Dropout layer:
               - dropout rate of 0.35
Step 20: ADD another LSTM layer:
               - 256 units
               - return sequences set to True
Step 21: ADD a Dropout layer:
               - dropout rate of 0.35
Step 22: ADD a GRU layer:
               - 256 units
               - return sequences set to True
Step 23: ADD a Dropout layer:
               - dropout rate of 0.35
Step 24: ADD another GRU layer:
               - 256 units
               - return sequences set to True
```

```
Step 25: ADD a Dropout layer:
         - dropout rate of 0.35
Step 26: ADD another GRU layer:
         - 256 units
         - return sequences set to True
Step 27: ADD a Dropout layer:
         - dropout rate of 0.35
Step 28: ADD another GRU layer:
         - 256 units
         - return sequences set to False
Step 29: ADD a Dropout layer:
         - dropout rate of 0.35
Step 30: ADD a Dense layer:
         - 5 units
         - softmax activation
Step 31: SET optimizer to Adam:
         - learning rate of 0.0001
Step 32: COMPILE the model with:
         - categorical cross-entropy loss
         - accuracy as the metric
END
```

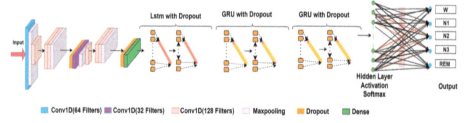

Figure 10.8: Visual representation of our proposed hybrid HySleep_Net model for automatic sleep stage detection.

Firstly, a sequence of Conv1D and Max-Pooling is added to help capture local patterns and extract relevant features from the input sequences. The first set of such layers, up to the first dropout layer, which is strategically inserted to mitigate overfitting, are there to extract the finer characteristics of the PSG sleep recording data, and the second set works towards capturing the coarse features of the same data. Max-pooling layers reduce spatial dimensions by selecting the maximum value from each group of two elements along the time axis. CNN layers are followed by dense layers with ReLU activation functions. Subsequently, Then, LSTM layers are introduced to capture the temporal dependencies of the sequence, allowing our model to detect patterns between successive data points. To mitigate overfitting, dropout layers are reinserted after each LSTM layer. To further increase the performance of the model, a set of GRU layers are added along with the corresponding dropout layers. The introduction of GRU layers results in fewer parameters, thus increasing the efficiency of the model without compromising performance. The final layer uses Softmax to provide a probability distribution for each sleep stage category. HySleep_Net is trained with training and validation sets to closely monitor and improve its performance over the epochs, using the Adam optimizer and the loss function: categorical cross-entropy.

The total number of parameters in HySleep_Net is 4,852,581. Of these, 4,852,581 are trainable and 0 are not trainable. With such a large number of trainable parameters, the model has more than enough capability to discern and learn complex patterns from the training data.

10.5 Results and discussion

10.5.1 Evaluation metric

The provided text explains the various metrics [44] used to evaluate the effectiveness of classification models. Here's a breakdown of the key concepts mentioned:

1. *Accuracy:*
   - The percentage of accurately predicted predictions out of all predictions.
   - *Accuracy = Number of Correct Predictions/Number of Total Predictions* $* 100\%$
2. *Precision (A):*
   - Out of all expected positives, precision is the number of true positive observations.

   Components:
   - True Positive (w): +ve results predicted correctly.
   - True Negative (x): -ve results predicted successfully.
   - False Positive (y): -ve outcomes classified as +ve.
   - False Negative (z): +ve outcomes classified as -ve.
   - Formula: *Precision* $= w/(w+y)$
3. *Recall (B):*
   - Definition: Recall measures a classifier's capacity to locate positive observations within a dataset.
   - Formula: *Recall* $= w/(w+z)$
4. *F1-score (C):*
   - Definition: A single statistic that offers a truthful assessment of a model's performance by combining precision and recall.
   - Formula: *F1 Score* $= 2AB/(A+B)$

5. *Confusion Matrix:*
   – Definition: A matrix that evaluates the performance of classification models by comparing predicted and actual values.

Each layer of the HySleep_Net model was carefully tuned to find the perfect balance between performance and efficiency. Table 10.2 describes the hyperparameters used the HySleep_Net model for the four datasets. For each dataset, we have employed the identical train-test split ratio of 70:30. Using the Adam optimizer allows us to converge to the result at a faster rate. The learning is kept at 0.0001, which produces the best results. We have used ReLU for all the CNN layers and the first dense layer to introduce nonlinearity in the model and used Softmax for the last dense layer as it is a multiclass classification model. We used an early stopping method to converge to the result faster with less number of epochs i. e. 18, 14, 19 and 17 for Sleep-EDF, Sleep-EDF 78, SHHS and ISRUC datasets, respectively. The batch size of 32 is chosen for the relatively smaller Sleep-EDF and ISRUC datasets, and the batch sizes of 64 and 128 are chosen for the relatively larger size Sleep-EDF 78 and SHHS datasets for efficient convergence.

Table 10.2: Hyperparameters used in the HySleep_Net model for the four datasets.

Parameter	Sleep-EDF	Sleep-EDF Expanded	SHHS	ISRUC
Train-test ratio	70:30	70:30	70:30	70:30
Optimization Algorithm	Adam	Adam	Adam	Adam
Learning-Rate	0.0001	0.0001	0.0001	0.0001
Activation Function(s)	ReLU, Softmax	ReLU, Softmax	ReLU, Softmax	ReLU, Softmax
# epoch	18	14	19	17
Batch size	32	128	64	32

The overall performance metrics for the four datasets are shown in Table 10.3. We have achieved exemplary results all across the board, with accuracies of 94 %, 89 %, 89 % and 90 % in Sleep-EDF, Sleep-EDF 78, SHHS and ISRUC, respectively, while having maintained efficiency by converging to these results in less than 20 epochs for all of the

Table 10.3: Overall performance report produced by the proposed hybrid model on four standard stress detection datasets.

Dataset	Accuracy (%)	Precision	Recall	F1-score	#Epochs	Batch Size
Sleep-EDF	94	0.94	0.94	0.94	18	32
Sleep-EDF Expanded	89	0.89	0.89	0.89	14	128
SHHS	89	0.89	0.89	0.89	19	64
ISRUC	90	0.90	0.90	0.90	17	32

four datasets. We obtained the maximum performance metrics for the Sleep-EDF dataset with an A of 0.94, a B of 0.94 and a C of 0.94 using only 18 epochs. We also exceeded the benchmark metrics for the other datasets.

10.5.2 Results on Sleep-EDF

For the Sleep-EDF dataset, the study aims to robustly classify the sleep stages of individuals, between 0 'Wake' and 4 'REM'. After 18 epochs, HySleep_Net achieves an astounding accuracy of 94 %. Figure 10.9 displays the model's sleep stage identification performance against the Sleep-EDF dataset. The class '0' (i. e. 'Wake') is seen to be the best performing class here, with an accuracy of 97 %, while the class '2' (i. e. 'NREM 2') has the lowest performance. The relatively lower performance of the class 'NREM 2' may be due to the high number of samples present in the original data compared to other classes, which may consist of additional noise. The model uses only 18 training epochs, since we don't find any further improvement in loss reduction, while also ensuring that the model doesn't fit too well to the training data as a regularization measure. The confusion matrix generated by our proposed HySleep_Net is depicted in Figure 10.10. It demonstrates that class 'NREM 2' has the most misclassifications with the class 'REM', which is 312 in number. Figure 10.11 depicts the class-wise ROC and AUC for the Sleep-EDF dataset, showing that the class '0' (i. e., 'Wake') and class 'NREM 3' give the best results, with AUC scores close to 1.00.

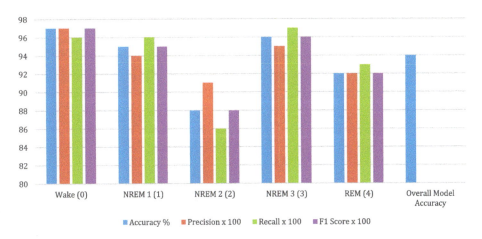

Figure 10.9: Summary of the performance evaluation produced against the Sleep-EDF dataset using the HySleep_Net model.

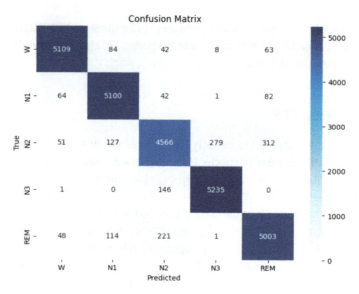

Figure 10.10: Confusion matrix obtained by the proposed method using HySleep_Net model on the *Sleep-EDF* dataset.

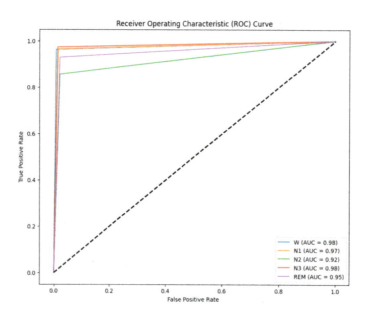

Figure 10.11: ROC Curve obtained by the proposed method using HySleep_Net model on the *Sleep-EDF* dataset.

10.5.3 Results for Sleep-EDF 78

Regarding the Sleep-EDF 78, we have already mentioned that it is the extended version of the previously mentioned Sleep-EDF dataset. Table 10.4 illustrates the effectiveness of the model in detecting different sleep stages using the Sleep-EDF 78 dataset. It is noteworthy that the class '3' (i. e. 'NREM 3') has the highest performance of all classes, with an accuracy of 95 %, followed closely by the 'Wake' and class 'REM' classes. Figure 10.12 shows the confusion matrix with the most misclassifications between class '2' (i.e 'NREM 2') and class '1' (i. e. 'NREM 1'). A total of 1008 misclassifications occur between these two classes. Figure 10.13 shows the class-wise ROC curve obtained by the model, which further shows the superior performance for the class 'NREM 3', with an AUC value close to 1.00. As this

Table 10.4: Summary of the performance evaluation produced against the *Sleep-EDF 78* dataset using the HySleep_Net model.

Class Labels	Accuracy %	Precision	Recall	F1-Score
Wake (0)	93	94	92	93
NREM 1 (1)	84	83	85	84
NREM 2 (2)	83	86	80	83
NREM 3 (3)	95	93	97	95
REM (4)	90	89	92	90
Overall Model Accuracy	89			

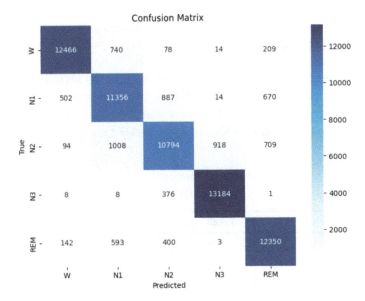

Figure 10.12: Confusion matrix obtained by the proposed method using HySleep_Net model on the *Sleep-EDF 78* dataset.

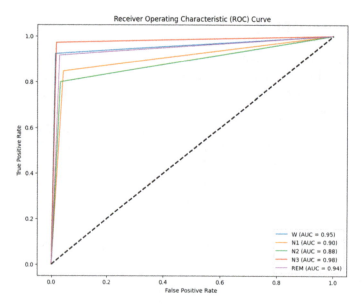

Figure 10.13: ROC Curve obtained by the proposed method using HySleep_Net model on the *Sleep-EDF 78* dataset.

is the extended version of the Sleep-EDF dataset, it also suffers from class imbalance, which consequently makes the class 'NREM 2' perform relatively weaker compared to the other classes.

10.5.4 Results on SHHS dataset

Another dataset with different input attributes is also used to check the performance against it. Using a similar procedure to that used for the above datasets, we have achieved an accuracy of 89 %. Table 10.5 outlines how well the model performs in distinguishing various sleep stages using the SHHS dataset. Notably, the 'NREM 1' class

Table 10.5: Summary of the performance evaluation produced against the SHHS dataset using the hybrid CNN + LSTM + GRU model.

Class Labels	Accuracy %	Precision	Recall	F1-Score
Wake (0)	92	0.93	0.91	0.92
NREM 1 (1)	95	0.92	0.98	0.95
NREM 2 (2)	78	0.87	0.70	0.78
NREM 3 (3)	90	0.86	0.95	0.90
REM (4)	89	0.87	0.91	0.89
Overall Model Accuracy	**89**			

emerges as the top-performing class in this context, with an accuracy of 95 % and the 'NREM 2' class on the other end of the spectrum.

This dataset also consists of the class 2 'NREM 2', which has much more samples compared to the other classes, which could be the reason for the slightly less robust performance of this class. The confusion matrix produced in the Figure 10.14 shows that most of the misclassifications for class '2' (i. e. 'NREM 2') have occurred with class '3' (i. e. 'NREM 3'), with a total of 3386 misclassifications. Figure 10.15 displays the ROC curve for each class obtained by the model, indicating outstanding performance for the class 1 'NREM 1', with an AUC of 0.98.

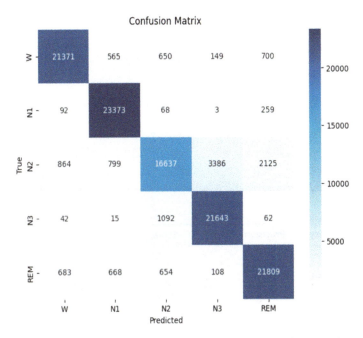

Figure 10.14: Confusion matrix obtained by the proposed method using HySleep_Net model on the *SHHS* dataset.

10.5.5 Results on the ISRUC dataset

Now we come to the last dataset we have worked on, the ISRUC dataset. We have tested our model using the same parameters and achieved an outstanding 90 % accuracy on the test data. This dataset also suffers from the same class 'NREM 2' problem. On the other hand, class 'NREM 1' has very few samples in the original dataset compared to the other classes, which may be the reason why these two classes have comparatively less robust results, as shown in Table 10.6, which describes the model's performance in classifying various sleep stages using the ISRUC dataset. The 'Wake' class and the 'REM' class yield the best results with accuracies of 95 % and 94 %, respectively, which is also evident

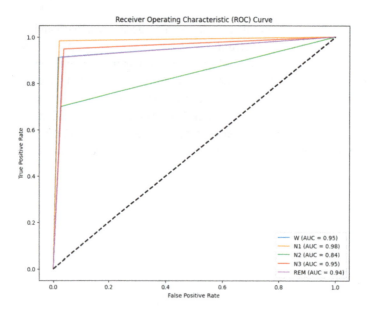

Figure 10.15: ROC Curve obtained by the proposed method using hybrid HySleep_Net model on the *SHHS* dataset.

Table 10.6: Summary of performance evaluation produced against ISRUC dataset using the hybrid CNN + LSTM + GRU model.

Class Labels	Accuracy %	Precision	Recall	F1-Score
Wake (0)	95	0.97	0.93	0.95
NREM 1 (1)	84	0.86	0.81	0.84
NREM 2 (2)	82	0.80	0.84	0.82
NREM 3 (3)	93	0.91	0.94	0.93
REM (4)	94	0.93	0.95	0.94
Overall Model Accuracy	**90**			

from the classification matrix and the ROC curve. As seen in the confusion matrix in Figure 10.16, class 'NREM 1' is misclassified as class 'NREM 2' a total of 90 times, which is the highest number. Figure 10.17 shows the ROC curve of the classes present in the ISRUC dataset, from which we can see that the class 'REM' performs exceptionally well, with an AUC close to 1.00.

10.5.6 Ablation study

We have employed three important modules in our HySleep_Net model, the convolutional layers for coarse feature extraction and the LSTM and GRU layers for analyzing

10 HySleep_Net: a hybrid DL model for automatic sleep stage detection from PSG signals — 175

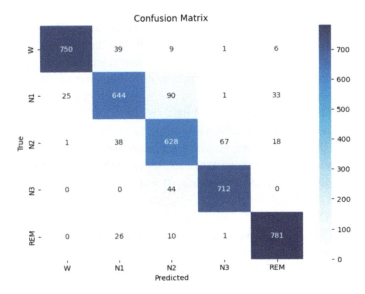

Figure 10.16: Confusion matrix obtained by the proposed method using hybrid HySleep_Net model on the *ISRUC* dataset.

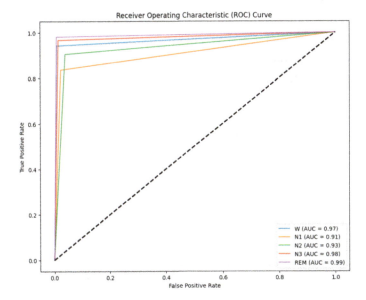

Figure 10.17: ROC Curve obtained by the proposed method using HySleep_Net model on the *ISRUC* dataset.

the temporal dependencies of the data. Let us take a look at the performance comparison between our HySleep_Net model, a model without the GRU layers and the coarse feature detection module (hereafter referred to as CNN+LSTM) and a model without the LSTM layers, the GRU layers and the coarse feature detection module (hereafter referred to as CNN Only). Table 10.7 shows the performance metrics of three different models: CNN Only, CNN+LSTM, and HySleep_Net on four distinct datasets: Sleep-EDF, Sleep-EDF 78, SHHS, and ISRUC. The HySleep_Net model consistently outperforms the other two models across all datasets, achieving the highest accuracy, precision, recall, and F1-scores. Specifically, HySleep_Net attains an impressive 94 % accuracy on the Sleep-EDF dataset, outperforming the CNN Only and CNN+LSTM models by 11 % and 7 %, respectively. Similarly, on the Sleep-EDF 78 dataset, HySleep_Net maintains a strong performance with 89 % accuracy, while the CNN Only and CNN+LSTM models lag behind by 8 % and 7 %, respectively. On the SHHS dataset, our HySleep_Net model achieves 89 % accuracy, demonstrating superior performance compared to the other two models, beating them by 8 % and 7 %, respectively. Finally, on the ISRUC dataset, HySleep_Net excels with an accuracy of 90 %, significantly higher than 79 % and 76 % accuracy of the CNN Only and CNN+LSTM models, respectively. These results highlight the robustness and efficacy of the HySleep_Net model and demonstrate the need for the CNN layers to extract coarse features and the GRU layers.

Table 10.7: Comparison of results produced using CNN-Only, CNN+LSTM and HySleep_Net models.

Model	Dataset	Accuracy %	Precision	Recall	F1-Score
CNN-Only	Sleep-EDF	83	0.83	0.83	0.82
CNN+LSTM	Sleep-EDF	87	0.87	0.87	0.87
HySleep_Net	**Sleep-EDF**	**94**	**0.94**	**0.94**	**0.94**
CNN-Only	Sleep-EDF 78	81	0.80	0.81	0.80
CNN+LSTM	Sleep-EDF 78	82	0.82	0.83	0.82
HySleep_Net	**Sleep-EDF 78**	**89**	**0.89**	**0.89**	**0.89**
CNN-Only	SHHS	81	0.79	0.81	0.79
CNN+LSTM	SHHS	82	0.82	0.83	0.82
HySleep_Net	**SHHS**	**89**	**0.89**	**0.89**	**0.89**
CNN-Only	ISRUC	79	0.80	0.79	0.79
CNN+LSTM	ISRUC	76	0.76	0.76	0.76
HySleep_Net	**ISRUC**	**90**	**0.90**	**0.90**	**0.90**

10.5.7 Comparison with existing sleep stage detection models

A comparative analysis of the proposed method against various publicly available works in the literature is shown in Tables 10.8, 10.9, 10.10 and 10.11. The evaluation is conducted using the Sleep-EDF, Expanded Sleep-EDF, SHHS, and ISRUC datasets, respectively. The comparison is made in terms of accuracy scores, showing how the proposed method performs in relation to other notable approaches in the field.

Table 10.8 renders the performance comparison of our model with some prominent contemporary proposals on the Sleep-EDF dataset. From Table 10.8, we can see that Qureshi et al. achieved a decent accuracy of 92.5 % using only a CNN-based model, while Michielli et al., using their LSTM-based model acquired an accuracy of 86.7 %. Our HySleep_Net model achieves an accuracy of 94 %, which combines the best of both worlds and thus outperforms the benchmark.

Table 10.8: Comparison of our proposed HySleep_Net model with some recently proposed models on the Sleep-EDF dataset.

Researchers	Year	Model	Dataset	Accuracy
Zhu et al. [16]	2020	Attention-based CNN		93.7 %
Qureshi et al. [17]	2019	CNN		92.5 %
Hsu et al. [18]	2013	Elman RNN		87.2 %
Michielli et al. [19]	2019	LSTM		86.7 %
Mousavi et al. [20]	2019	SleepEEGNet		84.26 %
Seo et al. [21]	2020	IITNet		83.9 %
Zhang et al. [22]	2020	DNN	Sleep-EDF	81.81 %
Supratak et al. [23]	2017	DeepSleepNet		82 %
Phan et al. [24]	2019	Multi-task CNN		81.9 %
Xu et al. [25]	2020	DNN		86.1 %
Vilamala et al. [45]	2017	CNN		81.3 %
Phan et al. [46]	2018	1-max CNN		79.8 %
Phan et al. [47]	2018	Attentional RNN		79.1 %
Proposed	**2024**	**HySleep_Net Model**		**94 %**

Similarly, Table 10.9 shows how our HySleep_Net model performs against some of the best peer works done on the Expanded Sleep-EDF dataset. Most of the work is based on CNN Only. The hybrid nature of HySleep_Net gives it an edge over previous works, achieving a +6.2 % accuracy over the benchmark model.

Table 10.9: Comparison of our proposed HySleep_Net model with some recently proposed models on the Expanded Sleep-EDF dataset.

	Year	Model	Dataset	Accuracy
Zhu et al. [16]	2020	attention CNN		82.8 %
Mousavi et al. [20]	2019	1D-CNN		80 %
Tsinalis et al. [26]	2016	2D-CNN	Expanded Sleep-EDF	74 %
Sokolovsky et al. [27]	2019	CNN		81 %
Proposed	**2024**	**HySleep_Net Model**		**89 %**

Table 10.10 denotes the comparison of our HySleep_Net model's performance with respect to other methods employed on the SHHS dataset. Sors et al. propose a CNN-based model that achieves a fairly decent accuracy of 87%. HySleep_Net beats this result, gaining a 2% accuracy over it, which may not seem much, but in the critical field of sleep stage detection, it can be a matter of life and death.

Table 10.10: Comparison of our proposed HySleep_Net model with some recently proposed models on the SHHS dataset.

Researchers	Year	Model	Dataset	Accuracy
Seo et al. [21]	2020	IITNet		86.7%
Sors et al. [28]	2018	CNN		87%
Fernández-Varela et al. [29]	2019	1D-CNN	SHHS	78%
Zhang et al. [30]	2019	CNN-LSTM		87%
Li et al. [31]	2018	CNN		65.9%
Proposed	2024	HySleep_Net Model		89%

Finally, Table 10.11 shows the performance comparison with respect to the ISRUC dataset. Although this dataset is the least used in research, it is still valuable in the field of sleep stage detection. Here we can see that a traditional machine learning approach i. e. Random Forest proposed by Li et al. achieves the highest accuracy of 84.7%. Still, it is evident that HySleep_Net outperforms this model by a wide margin.

Table 10.11: Comparison of our proposed HySleep_Net model with some recently proposed models on the ISRUC dataset.

	Year	Model	Dataset	Accuracy
Chen et al. [32]	2024	Multi-view fusion network		84.1%
Li et al. [33]	2023	Random Forest		84.7%
Ji et al. [34]	2023	3D CNN	ISRUC	83.2%
Giannakeas et al. [35]	2018	Random Forest		75.29%
Xiaopeng et al. [36]	2024	3D Convolutional + Graph Convolutional		83%
Proposed	2024	HySleep_Net Model		90%

10.6 Conclusion and future works

In the past, studies based on traditional machine learning models faced significant challenges in recognizing complex patterns in the PSG data, and researchers had to manually extract relevant features. Our study proposes a novel hybrid DL model, HySleep_Net, which combines CNN with both LSTM and GRU layers for automatic sleep stage classification. The HySleep_Net model achieved high accuracies of 94 %, 89.06 %, and 88.13 % and 90 % on the four datasets, while also having the capability of automatic feature extraction. These results outperformed many previously proposed CNN- or LSTM-based techniques. The performance of the model in identifying intricate temporal patterns in the sleep data is increased by adding GRU layers in addition to LSTM layers.

There are several ways we might further improve our work. Here are a few key areas for investigation:

- Currently, our model only uses PSG data. In the future, we can explore the effects of including physiological measures such as muscle activity (EMG) and respiratory patterns (e. g., airflow, thoracic, and abdominal movements). This will make the classification of sleep stages even more precise.
- The effectiveness of our model was assessed using four public datasets. We aim to include more standard datasets in our work. This could further validate the robustness of our model.
- The PSG data can be further processed into spectrogram or Gramian Angular Field (GAF) images [48] and then be used for training and testing purposes for better performance and efficiency [49].
- We can explore the potential of using an ensemble of different models to further improve the performance and robustness of our work. Ensemble learning combines the predictions of multiple models. It can often outperform individual models by mitigating their weaknesses and amplifying their strengths.

Bibliography

[1] Sleep Foundation – Physical health and sleep: how are they connected? https://www.sleepfoundation.org/physical-health.
[2] National Institutes of Health – The benefits of slumber. https://www.nhlbi.nih.gov/news/2013/benefits-slumber-why-you-need-good-nights-sleep.
[3] National Sleep Foundation – Stages of sleep: what happens in each. https://www.sleepfoundation.org/stages-of-sleep.
[4] Horie, K., Ota, L., Miyamoto, R., et al. (2022). Automated sleep stage scoring employing a reasoning mechanism and evaluation of its explainability. Sci. Rep., 12, 12799. https://doi.org/10.1038/s41598-022-16334-9.
[5] Institute of Medicine (US) Committee on Sleep Medicine and Research, Colten, H. R. & Altevogt, B. M. (Eds.), (2006). 3, Extent and health consequences of chronic sleep loss and sleep disorders. Sleep Disorders and Sleep Deprivation: An Unmet Public Health Problem. Washington (DC): National Academies Press (US). Available from: https://www.ncbi.nlm.nih.gov/books/NBK19961/.
[6] Kemp, B., Zwinderman, A. H., Tuk, B., Kamphuisen, H. A. C. & Oberyé, J. J. L. (2000). Analysis of a sleep-dependent neuronal feedback loop: the slow-wave microcontinuity of the EEG. IEEE Trans. Biomed. Eng., 47(9), 1185–1194.
[7] Zhang, G. Q., Cui, L., Mueller, R., Tao, S., Kim, M., Rueschman, M., Mariani, S., Mobley, D. & Redline, S. (2018). The National Sleep Research Resource: towards a sleep data commons. J. Am. Med. Inform. Assoc., 25(10), 1351–1358. https://doi.org/doi:10.1093/jamia/ocy064. PMID: 29860441; PMCID, PMC6188513.

[8] Khalighi, S., Sousa, T., Santos, J. M. & Nunes, U. (2016). ISRUC-Sleep: a comprehensive public dataset for sleep researchers. Comput. Methods Programs Biomed., 124, 180–192. ISSN 0169-2607. https://doi.org/10.1016/j.cmpb.2015.10.013.

[9] Marik, A., Chattopadhyay, S. & Singh, P. K. (2023). A hybrid deep feature selection framework for emotion recognition from human speeches. Multimed. Tools Appl., 82(8), 11461–11487). Springer Publishers (Special Issue: 1226 Deep-Patterns Emotion Recognition in the Wild).

[10] Sahoo, K. K., Ghosh, R., Mallik, S., Roy, A., Singh, P. K. & Zhao, Z. (2022). Wrapper-based deep feature optimization for activity recognition in the wearable sensor networks of healthcare systems. Sci. Rep., 13:(965), 1–18.

[11] Bhattacharya, D., Sharma, D., Kim, W., Ijaz, M. F. & Singh, P. K. (2022). Ensem-HAR: an ensemble deep learning model for smartphone sensor-based human activity recognition for measurement of elderly health monitoring. Biosensors, 12(6), 393, 1–25. MDPI Publishers.

[12] Paul, A., Khan, S., Mondal, D. & Singh, P. K. (2025). Recognizing human activities in ambient assisted environment from wearable sensor data using Gramian Angular Field and deep CNN. In Enabling Person-Centric Healthcare Using Ambient Assistive Technology, Volume 2: Personalized and Patient-Centric Healthcare Services in AAT (pp. 199–226). Cham: Springer Nature Switzerland.

[13] Das, A., Guha, S., Singh, P. Kr., Ahmadian, A., Senu, N. & Sarkar, R. (2020). A hybrid meta-heuristic feature selection method for identification of Indian spoken languages from audio signals. IEEE Access, 8, 181432–181449.

[14] Sheikh, K. H., Ahmed, S., Mukhopadhyay, K., Singh, P. Kr., Yoon, J. H., Geem, Z. W. & Sarkar, R. (2020). EHHM: electrical harmony based hybrid meta-heuristic for feature selection. IEEE Access, 8, 158125–158141.

[15] Halder, A., Gharami, S., Sadhu, P., et al. (2024). Implementing vision transformer for classifying 2D biomedical images. Sci. Rep., 14, 12567. https://doi.org/10.1038/s41598-024-63094-9.

[16] Zhu, T., Luo, W. & Yu, F. (2020). Convolution-and attention-based neural network for automated sleep stage classification. Int. J. Environ. Res. Public Health, 17, 4152.

[17] Qureshi, S., Karrila, S. & Vanichayobon, S. (2019). GACNN SleepTuneNet: a genetic algorithm designing the convolutional neuralnetwork architecture for optimal classification of sleep stages from a single EEG channel. Turk. J. Electr. Eng. Comput. Sci., 27, 4203–4219. CrossRef.

[18] Hsu, Y.-L., Yang, Y.-T., Wang, J.-S. & Hsu, C.-Y. (2013). Automatic sleep stage recurrent neural classifier using energy features of EEG signals. Neurocomputing, 104, 105–114. CrossRef.

[19] Michielli, N., Acharya, U. R. & Molinari, F. (2019). Cascaded LSTM recurrent neural network for automated sleep stage classification using single-channel EEG signals. Comput. Biol. Med., 106, 71–81. CrossRef.

[20] Mousavi, S., Afghah, F. & Acharya, U. R. (2019). SleepEEGNet: automated sleep stage scoring with sequence to sequence deep learning approach. PLoS ONE, 14, e0216456. [CrossRef] [PubMed].

[21] Seo, H., Back, S., Lee, S., Park, D., Kim, T. & Lee, K. (2020). Intra- and inter-epoch temporal context network (IITNet) using sub-epoch features for automatic sleep scoring on raw single-channel EEG. Biomed. Signal Process. Control, 61, 102037. CrossRef.

[22] Zhang, X., Xu, M., Li, Y., Su, M., Xu, Z., Wang, C., Kang, D., Li, H., Mu, X., Ding, X., et al. (2020). Automated multi-model deep neural network for sleep stage scoring with unfiltered clinical data. Sleep Breath., 24, 581–590. [CrossRef] [PubMed].

[23] Supratak, A., Dong, H., Wu, C. & Guo, Y. (2017). DeepSleepNet: a model for automatic sleep stage scoring based on raw single-channel EEG. IEEE Trans. Neural Syst. Rehabil. Eng., 25, 1998–2008. [CrossRef] [PubMed].

[24] Phan, H., Andreotti, F., Cooray, N., Chén, O. Y. & de Vos, M. (2019). Joint classification and prediction CNN framework for automatic sleep stage classification. IEEE Trans. Biomed. Eng., 66, 1285–1296. CrossRef.

[25] Xu, M., Wang, X., Zhangt, X., Bin, G., Jia, Z. & Chen, K. (2020). Computation-efficient multi-model deep neural network for sleep stage classification. In Proceedings of the ASSE '20: 2020 Asia Service

Sciences and Software Engineering Conference, Nagoya, Japan, 13–15 May 2020 (pp. 1–8). New York, NY, USA: Association for Computing Machinery. 86.1 EDF20.
[26] Tsinalis, O., Matthews, P. M., Guo, Y. & Zafeiriou, S. (2016). Automatic Sleep Stage Scoring with Single-Channel EEG Using Convolutional Neural Networks. London, UK: Imperial College London.
[27] Sokolovsky, M., Guerrero, F., Paisarnsrisomsuk, S., Ruiz, C. & Alvarez, S. A. (2019). Deep learning for automated feature discovery and classification of sleep stages. IEEE/ACM Trans. Comput. Biol. Bioinform., 17.
[28] Sors, A., Bonnet, S., Mirek, S., Vercueil, L. & Payen, J.-F. (2018). A convolutional neural network for sleep stage scoring from raw single-channel EEG. Biomed. Signal Process. Control, 42, 107–114.
[29] Fernández-Varela, I., Hernández-Pereira, E., Alvarez-Estevez, D. & Moret-Bonillo, V. (2019). A convolutional network for sleep stages classification. arXiv:1902.05748v1.
[30] Zhang, L., Fabbri, D., Upender, R. & Kent, D. T. (2019). Automated sleep stage scoring of the sleep heart health study using deep neural networks. Sleep, 42.
[31] Li, Q., Li, Q. C., Liu, C., Shashikumar, S. P., Nemati, S. & Clifford, G. D. (2018). Deep learning in the cross-time frequency domain for sleep staging from a single-lead electrocardiogram. Physiol. Meas., 39, 124005.
[32] Li, Y., Chen, J., Ma, W., Zhao, G. & Fan, X. (2024). MVF-SleepNet: multi-view fusion network for sleep stage classification. IEEE J. Biomed. Health Inform., 28(5), 2485–2495. https://doi.org/10.1109/JBHI.2022.3208314.
[33] Li, Y., Xu, Z., Zhang, Y., Cao, Z. & Chen, H. (2022). Automatic sleep stage classification based on a two-channel electrooculogram and one-channel electromyogram. Physiol. Meas., 43(7), 07NT02. https://doi.org/10.1088/1361-6579/ac6bdb.
[34] Ji, X., Li, Y. & Wen, P. (2023). 3DSleepNet: a multi-channel bio-signal based sleep stages classification method using deep learning. IEEE Trans. Neural Syst. Rehabil. Eng., 31, 3513–3523. https://doi.org/10.1109/TNSRE.2023.3309542.
[35] Giannakeas, N. (2018). EEG-based automatic sleep stage classification. Biomed. J. Sci. Tech. Res.. Biomedical Research Network, LLC. https://doi.org/10.26717/bjstr.2018.07.001535.
[36] Ji, X., Li, Y., Wen, P., Barua, P. & Rajendra Acharya, U. (2024). MixSleepNet: a multi-type convolution combined sleep stage classification model. Comput. Methods Programs Biomed., 244, 107992. https://doi.org/10.1016/j.cmpb.2023.107992.
[37] Goldberger, A., Amaral, L., Glass, L., Hausdorff, J., Ivanov, P. C., Mark, R., …, Stanley, H. E. (2000). PhysioBank, PhysioToolkit, and PhysioNet: components of a new research resource for complex physiologic signals. Circulation, 101(23), e215–e220.
[38] Rundo, J. V. & Downey, R. (2019). Polysomnography. In Handbook of Clinical Neurology (Vol. 160, pp. 381–392). https://doi.org/10.1016/B978-0-444-64032-1.00025-4. PMID 31277862.
[39] Kemp, B., Värri, A., Rosa, A. C., Nielsen, K. D. & Gade, J. (1992). A simple format for exchange of digitized polygraphic recordings. Electroencephalogr. Clin. Neurophysiol., 82(5), 391–393. ISSN 0013-4694. https://doi.org/10.1016/0013-4694(92)90009-7.
[40] Chawla, N. V., Bowyer, K. W., Hall, L. O. & Kegelmeyer, W. P. (2002). SMOTE: synthetic minority over-sampling technique. J. Artif. Intell. Res., 16(1), 321–357. 2002.
[41] He, H., Bai, Y., Garcia, E. A. & Li, S. (2008). ADASYN: adaptive synthetic sampling approach for imbalanced learning. In 2008 IEEE International Joint Conference on Neural Networks (IEEE World Congress on Computational Intelligence), Hong Kong (pp. 1322–1328). https://doi.org/10.1109/IJCNN.2008.4633969.
[42] Chung, J., Gulcehre, C., Cho, K. & Bengio, Y. (2014). Empirical evaluation of gated recurrent neural networks on sequence modeling.
[43] Hochreiter, S. & Schmidhuber, J. (1997). Long short-term memory. Neural Comput., 9, 1735–1780. https://doi.org/10.1162/neco.1997.9.8.1735.
[44] Yacouby, R. & Axman, D. (2020). Probabilistic extension of precision, recall, and F1 score for more thorough evaluation of classification models (pp. 79–91). https://doi.org/10.18653/v1/2020.eval4nlp-1.9.

[45] Vilamala, A., Madsen, K. H. & Hansen, L. K. (2017). Deep convolutional neural networks for interpretable analysis of EEG sleep stage scoring. In Proceedings of the 2017 IEEE 27th International Workshop on Machine Learning for Signal Processing (MLSP), Tokyo, Japan, 25–28 September 2017 (pp. 1–6). CrossRef.

[46] Phan, H., Andreotti, F., Cooray, N., Chen, O. Y. & de Vos, M. (2018). DNN filter bank improves 1-max pooling CNN for single-channel EEG automatic sleep stage classification. In Proceedings of the 2018 40th Annual International Conference of the IEEE Engineering in Medicine and Biology Society (EMBC), Honolulu, HI, USA, 18–21 July 2018 (pp. 453–456). CrossRef.

[47] Phan, H., Andreotti, F., Cooray, N., Chen, O. Y. & De Vos, M. (2020). Automatic sleep stage classification using single-channel EEG: learning sequential features with attention-based recurrent neural networks. In Proceedings of the 2018 40th Annual International Conference of the IEEE Engineering in Medicine and Biology Society (EMBC), Honolulu, HI, USA, 18–21 July 2018. Appl. Sci., 10, 8963 23 of 24.

[48] Duygu, S. T. (2022). Gramian Angular field transformation-based intrusion detection. Comput. Sci., 23. https://doi.org/10.7494/csci.2022.23.4.4406.

[49] Ghosh, S., Kim, S., Ijaz, M. F., Singh, P. K. & Mahmud, M. (2022). Classification of mental stress from wearable physiological sensors using image-encoding-based deep neural network. Biosensors, 12(12), 1153.

Debangshu Ghosh, Arundhuti Mukhopadhyay, and Radha Krishna Jana
11 Ambulance booking and tracking website

Abstract: MedWheels is a pioneering solution revolutionizing emergency medical transportation, inspired by the seamless efficiency of ridesharing services like Uber and Ola. MedWheels offers an intuitive web application that connects individuals in need with prompt and professional ambulance services. Users can quickly request an ambulance to their location, by simply specifying their destination. Our platform ensures every journey is conducted by certified medical professionals, in state-of-the-art ambulances outfitted with life-saving equipment. Real-time tracking provides users with transparency and peace of mind throughout the transport process. With options for specialized medical care, wheelchair accessibility, and efficient routing algorithms, MedWheels prioritizes user safety, comfort, and timely response. By leveraging technology and innovation, MedWheels aims to bridge the gap between medical assistance and those in need, making emergency healthcare more accessible and reliable for communities. Join us in our mission to create a safer, more efficient future for emergency medical transportation.

Keywords: Ambulance booking system, HealthTech innovations, real-time location services, emergency medical response, AI in healthcare logistics, healthcare app user interface, geolocation API integration, online medical assistance, healthcare mobile application, predictive analytics in emergency care

11.1 Introduction

In moments of crisis, access to timely and reliable emergency medical transportation can mean the difference between life and death. Recognizing the critical need for efficient healthcare services, we introduce MedWheels, an innovative solution that is poised to revolutionize the landscape of emergency medical transportation.

Inspired by the paradigm-shifting models of ridesharing services like Uber and Ola, MedWheels harnesses the power of technology to streamline and optimize the process of accessing ambulance services. With the simple tap of a button on our user-friendly web application, individuals facing medical emergencies can initiate a seamless journey to get the care they need.

The genesis of MedWheels stems from a deep-seated commitment to addressing the inherent challenges and shortcomings within traditional emergency medical trans-

---

Debangshu Ghosh, Department of Computer Science and Engineering, JIS University, 48, Shibtala Ghoshpara, Kolkata 700122, West Bengal, India, e-mail: shadebangshu155@gamil.com
Arundhuti Mukhopadhyay, Radha Krishna Jana, Department of Computer Science and Engineering, JIS University, Kolkata, India, e-mails: arnamukherjee4@gmail.com, radhakrishnajana@gmail.com

https://doi.org/10.1515/9783111504667-011

portation systems. Time and time again, individuals in distress have encountered obstacles in securing timely assistance, navigating complex dispatch procedures, and ensuring access to qualified medical professionals during transit. These inefficiencies not only exacerbate the severity of medical emergencies but also contribute to increased stress and uncertainty for patients and their loved ones.

MedWheels seeks to alleviate these burdens by offering a comprehensive, user-centered approach to emergency medical transportation. Our platform prioritizes accessibility, reliability, and patient-centered care, ensuring that individuals receive the prompt attention and support they deserve in critical moments.

Central to the MedWheels experience is our unwavering commitment to safety and quality. Every aspect of our service, from recruiting highly trained medical personnel to maintaining state-of-the-art ambulance fleets, is meticulously designed to meet the highest standards of professionalism and efficacy. Real-time tracking capabilities enable users to monitor the progress of their ambulance in transit, fostering transparency and confidence in our service delivery.

As we embark on this journey to redefine emergency medical transportation, we invite you to join us in realizing our vision of a world where access to life-saving care is not just a privilege but a fundamental human right. Together, let us pave the way towards a future where every individual can confidently rely on MedWheels to deliver compassionate and timely assistance in their time of need.

11.2 Background and literature survey

11.2.1 Background

Our platform is designed to transform the way ambulance services are booked and managed, offering a user-friendly experience that emphasizes efficiency, transparency, and safety. Through an intuitive interface, we simplify the process of booking and tracking ambulance services for both patients and drivers, ensuring that critical services are easily accessible during emergencies.

One of the standout features of our website is the ability to display nearby hospitals based on the user's current location. This allows users to not only book ambulances directly, but also visit or contact the hospital for additional support, thereby streamlining access to urgent care.

In addition, we enhance the quality of transportation by providing personalized medical assistance tailored to the patient's needs, ensuring a comfortable and safe journey. Leveraging cutting-edge technology, we prioritize customer satisfaction and aim to become the leading platform for reliable ambulance services, setting a benchmark for excellence in emergency medical transportation.

Our commitment to innovation extends to the integration of artificial intelligence (AI) and machine learning (ML). By analyzing accident data, we predict high-risk locations for emergencies. Ambulances are strategically pre-positioned in these areas, enabling faster response times and more effective emergency intervention.

In essence, we aim to be a trusted partner in critical moments, offering peace of mind and timely assistance when it matters most. Through technology-driven solutions and a focus on user safety, we are setting a new standard in the emergency medical services industry.

India's rapid urbanization and growing traffic issues have led to a critical need for efficient emergency medical transportation. Conventional ambulance services often face delays due to a lack of modern technology, inefficient communications, and minimal integration with healthcare providers, resulting in suboptimal emergency response.

Many regions suffer from fragmented communications and ineffective tracking systems, resulting in delayed medical response times. The lack of real-time updates creates confusion for both patients and caregivers, increasing the risk to patients during emergencies due to prolonged wait times.

MedWheels integrates advanced technologies such as geolocation, GPS, and ride-hailing services to streamline ambulance dispatch and route planning. This allows for quicker, more accurate responses. Real-time tracking improves transparency and reliability, enhancing the experience for both users and healthcare providers.

MedWheels leverages artificial intelligence (AI) and machine learning (ML) to forecast ambulance demand and optimize resource deployment. Key benefits include:

- Faster response times: AI helps pre-position ambulances in high-demand areas, reducing emergency response times.
- Optimized resource allocation: By identifying demand hotspots, AI ensures that ambulances are positioned where they are needed most.
- Improved coverage: Reduces gaps in service areas, ensuring patients get help faster.
- Data-driven decisions: Continuous data analysis enables strategic planning and better resource management.
- Increased efficiency: AI optimizes processes, minimizing user wait times and improving overall service performance.

MedWheels offers a comprehensive ambulance booking platform with three categories: *Basic Life Support* (BLS) for less urgent cases, *Advanced Life Support* (ALS) for critical emergencies, and *Intensive Care Unit* (ICU) ambulances for patients requiring advanced medical care. The platform features real-time tracking, secure OTP-based ride verification, and AI-driven driver dispatch to ensure fast, safe, and reliable service for patients.

MedWheels differentiates itself by combining cutting-edge technology with its three-tiered ambulance service options (BLS, ALS, ICU). Its geolocation-based booking system and hospital integration create a seamless user experience. The inclusion of AI and ML enhances the platform's operational efficiency by improving response times, resource allocation, and service delivery. Features such as OTP verification and automated feedback mechanisms ensure both security and quality in the user journey.

11.2.2 Literature survey

This paper proposes a mobile tracking application for emergency ambulance services that address the challenges of vehicle tracking and monitoring. The system sends alert messages in emergency situations and provides location information. Unlike conventional methods, where ambulances often arrive late due to traffic, this application enables real-time tracking. Ambulance drivers can update their availability and location, while users can book ambulances and view nearby options on Google Maps. The app also updates ambulance locations and helps navigate to hospitals, controlling traffic lights to ensure a clear route [1].

The growing number of vehicles in densely populated cities poses a significant challenge to traffic management. Delays in medical assistance due to traffic congestion result in a significant number of avoidable deaths daily, especially in urban regions. To address this issue, this paper explores existing literature on ambulance tracking systems and methods to reduce response times, aiming to provide a solution to minimize delays in medical assistance [2].

The growing population has led to an increase in accidents, highlighting the need for smart technology in healthcare. Delays in reaching hospitals due to traffic jams, road issues, or location problems can be fatal. To address this, a project has been proposed that leverages big data, IoT, and smart traffic management. The system aims to reduce mortality rates and travel time by controlling traffic lights, tracking the location of ambulances, and enabling drivers to select nearby hospitals [3].

India's densely populated cities face severe traffic congestion, resulting in delayed ambulance arrival and increased fatalities. To address this, a "smart ambulance" system is proposed that uses RF communication and Arduino technology to dynamically control traffic signals to ensure smooth ambulance movement. In addition, a medical record storage system will be developed, that allows for fingerprint-authenticated data retrieval and transmission to nearby hospitals via GPS, aiming to save lives by streamlining emergency response times [4].

A mobile app for real-time ambulance tracking is proposed to address the challenges of emergency vehicle tracking. The app sends alerts, provides location information, and enables users to book ambulances and view nearby options on Google Maps. Ambulance locations are tracked and shared with traffic police, who can control signals to provide a clear route. This system aims to reduce response times and save lives by streamlining emergency ambulance services [1].

11.2.3 Key functionalities

1. User registration and login:
   Users must first create an account and log in to access the ambulance booking features. This process ensures secure authentication and allows users to effectively manage their profiles.

2. Ambulance booking and availability:
   Once logged in, users can manually enter their pick-up location or use the geolocation API to automatically detect their current location. The destination drop-off location is then provided by the user. Three ambulance options are available:
   - *MedBLS:* Suitable for non-emergency transportation.
   - *MedALS:* Equipped with additional medical equipment and highly trained medical professionals capable of providing life-saving assistance in emergencies.
   - *MedICU:* Equipped with advanced life support systems, ventilators, cardiac monitors, infusion pumps, and other critical care equipment, these ambulances help transport critically ill patients who require intensive medical care.

   After selecting the type of ambulance, a booking request is submitted, and the system notifies drivers via email. If a driver accepts the request, the user can track the ambulance in real time, and an OTP is sent to confirm the ride.

3. Real-time tracking and driver details:
   After verifying the ride OTP, the user can monitor the ambulance's journey in real time, from the pick-up point to the destination. Driver details, including name and contact information, are also displayed for transparency and convenience.

4. Payment and feedback:
   Once the destination is reached, a payment page is displayed for both the user and the driver. After successful payment verification, users are prompted to provide feedback on their experience.

5. Driver registration and dashboard:
   Drivers can register and create an account, and once logged in, they can view their account details, earnings, and their last five rides. The dashboard also displays driver ratings, and allows drivers to update their personal information as needed.

6. Hospital page and nearby hospital feature:
   The hospital page accesses the user's current location to display nearby hospitals. From this page, users can book ambulances directly, call the hospitals, check OPD availability, or visit the hospital's website.

7. AI and ML-based accident prediction:
   Leveraging artificial intelligence and machine learning, the platform uses accident data to predict high-risk locations. Ambulances are strategically positioned in these areas, ensuring faster emergency response times when accidents occur.

8. Technology stack:
   - Frontend: HTML, CSS, JavaScript
   - Backend: Django, Python
   - Database: MySQL
   - APIs: Google Maps API for real time location tracking and route management

9. Focus:

9.1. Clarity:
MedWheels aims to fill significant gaps in ambulance access and response times within the Indian healthcare system. With a user base of over 30 million by 2024 and a rapidly expanding ambulance market, the demand for reliable emergency transportation is urgent. Research shows that real-time tracking and integrated technology can significantly improve emergency response efficiency and overall service quality.

9.2. Parallels:
MedWheels: A Solution
MedWheels integrates advanced technology into a structured framework to effectively address these issues. The platform offers three levels of ambulance services—Basic Life Support (BLS), Advanced Life Support (ALS), and Intensive Care Unit (ICU)—ensuring that patients receive appropriate care based on their specific needs.

- User-friendly Registration: The platform simplifies account creation with a robust OTP verification process to minimize user frustration.
- Real-time tracking: Using GPS and geolocation, users can efficiently track ambulance locations, reducing uncertainty during emergencies.
- Integrated medical support: MedWheels differentiates itself from standard ride-hailing services by including trained medical personnel and essential medical equipment, prioritizing patient care during transport.
- Multiple ambulance options: Med BLS, Med ALS, and Med ICU for customized emergency care.
- Easy booking: Geolocation and direct booking streamline the process.
- Efficient communication: Automated emails and OTP verification for smooth interactions.
- Hospital integration: Locate and contact nearby hospitals directly.
- Enhanced features: Drivers track earnings and rides, while users provide feedback.
- AI/ML integration: The platform uses artificial intelligence (AI) and machine learning (ML) to predict demand patterns and optimize resource allocation. This technology enables faster response times by pre-positioning ambulances in high-risk areas, improving coverage and efficiency while ensuring timely assistance to users.

11.3 Work performed

11.3.1 Workflow diagram

11 Ambulance booking and tracking website — **189**

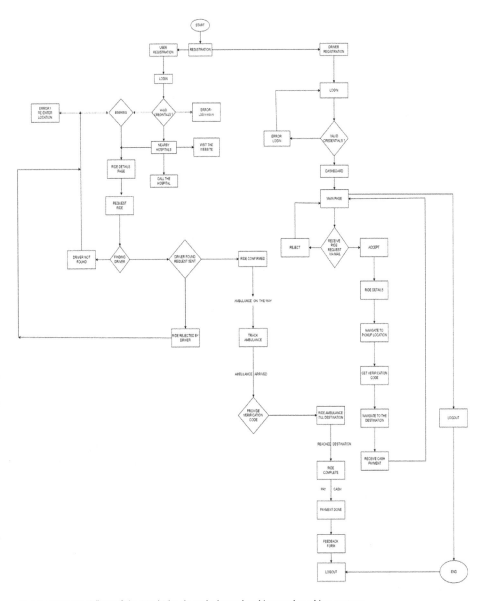

Figure 11.1: Workflow of the MedWheels ambulance booking and tracking system.

11.3.2 Algorithm

1. Start:
   – Begin the process.
2. User registration and login:
   – User registration: New users register by providing the required details.

- Login: Users log in to the system. If login fails due to an error (incorrect credentials), prompt the user to try again.
3. Driver registration and login:
    - Driver registration: New drivers register by providing the necessary details.
    - Login: Drivers log in to their dashboard. If login fails, prompt to correct the credentials.
4. Main functionality:
    - User path:
        - Booking:
            * Users manually enter or use geolocation for pick-up location.
            * Users enter drop-off location.
            * Users select ambulance type: MedBLS, MedALS, MedICU.
            * System notifies driver about the new ride request.
        - Driver response:
            * If the driver is available and accepts the request, proceed to ride details.
            * If no driver is found or ride is rejected, notify the user.
        - Ride confirmation:
            * If the ride is accepted, provide real-time tracking from pick-up to drop-off location.
            * Navigate the ambulance to the pick-up location.
            * Provide OTP for ride verification.
            * Navigate to the destination after verifying the OTP.
        - Payment and feedback:
            * On reaching the destination, the payment page is displayed.
            * After payment confirmation, prompt the user to fill out a feedback form.
        - Logout:
            * User logs out after completing the feedback.
    - Driver path:
        - After login, the driver sees their dashboard with account info, earnings, and ride history.
        - Drivers can edit their personal details.
    - Hospital page:
        - Access user's current location.
        - Display nearby hospitals where users can book ambulances directly, call the hospital, or visit the hospital's website.
5. End:
    - End of the process.

11.4 Experimental results and comparison

11.4.1 Experimental results

MedWheels operates as an on-demand ambulance booking platform. Users register and log in, then input their pick-up and drop-off locations to request an ambulance. The system validates these details and dispatches the request to nearby drivers. Upon acceptance, users receive a verification code and can track the ambulance in real time. Once the ambulance arrives, the user provides the code to the driver to verify the ride. The ride proceeds to the drop-off location, and upon completion, users can provide feedback. This process ensures efficient, transparent, and timely medical transportation, improving emergency response and user satisfaction.

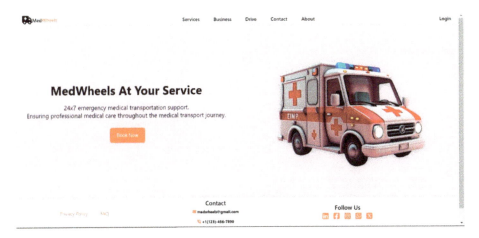

Figure 11.2: Homepage of the MedWheels platform.

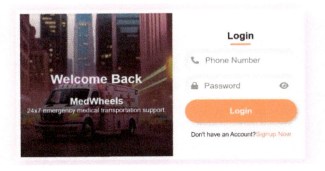

Figure 11.3: Login page for users on the MedWheels platform.

192 — D. Ghosh et al.

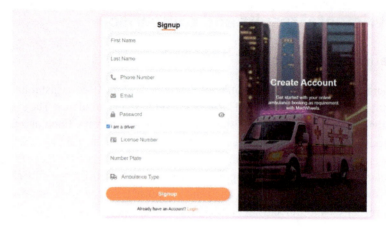

Figure 11.4: Signup/registration interface for new users.

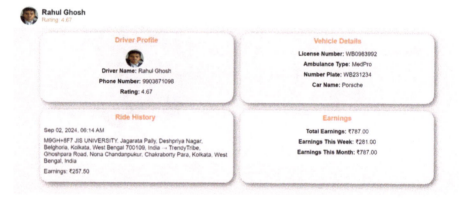

Figure 11.5: Driver dashboard showing ride status and earnings.

11 Ambulance booking and tracking website — 193

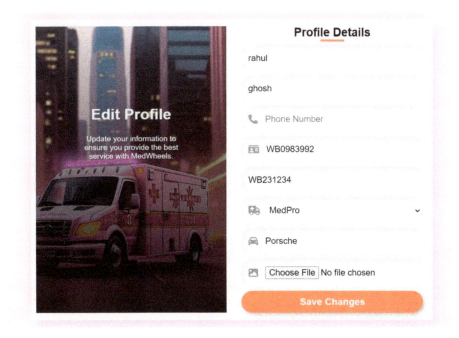

Figure 11.6: Driver profile edit page.

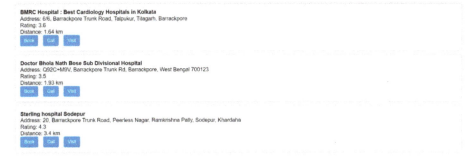

Figure 11.7: Nearby hospitals listing with booking/call options.

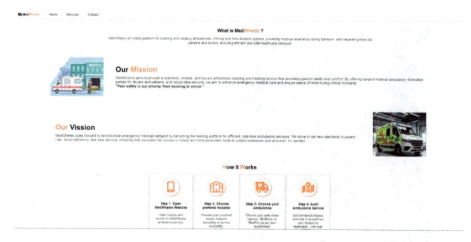

Figure 11.8: About page of the MedWheels platform.

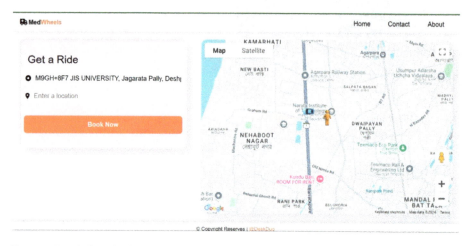

Figure 11.9: Ambulance booking interface for users.

11 Ambulance booking and tracking website — 195

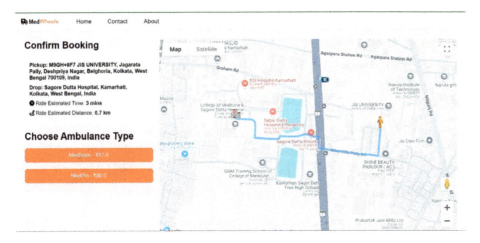

Figure 11.10: Ambulance confirmation screen.

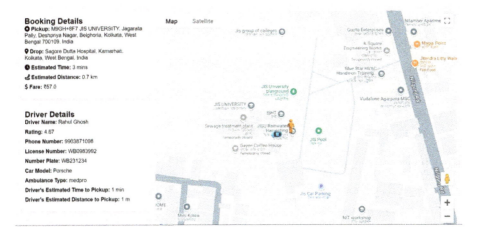

Figure 11.11: Booking summary and confirmation page.

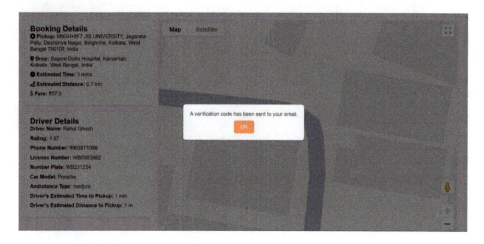

Figure 11.12: OTP verification prompt shown to users.

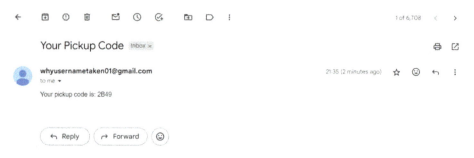

Figure 11.13: Email verification message sent to user.

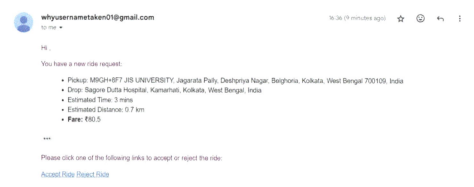

Figure 11.14: Driver receives booking request via email.

11 Ambulance booking and tracking website — 197

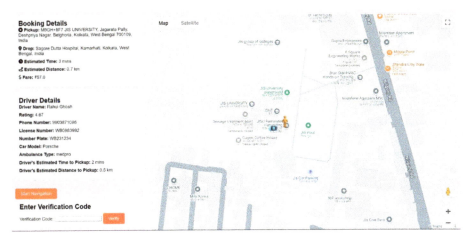

Figure 11.15: Page for entering verification code before ride starts.

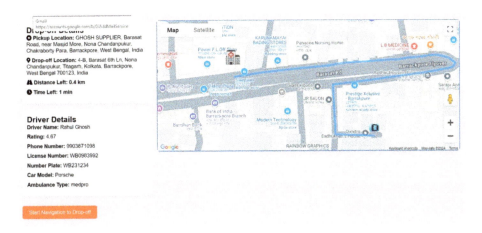

Figure 11.16: Real-time route tracking screen for drop-off.

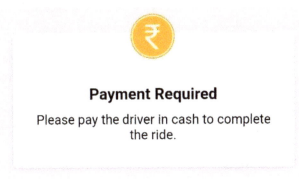

Figure 11.17: Payment interface after ride completion.

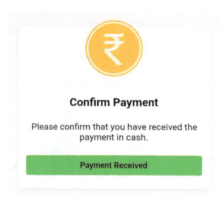

Figure 11.18: Confirmation of payment screen.

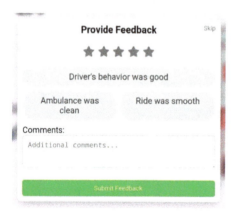

Figure 11.19: User feedback form after ride ends.

11.4.2 Comparison with existing ambulance services

1. Advantages of existing ambulance services:
   - User-friendly interfaces: Most platforms offer intuitive and accessible interfaces that simplify the ambulance booking process, making it easier for users to navigate the app or website.
   - Real-time tracking: Many platforms provide real-time tracking features that allow users to monitor the location of their ambulance, improving transparency and reducing anxiety during emergencies.
   - Variety of ambulance options: Platforms offer a range of ambulance types to meet different medical needs, ensuring that users can choose the most appropriate service for their situation.
   - Broad coverage areas: Companies leverage extensive networks to provide broad geographic coverage, increasing the likelihood of prompt ambulance availability in different locations.

2. Disadvantages of existing ambulance services:
   - OTP and registration issues: Many platforms, often encounter frequent OTP verification problems during user registration, leading to frustration and a lack of feedback mechanisms.
   - Service reliability concerns: Several services, have been reported for scams and unreliable service, often involving extra charges and unprofessional staff behavior.
   - Technical failures: Many apps suffer from frequent crashes and slow performance, which negatively impact effective ambulance tracking and overall user experience.
   - Pricing and payment challenges: Many platforms lack transparent pricing structures and experience frequent payment errors, discouraging potential users from using their services.
   - Location tracking failures: Inaccurate tracking and delays in map updates in apps hinder users' ability to locate ambulances in a timely manner, impacting emergency response times.
3. Benefits of MedWheels:
   - Enhanced accessibility: MedWheels provides a user-friendly platform for booking ambulances, making emergency medical transportation more accessible to a broader population, including integration with nearby hospitals for streamlined services.
   - Real time tracking: The integration of GPS and geolocation features allows users to track ambulance locations in real time, reducing anxiety during emergencies and improving overall transparency.
   - Tailored medical services: With specialized ambulance options (BLS, ALS, ICU), MedWheels ensures that patients receive appropriate care based on their medical needs, enhancing the quality of emergency services.
   - AI/ML optimization: The use of AI and machine learning enables predictive analytics for demand forecasting and efficient resource allocation, resulting in faster response times and better service delivery.
   - Secure booking process: MedWheels uses robust OTP verification and other security measures to ensure a safe and reliable booking experience, fostering user trust.

Conclusion:

MedWheels stands out by providing a comprehensive emergency ambulance service with real time tracking, optional medical staff and equipment. While similar services offer valuable insights, MedWheels aims to fill the specific gap in emergency medical transportation with features designed to improve both user experience and medical response efficiency. However, it must overcome scalability and infrastructure challenges to achieve widespread adoption and reliability.

11.4.3 Detailed market analysis

1. India's ambulance services market:
   Over the past five years (2019–2024), India's ambulance services sector has witnessed notable growth, primarily due to a surge in demand for emergency healthcare services. Factors such as increasing accident rates and the need for timely medical intervention have contributed to this expansion. The market has achieved a compound annual growth rate (CAGR) of approximately 7–8 %, and it is expected to maintain this upward trend due to ongoing technological advancements and improvements in healthcare infrastructure, *India*: 7–8 % CAGR.
2. Global ambulance services market:
   Globally, the ambulance services market has grown at a slightly faster pace, with a CAGR of approximately 8.7 %. Projections indicate that the global market could reach a valuation of approximately USD 68 billion by 2030. This growth is driven by factors such as the rising prevalence of cardiovascular disease, an aging population, and increased demand for emergency medical services. *Global*: 8.7 % CAGR.

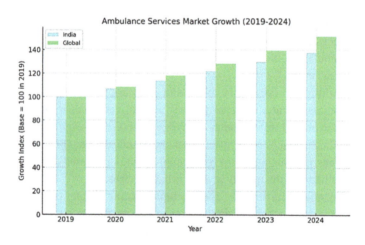

Figure 11.20: Ambulance Services Market Growth (2019–2024).

3. Indian customer base growth:
   The ambulance services market in India has experienced significant growth, increasing at a CAGR of 7–8 % from 2019 to 2024, driven by rising healthcare demands and the inefficiencies in public services. Delayed ambulance responses have led to preventable fatalities, emphasizing the critical need for system improvements. A 2020 report from AIIMS-NITI Aayog revealed that 90 % of ambulances lack essential medical equipment, highlighting the need for comprehensive service improvements.

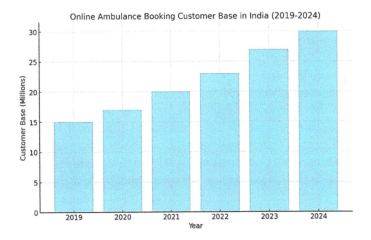

Figure 11.21: Online Ambulance Booking Customer Base in India (2019–2024).

4. Mortality rate due to ambulance arrival:
   In 2020, approximately 45 % of deaths in India occurred without access to medical care, a significant increase from 34.5 % in 2019. This increase can be partly attributed to the disruption caused by the COVID-19 pandemic. Traffic accidents also played a major role, with over 160,000 fatalities reported in 2023, many of which could have been prevented with timely emergency care, including access to ambulance services.
   Research indicates that up to 50 % of traffic accident deaths in India could be prevented if victims received medical attention during the critical "golden hour." However, the country's emergency response system has notable shortcomings. In 2020, more than 90 % of road ambulances lacked necessary equipment, and many were operated by untrained personnel.

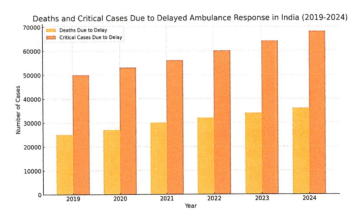

Figure 11.22: Death and critical Cases Due to Delayed Ambulance Response in India (2019–2024).

This data highlights the urgent need to overhaul India's emergency medical services, especially in rural areas and on highways, where ambulance delays have had severe consequences.

5. Ambulance sector growth in India:
   In 2019, private ambulance services held approximately 35–40 % of the market. By 2024, their market share increased significantly, with estimates suggesting that private operators now control around 50–55 % of the market. This growth is largely attributed to the inefficiencies within public ambulance services, such as outdated equipment and insufficient staff. Companies such as Ziqitza Healthcare and newer entrants such as StanPlus have capitalized on this opportunity by expanding their fleets, incorporating advanced technology, and offering better equipped ambulances. Meanwhile, government ambulance services continue to play an essential role, though their expansion has been slower in comparison.

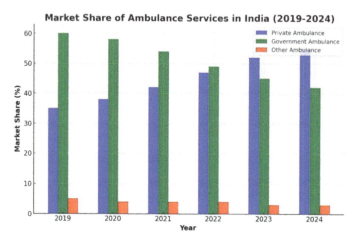

Figure 11.23: Market Share of Ambulance Services in India (2019–2024).

11.5 Conclusion, summary and future scope

11.5.1 Conclusion

MedWheels stands at the forefront of emergency medical transportation innovation, integrating advanced features that significantly enhance service delivery. Using AI and ML for predictive analytics, the platform can identify accident prone areas and optimize ambulance positioning. This, coupled with various specialized ambulance options—including Med BLS, Med ALS, and Med ICU—real time tracking, OTP verification, and seamless hospital integration, addresses both routine and critical medical needs. MedWheels not only improves response times but also increases overall reliability and efficiency.

Key points:
- Comprehensive service integration: Combines ambulance booking, real-time tracking, hospital services, and AI/ML capabilities into one cohesive solution.
- Enhanced security: Implements OTP verification to ensure secure ride confirmations.
- Data-driven insights: Leverages historical and real-time data for informed decision-making and improved resource management.
- User-centric design: Features an intuitive interface and streamlined booking process for an optimal user experience.
- Feedback mechanism: Encourages user ratings and reviews to continuously enhance service quality.
- Overall, MedWheels effectively fills existing gaps in emergency medical services, provides a superior user experience and sets a new standard for reliability and efficiency.

11.5.2 Summary

MedWheels is revolutionizing emergency medical transportation through its integrated and user-friendly platform. Users can easily create accounts, book ambulances, and track their rides in real time. The platform provides a variety of specialized ambulance options, including Med BLS, Med ALS, and Med ICU, tailored to meet different medical needs. Key features also include secure OTP verification for ride confirmation and direct integration with nearby hospitals for additional services.

Key points:
- Integrated services: Combines ambulance booking, real-time tracking, OTP verification, hospital connectivity, and AI/ML analytics into a unified system.
- Specialized ambulance options: Offers tailored services (Med BLS, Med ALS, Med ICU) to meet diverse medical requirements.
- Predictive analytics: Leverages historical data and real-time traffic information to enhance resource allocation and response times.
- User and driver features: Includes a detailed driver dashboard and a feedback system to facilitate continuous service improvement.
- Security and usability: Focuses on secure transactions and an intuitive user experience.
- This platform significantly improves the efficiency of medical transportation, addresses current service gaps and increases overall user satisfaction.

11.5.3 Future scope

Expanded service offerings:
- Specialized medical equipment: Integrates advanced medical devices, such as portable ventilators and diagnostic tools, to improve on-site care.
- Enhanced telemedicine: Develops integrated telemedicine features for real time consultation with healthcare professionals during transport.
- Advanced technology integration:
  - AI and machine learning: Continues to enhance AI capabilities for predictive analytics, optimizes ambulance positioning based on historical and real-time data, and improves overall response times.
  - Advanced GPS and navigation: Implements sophisticated GPS systems for precise tracking and real-time traffic updates to further enhance service reliability.
- Broader geographic reach:
  - Regional expansion: Extends services to additional cities and rural areas, improving accessibility in different regions.
  - International expansion: Explores opportunities to adapt and implement the platform in other countries.
- User experience enhancements:
  - Personalization: Develops customized features, such as user profiles with medical history and preferences, for a more customized experience.
  - Voice assistance: Integrates voice command capabilities to simplify booking and navigation, particularly for users with disabilities.
- Improved data analytics:
  - Advanced reporting: Provides in-depth analytics for hospitals and drivers to track performance, patient outcomes, and operational efficiency.
  - Feedback analytics: Uses sentiment analysis tools to better understand user feedback, driving data-driven improvements.
- Regulatory compliance and safety:
  - Compliance updates: Regularly update the platform to meet evolving healthcare regulations and standards.
  - Safety features: Implements emergency alert buttons and automated incident reporting to enhance user safety.
- These future developments will expand MedWheels' capabilities, increase its impact, and further improve the overall efficiency and user experience of medical transportation services, particularly through the integration of AI/ML for predictive insights and improved hospital connectivity.

Bibliography

[1] Sasipriya, S., Arfana Suraiba R, Ajaai R & Harini S (2021). Accident alert and ambulance tracking system. In 2021 6th International Conference on Communication and Electronics Systems (ICCES), Coimbatore, India (pp. 1659–1665). https://doi.org/10.1109/ICCES51350.2021.9489078.

[2] Pradeepa, R., Mohan, P. & Joy, S. I. (2023). A review on ambulance tracking system using GPS technology integrated with an Android application. In 2023 3rd International Conference on Innovative Mechanisms for Industry Applications (ICIMIA), Bengaluru, India (pp. 1296–1300). https://doi.org/10.1109/ICIMIA60377.2023.10425940.

[3] Kumar, P., Mohan, A., Raju, K., Ahmed, S. & Mehta, A. (2022). Smart ambulance for traffic control and tracking by GPS through IoT. In 2022 International Conference on Smart Technologies and Systems for Next Generation Computing (ICSTSN), Villupuram, India (pp. 1–5). https://doi.org/10.1109/ICSTSN53084.2022.9761369.

[4] Thirumoorthi, P., Deeparasi, M., Hariprakash, J., Meena, A. & Premalatha, K. (2021). Development of smart system for ambulance. In 2021 International Conference on Advancements in Electrical, Electronics, Communication, Computing and Automation (ICAECA), Coimbatore, India (pp. 1–5). https://doi.org/10.1109/ICAECA52838.2021.9675577.

Amalendu Si
12 Entropy based emergency rescue location selection with uncertain travel time

Abstract: Rescuers find it very challenging to select the ideal location for the rescue centers in order to conduct the rescue operation effectively during any emergency caused by natural disasters. An effective Emergency Rescue Model (ERD) is required to assist the rescuers in determining the optimal path to reach the affected locations. To address this issue, the ERD model is crucial for emergency rescue management since it can reduce the number of casualties and financial damages of a disaster. The ERD model consists of a set of rescue centers (RC) and a collection of demand points (DP). The RCs are used to schedule and distribute the resources among the DPs and the DPs provide the service within the communities. Therefore, choosing the best location to build the RC is essential for dealing with the unpredictable travel times caused by congestion and breakdowns as well as the unpredictable demand for logistics among DPs. The proposed ERD model considers the principles of interval analysis and entropy measurement. The uncertainty of the RCs is estimated through the entropy and the lower entropy value of the RC is selected for the final construction. The expected travel time is extracted from the uncertain interval travel time from RC to DP using interval analysis. The total cost of building a RC consists of a fixed established cost and an uncertain transportation cost based on the distance and travel time between RC and DP. Finally, we give an example of our recommended approach for the locations where an emergency rescue center is planned to be established with the lowest cost. Moreover, a comprehensive sensitivity analysis is performed to verify the stability and effectiveness of the proposed methodology.

Keywords: Rescue center, entropy, interval number, expected value

12.1 Introduction

Earthquakes, tsunamis, typhoons, and other natural disasters have become more frequent all over the world in recent decades. Simultaneously, human-made and artificially caused disasters, such as the World Trade Center terrorist attacks, are increasing worldwide [1]. These disasters have resulted in significant property loss, and post-disaster activities (whether caused by human actions or natural events) are crucial for reducing the causality rate and financial losses. Therefore, it is vital to conduct research on the logistics system and emergency management for unexpected disasters.

Amalendu Si, Department of Computer Applications, Maulana Abul Kalam Azad University of Technology, NH-12, Simhat, Nadia 741249, West Bengal, India, e-mail: siamalendu@gmail.com

https://doi.org/10.1515/9783111504667-012

Identifying the location of emergency rescue centers is a significant issue in emergency logistics management [1], and it is also a key component in the efficient distribution and scheduling of rescue resources following a disaster. The location of an emergency rescue center is different from the location of a typical site. The demand for the disaster area is unpredictable, and the need for rescue is urgent. Large-scale disaster rescue requires the mobilization of large-scale emergency resources. Reducing the number of casualties requires effective emergency rescue. However, in the event of a major disaster, people will need to quickly move a large number of rescuers and humanitarian supplies to the disaster site. In order to ensure the successful functioning of the entire emergency rescue network, it is necessary to optimize emergency location planning due to the suddenness and unpredictability of disasters, as well as the urgent need for emergency supplies [2].

Over the pas few decades, many researchers have been focusing on the emergency location problem, and consequently a number of research works have been conducted and achieved considerable success. Cooper's [13] solution to the facility location allocation problem has been widely applied to the emergency location field. Roth [14], Toregas and Swaim [15], and Murali et al. [16] addressed the emergency logistics facility location problem with capacity restrictions and produced the maximum coverage site model based on the assumption of covering all demand point consumers. The facility location allocation model with capacity limits was explored by Murtagh and Niwattisyawong [17]. Aran Jotshi et al. [18] studied the optimization of disaster relief resources; the objectives of the model were to reduce the time of transportation of injured people and to increase the probability of their survival. Wang Shao-ren [19] developed a two-stage triangular heuristic algorithm and a double-layer location-transportation model, then examined the complexity of the method and compared it with an improved genetic algorithm. In the rescue cover problem, Harewood [20] computed the probability of emergency rescue using the queuing theory and examined the emergency rescue problem at the lowest possible cost. Brotcorne et al. [21], Goldberg [22], Alsalloum and Rand [23], and Tovia [44] have examined the time and cost sensitive emergency location problem. Fang and He [25] proposed the least total cost model under the assumption that it fulfills the urgency of the rescue time. An embedded heuristic genetic algorithm was used to solve the emergency rescue center location model proposed by Wang and Zhang [26]. The model was based on the probability of disasters, the spread function of disasters, and the rescue function. In [24], the author introduced the model emergency rescue location problem with uncertain rescue time and minimized the estimated cost of developing the emergency rescue centers. Ma et al. [27] investigated three time-satisfying problems: the covering location problem, the set covering location problem, and the maximum covering location problem. Each of these problems was addressed using a different technique. The general rescue management model was shown with a logical structure (Fig. 12.1). The rescue points provide various types of services among the rescue points based on the requirement of selected demand points.

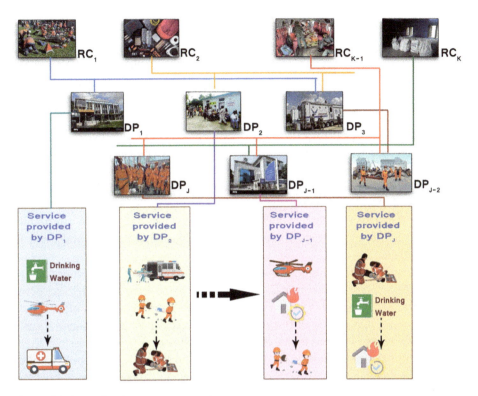

Figure 12.1: Conventional rescue management.

Although deterministic assumptions have been used extensively in studies of the emergency rescue locating problem, the real world abounds in nondeterministic elements. Uncertainty can take many different forms, including randomness, fuzziness, and fuzzy randomness [28]. Many researchers have experimented to address the ambiguity surrounding the emergency location dilemma to deal with the uncertainty of emergency situations. Facility location allocation problems with stochastic and fuzzy needs have been proposed by Zhou and Liu [29, 30]. The Benders decomposition technique was developed by Ren et al. [31] and a two-stage stochastic programming model of the unpredictable customer demand was constructed. Location problems with ambiguous criteria have been researched by Averbakh and Berman [32] using robust optimization techniques. Under a range of potential calamities, Mete and Zabinsky [33] suggested a stochastic optimization strategy for reserves and distribution. For hurricanes and other unpredictable disasters, Rawls and Turnquist [34] presented a two-stage stochastic mixed-integer programming model. To consider the event of insufficient knowledge about significant natural catastrophes, Sheu [35] presented a dynamic emergency rescue demand management model. Guo and Qi [36] provided the emergency material storage placement concept and technique in fuzzy environment by defining trapezoidal fuzzy number sorting criterion. A robust optimization model was used by Ben-Tal et al. [37] to address an emergency rescue location problem with unknown demand. A distribution center placement model with fuzzy variables was developed by Luo et al. [38] for the cases of factory supply capacity and consumer demand.

Probability theory is considered to be useful for managing objective uncertainty, while subjective uncertainty is well managed by fuzzy sets. We need a new tool if the uncertainty doesn't behave in a random or fuzzy way. Liu established uncertainty theory in 2007 [39] and redefined it in 2010 [40] to capture this kind of uncertainty. A subfield of axiomatic mathematics known as uncertainty theory is used to represent uncertainty in people. Numerous researchers have produced numerous important works in this field. According to Liu [41], the anticipated value operator is linear. A formula created by Liu and Ha [42] can be used to quickly determine the anticipated values of monotone functions with unknown variables. Liu [43] made a significant contribution by introducing uncertain programming, a type of mathematical programming using uncertain variables.

To summarize the aforementioned studies, it can be said that academics and researchers have focused more on logistics management, particularly the delivery of rescue supplies, which has been extensively researched. Disasters typically affect a large area, thus when one occurs, all rescuers should be dispatched to the affected areas to conduct the rescue as soon as feasible and minimize the loss as much as possible. Therefore, the best rescuer allocation strategy, which ensures that rescuers perform their tasks successfully and efficiently, is extremely important. However, there is relatively little research on this topic.

In this paper, we introduce the decision making model denoted as Emergency Rescue Model (ERD), which is based on the concepts of interval value analysis. The emergency rescue model is presented and solved through entropy-based emergency rescue center (RC) selection. The proposed model can effectively find the location to establish the rescue centers with minimum establishment cost, less distance from demand points (DPs), less traveling expenses and provide better service. The objective of the work is as follows:
– An entropy concept is introduced among the rescue centers to measure the uncertainty related to the demand points.
– An interval analysis is incorporated to estimate the probable travel time with respect to the uncertain travel time.
– An example is given to find the location for establishing the rescue centers to provide the service among the demand points, where the demand points distribute the logistics within the victim communities.
– Comparison and sensitivity assessment are performed to interpret the outcomes.

This paper is organized as follows. Section 12.2 introduces basic concepts of entropy and properties of uncertainty theory. Section 12.3 discusses about the interval number and expectation estimation. The emergency rescue center location model with uncertain rescue transport time and the appropriate decision matrix form are given in Section 12.4.

A numerical example is presented in Section 12.5. In Section 12.6, we perform the comparative study and sensitivity analysis. The conclusion is given in the last section.

12.2 Entropy and its related uncertainty

This section briefly discusses entropy, which has been used to measure uncertainty in order to compare different uncertain systems or events. In the entropy literature, the usual expected value of the information gain values is used to represent the entropy value of an uncertain system [54].

For the probabilistic processes where there are n probable outcomes, if $n = 2$, this might be as straightforward as a coin toss (p_1(head) = p_2(tell) = 0.5) and would follow the axiomatic properties of probability. Similarly, when $n > 2$, we assume that each of the n possibilities has a probability of $p_1, p_2, \ldots p_n$ and $p_1 = p_2 = \cdots = p_n = 1/n$, making all n outcomes equally probable. However, there are situations with maximum randomness, which are unpredictable and exhibit different degrees of randomness. Therefore, we should rank the objects according to uncertainty-based complexity. In this regard, entropy provides scientific information about the uncertainty of an event [45]. The entropy $H(p_i)$ is a function of the uncertainty of occurrence P_i, and this represents an approximation of the real likelihood of choice. In this study, we select n service-providing rescue centers to provide services among the demand points with least cost and minimum transportation time.

Definition. Consider a process with n possible outcomes with probabilities $p_1, p_2, p_3, \ldots, p_n$ respectively. Then the uncertainty $H(p_i)$ of the ith outcome and total uncertainty ($H(p)$) of the system are respectively defined by

$$H(p_i) = -p_i * \log(p_i), \qquad (12.1a)$$

$$H(p) = -\sum_{i=1}^{n} p_i * \log(p_i). \qquad (12.1b)$$

According to the definition, entropy satisfies the properties like continuity, symmetry, maximum, and additivity. The amount of information based on entropy could be summarized as follows:
- $H(p_i)$ is a monotonic decrease in p_i.
- $H(p_i) \geq 0$ information is a non-negative quantity (for two events $0 \leq H(p_i) \leq 1$).
- The uncertainty of $H(p_i) = 0$ is zero, in other words, the event always occurs.
- $H(p_1, p_2) = H(p_1) + H(p_2)$. This property is crucial and is verified with the maximum entropy demonstrated above ($p_1 = p_2 = 0.5$).

Example. Consider a dataset with 10 data instances, of which 6 belong to the positive class and 4 belong to the negative class. The entropy $H(p)$ is calculated as follows:

$$H(p) = -\left[\frac{6}{10}\log_2\frac{6}{10} + \frac{4}{10}\log_2\frac{4}{10}\right].$$

12.3 Basic concepts of interval analysis

In this section, we study the interval analysis to deal with the interval number in the decision making methods. An uncertain outcome in the interval-based method of the decision making has a lower and an upper bound, but the decision maker is unaware of any other information regarding the outcome.

An ordered pair of real number of the form of $A = [al, au]$ ($al, au \in R$ and $au \geq al$) is known as an interval number where al and au are the lower and upper bounds on the interval number A, respectively. Then A and B are the two interval numbers $A = [al, au]$ and $B = [bl, bu]$, two variables ma, mb are the mean values of the intervals as well as da and db are the distances of the interval number, respectively, has been used to compare two interval numbers [3, 4, 5]. For the operations related to the interval numbers see the references [6, 7, 8, 9].

Barker and Wilson [10] proposed the five rules for making decisions with intervals. For comparing the two interval numbers $A = [a, b]$ and $B = [c, d]$, where $a \leq b$ and $c \leq d$, assume that the decision maker prefers to either maximize or minimize the outcome depending on the problem types. The decision maker should favor interval $[a, b]$ to interval $[c, d]$ for each of the five rules.

- Worst case rule: $a > b$;
- Best case rule: $b > d$;
- Laplace rule: $a + b > c + d$;
- Minimum regret rule: $d - a < b - c$;
- Hurwicz's rule: $\alpha a + (1 - \alpha)b > \alpha c + (1 - \alpha)d$, where $\alpha \in [0, 1]$.

The decision maker should always prefer the interval number A over B for each of the five choice rules and for each value of $\alpha \in [0, 1]$ in the Hurwicz rule if $a > c$ and $b > d$. If the goal is to maximize the result, A can be said to dominate B in the case of two intervals shown in Figure 12.2. The decision maker should always choose B over A for any choice rule if $c > a$ and $d > b$. The preference link is weak if both of the greater-than inequalities are changed to greater-than-or inequalities. To avoid the trivial case where one interval is always preferred over another interval, the mathematical arguments always assume $c < a < b < d$ [12].

Each of these five interval decision rules can be simplified to the Hurwicz rule, as demonstrated by Cao [11]. It is possible to define the parameter as a compromise between the best case (optimism) and the worst case (pessimism). The Hurwicz rule is equivalent to the expected value of a uniform distribution only if $\alpha = 0.5$, because the expected value of a uniform distribution is equal to the midpoint. With an exponential utility function and a risk preference parameter selected to match α, the uniform distribution

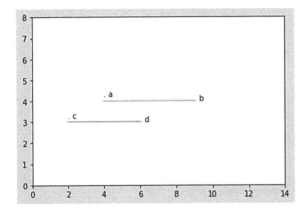

Figure 12.2: Representation of two interval numbers $[a, b]$ and $[c, d]$.

is employed. Then, the expected value (EV) according to the Hurwicz decision rule of the interval number $E = (a, b)$ can be estimated by the following equation:

$$EV(E) = 2b - a - 3\alpha(b - a), \quad \text{s.t. } a \le EV \le b \qquad (12.2)$$

12.4 Problem descriptions

Here we assume that there is a collection of service providing demand points. Each of the demand points has a specific location and population. We will build a collection of emergency rescue centers in the appropriate places to satisfy the requirement of demand points. A single emergency rescue center can serve several rescue demand points, and numerous emergency rescue centers can supply one demand point. We present the model parameters and decision factors that must be considered in order to solve this issue.

12.4.1 Index of the sets

i: index of emergency rescue centers.
j: index of demand points.

12.4.2 Model parameters

C_i: construction cost of emergency rescue center ($i = 1, 2, \ldots, n$).
E_{ij}: uncertain travel time interval between emergency rescue center i and demand point j

$(i = 1, 2, \ldots, n, \quad j = 1, 2, \ldots, m)$.

c_{ij}:   transportation cost between emergency rescue center i and demand point j

$(i = 1, 2, \ldots, n, \quad j = 1, 2, \ldots, m)$.

d_{ij}:   distance between emergency rescue center i and demand point j

$(i = 1, 2, \ldots, n, \quad j = 1, 2, \ldots, m)$.

T_j: time limit of demand point $(j = 1, 2, \ldots, m)$.
R: maximum number of emergency rescue center.
r_i: maximum number of demand point cover by each emergency rescue center $(i = 1, 2, \ldots, n)$.
Ent_i: entropy value of the emergency rescue center $(i = 1, 2, \ldots, n)$.
$EV(E_{ij})$: expected value of uncertain travel time interval of E_{ij} $(i = 1, 2, \ldots, n, j = 1, 2, \ldots, m)$.

12.4.3 Decision variable

sr_i: selected the emergency rescue center
- R number of rescue center selected with lower entropy and selected rescue center r_i denoted as sr_i.

ur_{ij}: rescue center RC_i providing service to demand point DP_j.
- If $EV(E_{ij}) < T_j$ then the demand point DP_j under the emergency rescue center r_i.

$$sr_i = \begin{cases} 1, & \text{if rescue centre } r_i \text{ is selected,} \\ 0, & \text{otherwise.} \end{cases}$$

$$ur_{ij} = \begin{cases} 1, & \text{if rescue centre } i \text{ provide service to demand point } j. \\ 0, & \text{otherwise.} \end{cases}$$

12.4.4 Emergency rescue model

The estimated variable Z represents the total cost, which includes transportation and construction costs.

$$Z = \sum_{i=1}^{n} C_i sr_i + \sum_{i=1}^{n}\sum_{j=1}^{m} c_{ij} ur_{ij} d_{ij} \tag{12.3}$$

In the decision-making process, we try to minimize the total cost. By the definition of the entropy, we consider the lower value of entropy of the emergency rescue center for providing the service to the demand points. Here, the rescue center RC$_i$ should be selected as the service provider to the demand point DP$_j$ if the expected travel time between RC$_i$ and DP$_j$ is less than the maximum time limit (T_j). Alternatively, consider the demand point DP$_j$ under the rescue center RC$_i$ if the expected travel time EV(E_{ij}) is less than the time limit T_j. Then, measure the entropy of each emergency rescue center based on the number of services providing demand points under of each rescue center (RC$_i$). Select the maximum number of rescue points (R) with lower entropy value. Based on the analysis of the decision making process, the Emergency Rescue Model (ERM) can be stated as follows:

$$\min Z(C, c, d) = \sum_{i=1}^{n} C_i \text{sr}_i + \sum_{i=1}^{n}\sum_{j=1}^{m} c_{ij} \text{ur}_{ij} d_{ij} \tag{12.4}$$

$$\text{s.t.} \sum_{i=1}^{n} \text{sr}_i \leq R \tag{12.5}$$

$$\sum_{i=1}^{n} \text{ur}_{ij} \leq r_i \tag{12.6}$$

$$\text{sr}_i, \text{ur}_{ij} \in \{0, 1\} \tag{12.7}$$

The goal of the objective function (12.4) is to minimize the total establish cost of the emergency rescue centers. Constraint (12.5) represents the maximum number of rescue centers are to be considered. Similarly, the constraint (12.6) denotes the maximum limit of demand points controlled by the individual emergency rescue center. Eq. (12.7) expresses the working emergency rescue center and demand point.

12.5 The numerical example

After our model is created and a conceptual approach is discovered, a practical question is how our model performs when the actual data is provided. The following tables give an example of a collection of demand points (DP$_i$) and the locations where emergency rescue centers (RC$_i$) are expected to be built. Additionally included are the distances between the locations, the costs associated with construction and transportation, as well as any efficiency limitations. In this example, we considered 5 emergency rescue centers and 20 demand sites. To represent the probable travel time as an interval number, we consider expert opinion as the dataset, which is represented in the three tables. Subsequently, Table 12.1 contains the information of surface-based travelling distance from each demand point to all rescue centers. Similarly, the travelling cost from each demand point to all rescue centers and establishment cost of each rescue center are represented in Table 12.2. The experts were unable to provide the actual travel time from all rescue centers to all demand points and instead used interval numbers to represent the uncertain travel time, which is shown in Table 12.3.

Table 12.1: Travelling distance from rescue center to demand points.

	R_1	R_2	R_3	R_4	R_5
DP_1	13.7	5.2	9.3	12	7.2
DP_2	19	13.1	8.4	3.2	7.6
DP_3	12	3.3	4.9	8	4.3
DP_4	14.5	8	3.6	2.5	3.8
DP_5	5.8	3.4	3.8	12.7	11.2
DP_6	6.7	4.3	4.1	19.3	9.8
DP_7	11.7	9.2	3.8	5.6	9.2
DP_8	6	7.9	6.3	10.9	12.6
DP_9	21	15	12.3	11.2	8.5
DP_{10}	13	5.2	8.4	10	21
DP_{11}	3.5	8.6	5.3	6.2	7.5
DP_{12}	20	16.5	13.1	12.1	5.7
DP_{13}	11.2	3.8	5.7	9.8	8.4
DP_{14}	14.3	8.9	7.5	12.5	10
DP_{15}	2.5	3.8	1.8	5.9	9.8
DP_{16}	15.6	5.6	4.8	12.3	21
DP_{17}	3.2	4.3	18.6	9.7	8.5
DP_{18}	7.8	19.3	8.5	3.2	12.8
DP_{19}	4.9	12.9	8.9	13.5	21
DP_{20}	15.6	6.5	13.8	4.2	10

In this problem, a maximum of three rescue centers (R) must be selected, and each rescue center can provide services to at most fifteen demand points ($r_{s1} = r_{s2} = r_{s3} = 15 \mid s1, s2, s3 \in [1, 5]$). According to this problem, it is necessary to evaluate the location selection vector, which represents the selected rescue centers, and develop the final cover matrix, which shows the selected demand points under selected rescue centers for estimating the minimum objective value. It is also justified whether the generated solution acceptable is acceptable and whether it satisfies all constraints. Moreover, sensitivity analysis was performed to understand the effect of the parameters on the evaluation of the objective function.

Initially, we calculated the expected travel time from the uncertain interval travel time based on the contents of Table 12.3, using Eq. (12.2) and developed the cover matrix that is represented in Table 12.4, where 0 and 1 indicate whether the expected travel time greater than or less than of the maximum time limit, respectively, according to Table 12.3. We use the concept of entropy to select the emergency rescue centers according to their estimated entropy values. A lower entropy value indicates less uncertainty, therefore, we choose the three rescue centers with the lowest associated entropy values. The evaluated entropy values of each rescue center are presented in the last row of Table 12.4. According to the three lowest entropy values, we create the emergency rescue location selection vector [0, 1, 1, 0, 1], which indicates that the emergency rescue centers r_2, r_3 and r_5 are selected to provide service among the demand points. Finally, based on

Table 12.2: Transportation cost per unit distance from rescue center to demand points.

	R_1	R_2	R_3	R_4	R_5
DP_1	2.1	2.2	2.3	2	2
DP_2	2.3	1.8	2.5	1.7	1.5
DP_3	1.9	1.9	1.6	2.4	3
DP_4	1.8	1.5	1.9	2.1	2.1
DP_5	1.7	2.5	1.5	2.3	3
DP_6	2.1	1.7	2.5	2.2	2.4
DP_7	2.3	1.6	2.1	2.4	2.1
DP_8	2.4	1.4	1.8	2.1	2
DP_9	2.5	2	1.7	2.5	2
DP_{10}	3	2.3	1.2	2.6	2.1
DP_{11}	1.8	1.3	1.3	3	2.6
DP_{12}	1.4	1.8	2	1.3	2.5
DP_{13}	2	1.6	2.1	1.8	2.8
DP_{14}	1.8	1.9	2.5	1.9	1.2
DP_{15}	1.6	2.1	2.4	1.5	1.6
DP_{16}	2.1	2.3	1.2	1.4	1.8
DP_{17}	2.6	1.1	2.3	2.6	1.7
DP_{18}	2.2	0.9	2.2	2.5	3
DP_{19}	1.6	1.6	2.2	2.2	1.9
DP_{20}	1.8	1.7	1.8	2.1	2.2
Establishment Cost	98	97	94	101	96

the proposed model and the information of the Table 12.5, the emergency rescue center r_2 can provide services to the demand points 1, 3, 5, 6, 7, 8, 10, 11, 13, 14, 15, 16, 17 and 20. Similarly, the rescue center r_3 provides services to the demand points 2, 3, 4, 5, 6, 7, 8, 9, 10, 11, 14, 15, 16, 17, 18 and 19. The demand points 1, 2, 3, 4, 7, 9, 11, 12 and 14 are under the service providing of rescue center r_5. The estimated objective value is 430.9.

12.6 Sensitivity analysis and validation of the results

After obtaining the initial results in the optimization model, the question arises of how subjectively defined input parameters affect the model results and what results are obtained by applying other minimization models [46]. Therefore, an indispensable step in the optimization technique is to check the robustness of the results and to analyze the sensitivity of the obtained results to changes in the input parameters of the optimization model [47]. Considering the recommendations of the literature [48, 49, 50, 51, 52, 53], in the following three sections present the sensitivity analysis and the validation of the results. In the first section, the effect of time limit changes of each demand point on establishment costs has been analyzed. In the second section, the analysis of the impact

Table 12.3: Rescue center based uncertain travel time of demand points with time limit.

	R_1	R_2	R_3	R_4	R_5	Time Limit
DP_1	(7.0,9.1)	(5.2,8.1)	(5.8,8.3)	(6.9,10.2)	(2.1,3.4)	6
DP_2	(8.2,13.3)	(8.1,12.2)	(4.6,8.1)	(1.7,2.8)	(2.5,3.9)	6
DP_3	(6.6,8.7)	(1.9,2.6)	(1.6,2.6)	(7.2,11.4)	(1.3,2.1)	3
DP_4	(7.1,9.8)	(3.1,4.5)	(1.9,3.2)	(1.2,2.1)	(1.2,2.1)	3
DP_5	(2.7,4.8)	(1.2,2.5)	(1.5,2.6)	(7.2,9.3)	(4.3,6.3)	4
DP_6	(3.2,5.1)	(1.1,1.7)	(1.2,2.5)	(8.2,13.2)	(3.2,5.4)	4
DP_7	(6.2,8.3)	(4.1,5.6)	(2.1,3.2)	(2.4,4.4)	(3.2,4.7)	5
DP_8	(2.4,4.7)	(3.4,6.2)	(3.8,5.9)	(3.6,6.2)	(4.7,7.2)	5
DP_9	(6.2,8.5)	(5.2,8.0)	(5.1,7.7)	(6.2,11.5)	(2.5,3.8)	6
DP_{10}	(8.3,12)	(4.7,8)	(4.6,9.6)	(7.2,11.6)	(3.2,6.9)	7
DP_{11}	(7.1,18)	(5.7,9.0)	(9.0,12.3)	(8.3,11)	(3.2,6.9)	7
DP_{12}	(10.4,13.9)	(4.8,9)	(8.2,10.8)	(6.5,10.3)	(2.5,4.1)	8
DP_{13}	(11.2,13.8)	(3.6,8.0)	(5.8,10.2)	(6.6,11.8)	(6.2,9.8)	7
DP_{14}	(9.1,12.8)	(5.1,8.9)	(5.0,9.0)	(6.6,12.1)	(5.4,9.8)	8
DP_{15}	(2.1,5.0)	(2.1,5.5)	(1.2,3.4)	(5.0,8.0)	(5.4,9.8)	4
DP_{16}	(8.2,11.1)	(2.3,6.2)	(2.2,5.6)	(6.8,11.4)	(10.1,13)	7
DP_{17}	(2.6,4.5)	(3.5,6.1)	(9.2,12.3)	(7.6,11.1)	(7.1,9.7)	6
DP_{18}	(6.6,10.6)	(12.9,14.6)	(6.2,11.2)	(2.5,4.6)	(7.3,11.4)	8
DP_{19}	(3.6,6.2)	(10.6,13.7)	(6.2,11.2)	(9.2,14.2)	(9.0,13.9)	8
DP_{20}	(9.8,13.6)	(4.5,10.7)	(9.8,11.7)	(3.1,4.7)	(7.2,11.2)	7

of changing the interval of uncertain travel times on the calculation of the expected travel time for the development of the coverage matrix as well as the calculation the entropy value was performed. In the third section, the robustness behavior in terms of demand point and rescue center of the final optimization value was justified by parameters involved in the final objective function. After that, in Subsection 12.6.4, the effect of changing travel cost and travel time on the minimization value of the objective function has been justified. Finally the robustness of the given solution was tested by comparing it with different minimization methods.

12.6.1 Effect of final cost due to change the time limit

The eligible demand points (r) will be increase if the time limit (T) of each demand point increases. This equality relation has a great impact within this location selection problem. Initially, additional number of demand points are eligible by increasing the time limit (T), after that the entropy values (Ent) will be changed due to increasing the number of demand points. The entropy value is the pivot point of the rescue center selection process.

Table 12.4: Entropy based coverage matrix.

	R_1	R_2	R_3	R_4	R_5
DP_1	0	1	1	0	1
DP_2	0	0	1	1	1
DP_3	0	1	1	0	1
DP_4	1	0	0	0	0
DP_5	0	0	0	1	1
DP_6	0	0	0	1	0
DP_7	1	0	0	0	0
DP_8	0	0	0	0	1
DP_9	1	1	1	1	0
DP_{10}	1	0	0	0	1
DP_{11}	0	0	0	0	0
DP_{12}	1	1	1	1	0
DP_{13}	1	0	0	0	0
DP_{14}	1	0	0	1	0
DP_{15}	0	0	0	0	0
DP_{16}	1	0	0	1	1
DP_{17}	0	0	1	0	0
DP_{18}	0	1	0	0	1
DP_{19}	0	1	0	1	1
DP_{20}	1	0	1	0	0
Entropy	0.24	0.12	0.15	0.27	0.17

Table 12.5: Requirements coverage matrix.

	DP_1	DP_2	DP_3	DP_4	DP_5	DP_6	DP_7	DP_8	DP_9	DP_{10}	DP_{11}	DP_{12}	DP_{13}	DP_{14}	DP_{15}	DP_{16}	DP_{17}	DP_{18}	DP_{19}	DP_{20}
R_1	0	0	0	0	0	0	0	0	0	0	0	0	0	0	0	0	0	0	0	0
R_2	1	0	1	0	1	1	1	1	0	1	1	0	1	1	1	1	1	0	0	1
R_3	0	1	1	1	1	1	1	1	1	0	1	0	0	1	1	1	1	1	1	0
R_4	0	0	0	0	0	0	0	0	0	0	0	0	0	0	0	0	0	0	0	0
R_5	1	1	1	1	0	0	1	0	1	0	1	1	0	1	0	0	0	0	0	0

12.6.2 Effect of changing the interval of uncertain travel times on the estimated final cost

The expected travel time (EV) between the rescue center and demand points is evaluated using the interval number analysis of the uncertain time interval (E). The expected value increases or decreases when the range of the interval changes either in the upper or lower direction, respectively. The expected travel time is the key parameter to develop the cover matrix and calculate the entropy of the rescue centers.

12.6.3 Influence of changing the number of rescue centers and demand points to estimating the final cost

The objective function $Z(C, c, d)$ depends on the distance (d) between rescue centers and demand points and the traveling cost (c) as well as the establishment cost (C) of each rescue center. Then the maximum number of rescue centers (R) and demand points (r) has no direct effect on estimating the establishment cost. So, the system can consider any number of rescue centers as well as demand points according to the intensity of the disaster. But if both the quantities of travel cost and distance are increased, the computational complexity increases as well.

12.6.4 Importance of the cost estimation of the travel cost and distance

The minimization function $Z(C, c, d)$ depends on the three factors: establishment cost (C), travel cost (c) and travel distance (d). These parameters are directly proportional to the objective function (Z). But the lower value of travel distance and travel cost can reduce the objective value up to a certain limit due to restrictions of maximum number of rescue centers and demand points.

12.6.5 Comparative study

In this subsection, we perform a comparative study with the previously introduced method [24]. The article [24], which presents a location selection model under uncertain rescue time, uses the same datasets, and the resulting selection vector is [01101]; service-providing demand points are shown in Table 12.6. The total optimal cost is 672.295. In our proposed model, the resulting selection vector is [01101], which is equivalent to the previous model, while the service providing demand points are different, as represented in Table 12.6. Finally, the estimated total cost is 430.9, which is better than previously introduced model.

Table 12.6: Outcome based comparison study.

Model	Selection Vector	Total cost	Service providing Demand Points
Emergency Rescue Location Model [24]	[01101]	672.295	R2-1, 4, 5, 7, 8, 10, 11, 12, 13, 14, 15, 16, 17, 18, 19, and 20. R3-2, 3, 4, 5, 6, 7, 8, 10, 13, 15, 16, 18, 19, and 20. R5-1, 2, 3, 4, 7, 9, 10, 11, 12, 14, and 17
Our proposed model	[01101]	430.9	R2-1, 2, 3, 5, 7, 8, 10, 13, 15, 16, 18, 19 and 20. R3-2, 3, 5, 6, 8, 9, 10, 11, 14, 15, 17 and 19. R5-1, 4, 5, 6, 8, 7, 9, 12, 13, 17 and 18

12.7 Conclusions

The issue of emergency rescue sites is crucial to emergency service providing system. In this paper, a location model for emergency rescue in a hazy environment is proposed. To explain the travel time between emergency rescue facilities and rescue demand sites, an unknown variable is included. The analysis of interval numbers is used to calculate expected travel time from the uncertain time interval. An uncertain anticipated cost minimization model was proposed based on the notion of uncertain time intervals. Here, we incorporated entropy to measure the uncertainty of the distance between emergency rescue centers and demand points for selecting a service provider. The usefulness of the approach has also been demonstrated using a numerical example.

Future study is suggested in a few places. To make this model more useful in emergency rescue management, we may add more uncertain factors to it or create a dynamic uncertainty model. Also, consider the machine learning approaches based on historical datasets.

Bibliography

[1] Chen, X. & Wang, C. X. (2012). Optimization model of location for emergency relief centers under fuzzy random demand. Oper. Res. Manag. Sci., 21(5), 73–77.
[2] Dai, J. & Guan, X. J. (2014). Literature review on robust optimization of location allocation of mass emergency rescue resources distribution nodes. Logist. Technol., 33(1), 8–11.
[3] Dubois, D. & Prade, H. (1989). The mean value of a fuzzy number. Fuzzy Sets Syst., 24(3), 279–300.
[4] de Campos Ibáñez, L. M. & Muñoz, A. G. (1989). A subjective approach for ranking fuzzy numbers. Fuzzy Sets Syst., 29(2), 145–153.
[5] Ishibuchi, H. & Tanaka, H. (1990). Multiobjective programming in optimization of the interval objective function. Eur. J. Oper. Res., 48(2), 219–225.
[6] Chanas, S. & Kuchta, D. (1996). Multiobjective programming in optimization of interval objective functions—a generalized approach. Eur. J. Oper. Res., 94(3), 594–598.
[7] Heilpern, S. (1997). Representation and application of fuzzy numbers. Fuzzy Sets Syst., 91(2), 259–268.
[8] Yao, J. S. & Wu, K. (2000). Ranking fuzzy numbers based on decomposition principle and signed distance. Fuzzy Sets Syst., 116(2), 275–288.
[9] Asady, B. & Zendehnam, A. (2007). Ranking fuzzy numbers by distance minimization. Appl. Math. Model., 31(11), 2589–2598.
[10] Barker, K. & Wilson, K. J. (2012). Decision trees with single and multiple interval-valued objectives. Decis. Anal., 9(4), 348–358.
[11] Cao, Y. (2014). Reducing interval-valued decision trees to conventional ones: comments on decision trees with single and multiple interval-valued objectives. Decis. Anal., 11(3), 204–212.
[12] Sivaprasad, S. (2017). What does decision making with intervals really assume? The relationship between the Hurwicz decision rule and prescriptive decision analysis. Diss. Iowa State University.
[13] Cooper, L. (1963). Location-allocation problems. Oper. Res., 11, 331–343.
[14] Roth, R. (1969). Computer solution to minimum cover problem. Oper. Res., 17(3), 455–465.
[15] Toregas, C. & Swaim, R. (1971). The location of emergency service facilities. Oper. Res., 19(6), 1363–1373.

[16] Murali, P., Ordóñez, F. & Dessouky, M. M. (2012). Facility location under demand uncertainty: response to a large-scale bio-terror attack. Socio-Econ. Plan. Sci., 46(1), 78–87.
[17] Murtagh, B. A. & Niwattisyawong, S. R. (1982). Efficient method for the multi-depot location-allocation problem. J. Oper. Res. Soc., 33(7), 629–634.
[18] Jotshi, A., Gong, Q. & Batta, R. (2009). Dispatching and routing of emergency vehicles in disaster mitigation using data fusion. Socio-Econ. Plan. Sci., 43(1), 1–24.
[19] Shao-ren, W. & Zu-jun, M. (2011). Location-routing problem in emergency logistics system for post-earthquake emergency relief response. Syst. Eng. Theory Pract., 31(8), 1497–1507.
[20] Harewood, S. I. (2002). Emergency ambulance deployment in Barbados: a multi-objective approach. J. Oper. Res. Soc., 53(2), 185–192.
[21] Brotcorne, L., Laporte, G. & Semet, F. (2003). Ambulance location and relocation models. Eur. J. Oper. Res., 147(3), 451–463.
[22] Goldberg, J. B. (2004). Operations research models for the deployment of emergency services vehicles. EMS Manag. J., 1(1), 20–39.
[23] Alsalloum, O. I. & Rand, G. K. (2006). Extensions to emergency vehicle location models. Comput. Oper. Res., 33(9), 2725–2743.
[24] Guan, J. Emergency rescue location model with uncertain rescue time. Mathematical Problems in Engineering. https://doi.org/10.1155/2014/464259.
[25] Fang, L. & He, J. M. (2004). Optimal location model of emergency systems by a given deadline. J. Ind. Eng. Eng. Manag., 18(1), 48–51.
[26] Wang, D.-W. & Zhang, G.-X. (2005). Model and algorithm to optimize location of catastrophic rescue center. J. Northeast. Univ., 26(10), 953–956.
[27] Ma, F. Y., Liu, Y. & Yang, C. (2006). Time-satisfaction-based set covering location problem and applications of greedy algorithms. J. Wuhan Univ. Sci. Technol., 29(6), 631–635.
[28] Dai, J. & Guan, X. J. (2014). Literature review on robust optimization of location allocation of mass emergency rescue resources distribution nodes. Logist. Technol., 33(1), 8–11.
[29] Zhou, J. & Liu, B. (2003). New stochastic models for capacitated location-allocation problem. Comput. Ind. Eng., 45(1), 111–125.
[30] Zhou, J. & Liu, B. (2007). Modelling capacitated location-allocation problem with fuzzy demands. Comput. Ind. Eng., 53(3), 454–468.
[31] Ren, M. M., Yang, C. & He, B. (2007). An integrated optimal approach for facility location and its size decision with uncertain demand. Syst. Eng., 25(6), 1–5.
[32] Averbakh, I. & Berman, O. (2000). Minmax regret median location on a network under uncertainty. INFORMS J. Comput., 12(2), 104–110.
[33] Mete, H. O. & Zabinsky, Z. B. (2010). Stochastic optimization of medical supply location and distribution in disaster management. Int. J. Prod. Econ., 126(1), 76–84.
[34] Rawls, C. G. & Turnquist, M. A. (2010). Pre-positioning of emergency supplies for disaster response. Transp. Res., Part B, Methodol., 44(4), 521–534.
[35] Sheu, J. B. (2010). Dynamic relief-demand management for emergency logistics operations under large-scale disasters. Transp. Res., Part E, Logist. Transp. Rev., 46(1), 1–17.
[36] Guo, Z. X. & Qi, M. R. (2010). Location model and its algorithm for emergency material storage under fuzzy environment. Comput. Eng. Appl., 46(25), 214–216.
[37] Ben-Tal, A., Chung, B. D., Mandala, S. R. & Yao, T. (2011). Robust optimization for emergency logistics planning: risk mitigation in humanitarian relief supply chains. Transp. Res., Part B, Methodol., 45(8), 1177–1189.
[38] Luo, H. X., Yuan, Z. Z. & Peng, S. S. (2012). Distribution center location with uncertain supply and demand. Sci. Technol. Eng., 12(30), 8100–8102.
[39] Liu, B. (2007). Uncertainty Theory (2nd edn.). Berlin, Germany: Springer.
[40] Liu, B. (2010). Uncertainty Theory: A Branch of Mathematics for Model Human Uncertainty. Berlin, Germany: Springer.

[41] Liu, B. (2009). Some research problems in uncertainty theory. J. Uncertain Syst., 3(1), 3–10.
[42] Liu, Y. H. & Ha, M. H. (2010). Expected value of function of uncertain variables. J. Uncertain Syst., 4(3), 181–186.
[43] Liu, B. (2009). Theory and Practice of Uncertain Programming (2nd edn.). Berlin, Germany: Springer.
[44] Tovia, F. (2007). An emergency logistics response system for natural disasters. Int. J. Logist. Res. Appl., 10(3), 173–186.
[45] Leipnik, R. (1959). Entropy and the uncertainty principle. Inf. Control, 2(1), 64–79.
[46] Kaya, S. K. (2020). Evaluation of the effect of COVID-19 on countries' sustainable development level: a comparative MCDM framework. Oper. Res. Eng. Sci. Theory Appl., 3(3), 101–122.
[47] Zolfani, S., et al. (2020). A VIKOR and TOPSIS focused reanalysis of the MADM methods based on logarithmic normalization. arXiv preprint arXiv:2006.08150.
[48] Wendell, R. E. (1992). Sensitivity analysis revisted and extended. Decis. Sci., 23(5), 1127–1142.
[49] Saaty, T. L. (1994). Fundamentals of Decision Making and Priority Theory with the Analytic Hierarchy Process. RWS publications.
[50] Simanaviciene, R. & Ustinovicius, L. (2012). A new approach to assessing the biases of decisions based on multiple attribute decision making methods. Elektron. Elektrotech., 117(1), 29–32.
[51] Mukhametzyanov, I. & Pamucar, D. (2018). A sensitivity analysis in MCDM problems: a statistical approach. Decis. Mak. Appl. Manag. Eng., 1(2), 51–80.
[52] Ecer, F., et al. (2019). Sustainability assessment of OPEC countries: application of a multiple attribute decision making tool. J. Clean. Prod., 241, 118324.
[53] Pamucar, D. & Ecer, F. (2020). Prioritizing the weights of the evaluation criteria under fuzziness: the fuzzy full consistency method–FUCOM-F. Facta Univ., Mech. Eng., 18(3), 419–437.
[54] Aggarwal, M. (2021). Attitude-based entropy function and applications in decision-making. Eng. Appl. Artif. Intell., 104, 104290.

Anomitro Das, Shayambhu Chaudhuri, Ashfaq Murshed, Rohini Basak, and Pawan Kumar Singh

13 Performance comparison of different deep learning ensemble models for sentiment classification of movie reviews

Abstract: Sentiment analysis is a common task in natural language processing that aims to detect the polarity of a text document. In the simplest situation, we distinguish only between positive and negative sentiment, turning the task into a standard binary classification problem. Sentiment classification can be useful in business intelligence by quickly summarizing consumer sentiment as feedback for a particular product. Movie reviews are of great importance as they can help viewers get an overview of the movie and also give producers and directors feedback on their work based on the public's opinion. However, manually analyzing the sentiments in reviews becomes tedious due to the large amount of corpuses present in multiple movie review sites. In this project, we investigate various deep learning algorithms for sentiment classification and try to implement different ensemble models over three sequential models on the IMDb movie review dataset. The results of this research show that the ensemble models achieve higher accuracy than their base learners, the highest being 90.4 % on the IMDb dataset, which is on par with state-of-the-art research and our proposed model. These results demonstrate that ensemble learning methods can be used as a viable method for sentiment classification. Our results are easily reproducible, as we publish the code/notebooks of our experiment.

Keywords: Ensemble learning, IMDb dataset, machine learning, natural language processing, sentiment classification

13.1 Introduction

NLP, or natural language processing, is a significant area of artificial intelligence that studies how computer and human languages (including text and speech) interact [1].

Anomitro Das, Shayambhu Chaudhuri, Ashfaq Murshed, Rohini Basak, Department of Information Technology, Jadavpur University, Jadavpur University Salt Lake Campus, Plot No. 8, Salt Lake Bypass, LB Block, Sector III, Salt Lake City, Kolkata 700106, West Bengal, India, e-mails: anomitro02@gmail.com, shayambhuchaudhuri7@gmail.com, ashfaqmurshed.2024@gmail.com, visitrohinihere@gmail.com
Pawan Kumar Singh, Department of Information Technology, Jadavpur University, Jadavpur University Salt Lake Campus, Plot No. 8, Salt Lake Bypass, LB Block, Sector III, Salt Lake City, Kolkata 700106, West Bengal, India; and Shinawatra University, 99, Moo 10, Bang Toei, Sam Khok, Pathum Thani, Thailand, 12160, e-mail: pawansingh.ju@gmail.com, https://orcid.org/0000-0002-9598-7981

https://doi.org/10.1515/9783111504667-013

With the advent of social media, several NLP applications have emerged, one of which is sentiment analysis.

Sentiment analysis (shown in Figure 13.1) is the automated recognition and classification of sentiment in written text. Sentiment analysis has become an essential technique for understanding public sentiment in a variety of fields, including business and politics, due to the exponential expansion of social media and the greater availability of public ideas and feelings [2]. It is widely applied to reviews left by survey respondents, reviews posted on social media and in online forums, and product reviews left in online e-stores. Marketing, advertising, and social behavior analysis are among the fields that have employed sentiment analysis [3], and it could prove to be instrumental in the creation of AI-based bots or assistants [4].

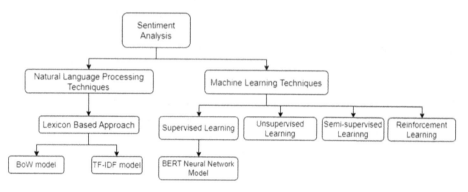

Figure 13.1: Various types of sentiment analysis [10].

Since the publication of Pang et al. [5], a number of improvements, strategies, and methodologies have been proposed for the sentiment analysis problem in a variety of applications and at different levels. Nevertheless, there is still no academic consensus on a unified approach to constructing an appropriate sentiment analysis model [6].

In terms of methodologies, sentiment analysis can be divided into two primary forms:
- Lexicon-based approach: This is an unsupervised method. The dictionary and corpus-based techniques are its two primary categories. The following are the general steps of this method. The text reviews are used to extract data. The retrieved data is then subjected to preprocessing procedures. Finally, a lexicon is applied to the processed data to determine the polarity of the document [7].
- Machine learning-based approach: Three different ML techniques are frequently used for SA: semi-supervised, unsupervised, and supervised. The availability of labeled data determines the strategy [8].

Some of the types of sentiment analysis based on usage are mentioned below:

- Fine-grained sentiment: When assessing sentiments, conventional categories such as positive, neutral, and negative are used. This includes rating "from 1 to 5" or "from 1 to 10".
- Emotion detection sentiment analysis: This is a more advanced approach for detecting feelings in text. This type of study can help identify and comprehend people's emotions, ranging from fear and anxiety to rage, despair, joy, and impatience.
- Aspect-based analysis: This type focuses primarily on a specific aspect of the service. Consider the following scenario: a company or organization that sells products or serves customers. Businesses may find it useful to automatically filter and analyze customer data with aspect-based sentiment analysis. Additionally, it can automate customer support tasks, resulting in insightful data [9].

13.1.1 Research goal

The primary objectives of the project can be stated as follows:
- Selecting, extracting, and executing data visualization to perform an exploratory study of the collected data.
- Dividing the data into sets for training, validation, and testing; then using and developing the selected algorithms after training the deep learning algorithms on the training data.
- Comparing the models on the test set using performance metrics such as accuracy, precision, recall, F1 scores, and the area under the accuracy and loss curves (described in Section 13.4.2).
- Performance metrics such as accuracy are considered while comparing the effectiveness of ensemble learning approaches such as majority voting, weighted averaging, and stacking with meta-learners (support vector machines and logistic regression) on the test set (see Section 13.4.3).

And then, based on the results of the evaluation, the most efficient algorithm is identified.

13.2 Related works

There have been several works based on sentiment analysis with varying degrees of success. The IMDB dataset has been widely used as a benchmark dataset for sentiment analysis classifiers. In this section, we will discuss some of the major works and publications in this field using this dataset.

Nasukawa et al. [11] provide a method for sentiment analysis to identify feelings in a document that are connected to positive or negative polarity for specific topics. The main challenge is to identify how sentiments are expressed in texts and whether these expressions indicate positive or negative opinions about the topic. To improve accuracy, it is essential to identify the semantic relationships between sentiment expressions and the subject. Using a syntactic parser and a sentiment lexicon in semantic analysis, their prototype system recognizes sentiments in news items and web pages with high accuracy (75–95 %, depending on the data). Reddy et al. [12] present a modified logistic regression technique for the classification and analysis of user reviews, a critical aspect of sentiment analysis. The study addresses the challenge of accurately determining the polarity of reviews—positive, negative, or neutral—expressed by different sentiments, ratings, and comments. Their proposed technique improves classification accuracy by using support count estimation and considering multiple independent words with similar meanings in parallel. Using a movie review dataset, their method achieves significant performance improvements, with classification accuracy, precision, recall, and f-measure at 90 %, 78.6 %, 75.6 %, and 76.5 %, respectively.

Sulthana et al. [13] investigate sentiment analysis in movie reviews using support vector machines (SVM) and ensemble learning approaches. The study classifies text data using machine learning and natural language processing techniques. The proposed approach consists of three main contributions: 1) applying a chi-square selector to select the k-best features, 2) using SVM for review classification with hyperparameters tuned via GridSearch, and 3) implementing a bagging algorithm with a base classifier over the SVM classifier. The number of base classifiers in the bagging algorithm is varied. Their results show that this technique outperforms previous systems in terms of classification accuracy and effectiveness, with an accuracy of 93 %. Parveen et al. [14] examined the supervised machine learning methods, with an emphasis on ensemble learning and voting algorithm approaches, for the sentiment categorization of movie reviews. The study used a total of 1000 files of two categories—positive and negative—of movie reviews obtained from community corpora. Numerous classifiers such as MultinomialNB, GaussianNB, and BernoulliNB are used in conjunction with a variety of classification techniques such as NaiveBayes, SkLearn, and Support Vector Machine. Different feature selection methods were employed to assess accuracy levels of the different algorithms. Ensemble learning is used to combine multiple classifiers, and a voting algorithm is implemented to determine the best accuracy, achieving an accuracy of 91 %. The study extends previous research by experimenting with various classifiers and feature selection techniques, providing insights into sentiment analysis in movie reviews. Sultana et al. [15] investigate ensemble learning based on meta-classifiers for sentiment categorization, aiming to extract emotional information from social media reviews. They highlight the importance of sentiment analysis in understanding customer opinions and satisfaction levels, especially in the era of big data from social networks. By integrating the meta-level characteristics of base classifiers with ensemble learning, the study explores the effectiveness of this combined approach. Seven supervised machine learning algorithms are selected for sentiment classification, including Naïve Bayes, Logistic Regression, SVM, SGD, KNN, and MLP. Ensemble techniques such as bagging, boosting, and stacking are used, with majority voting used for final sentiment prediction. The study focuses on binary sentiment classification (positive and negative) and presents experimental results to compare individual classifiers with the ensemble approach.

Mohammed et al. [16] present a detailed review of ensemble deep learning, highlighting the prospects and problems of the field. Ensemble learning, which integrates multiple base models, and deep learning, with its predictive accuracy, outperform traditional algorithms. While the success of ensemble methods depends on training and combining base models, deep learning requires expertise in optimizing hyperparameters. Recent research combines ensemble learning with deep learning to address this challenge, but mostly with simplistic methods. This review paper examines ensemble learning strategies, factors that influence their success, and research employing ensemble learning in various domains. Yenter et al. [17] propose several architectural variations to improve accuracy and minimize overfitting in sentiment analysis. They create five high-performing models by experimenting with different kernel sizes, network architectures, and regularization strategies. These models achieve over 89 % accuracy in predicting the polarity of IMDb reviews. Their best model outperforms previous models and significantly outperforms the baseline CNN+LSTM model. The combined kernel of the CNN-based LSTM architecture shows potential for other sentiment analysis or text classification tasks. Gupta et al. [18] propose an LSTM model with attention, 'Senti_ALSTM', which improves neural networks by assigning memory and mitigating the vanishing gradient problem in recurrent neural networks. Senti_ALSTM incorporates attention mechanisms to consider the input sequence information, thereby preserving the context and establishing the relationship between input and output sequences, achieving an accuracy of 87.32 %. Dang et al. [19] determine whether if hybrid models outperform single models in different domains and datasets. They create and evaluate hybrid sentiment analysis models by fusing support vector machines (SVM), convolutional neural networks (CNN), and long short-term memory (LSTM) networks on eight datasets of tweets and reviews. Compared to single models (SVM, LSTM, and CNN), hybrid models, especially those combining deep learning with SVM, show increased accuracy and significantly higher reliability with a record-breaking accuracy of 93.4 % on the IMDb dataset. Shiri et al. [20] conducted a comprehensive survey of deep learning models, such as Deep Reinforcement Learning (DRL), Deep Transfer Learning, Generative Models, Convolutional Neural Networks (CNNs), and Recurrent Neural Networks (RNNs). It examines the characteristics, applications, benefits, and limitations of each model. Additionally, the study contrasts the outcomes of three publicly accessible datasets—IMDb, ARAS, and Fruit-360—using six well-known deep learning models: CNN, Simple RNN, Long Short-Term Memory (LSTM), Bidirectional LSTM, Gated Recurrent Unit (GRU), and Bidirectional GRU. Singla et al. [21] employed a variety of models such as Naive Bayes, Logistic Regression, LSTM, LSVM, Decision Tree, and BiLSTM to conduct a sentiment analysis study on the IMDB dataset. The study evaluates the performance of these models in categorizing movie reviews as positive or negative, and examines the effects of data preprocessing and hyperparameter tuning on accuracy. In terms of recall, precision, and accuracy, the BiLSTM model outperforms the others, with LSTM, Logistic Regression, LSVM, Decision Tree, and Naive Bayes following close behind. The work highlights the importance of preprocessing methods and hyperparameter tuning, as well as the application of deep learning models, namely BiLSTM, in sentiment analysis.

13.2.1 Motivation

The motivation behind this thesis is twofold: to contribute to the academic understanding of deep learning applications in sentiment analysis and to provide a practical solution that can be implemented in real-world scenarios using various ensemble learning techniques.

In today's digital age, individuals frequently share movie reviews online, making it essential to understand, mine, and analyze this data. The explosive growth of big data requires the use of machine learning and deep learning models, as traditional models are unable to handle the amount of data collected.

The proposed advanced deep learning sentiment analysis model aims to address these challenges through novel architectural improvements and through the use of various ensemble techniques. This approach attempts to increase the accuracy of sentiment classification while remaining efficient in the face of the vast volume of textual material available on the internet.

13.3 Proposed methodology

13.3.1 Data collection

The IMDb dataset from kaggle.com is used for this study. It consists of 50,000 sequences, each labeled with binary labels for positive or negative. The preprocessing steps included tokenization, padding/truncation to a fixed length, and normalization.

This preprocessing ensured that the input data was in a suitable format for embedding layers and subsequent model training.

13.3.2 Feature engineering

Feature engineering was critical in transforming raw sequence data into formats suitable for machine learning models.

Embedding layers: Each input sequence has been transformed into dense vector representations using an embedding layer. This layer maps tokens in the sequences into high-dimensional space, capturing semantic similarities between words. For instance, words with similar meanings are placed closer together in this space. The embedding layer was initialized with random weights, which were then fine-tuned during the training process to capture the context-specific relationships in the data.

13.3.3 Model architectures

13.3.3.1 BiLSTM-CNN model

The BiLSTM-CNN model combines the strengths of both Bidirectional Long Short-Term Memory (BiLSTM) networks and CNNs to leverage both temporal and spatial features of the data.
- Embedding layer:
  - Input: The embedding layer takes as input of sequences of integers representing words in a vocabulary of size 10,000.
  - Output: It outputs dense vectors of a specified dimension (100), that capture the semantic meaning of the words.
- Bidirectional LSTM (BiLSTM):
  - The BiLSTM layer (shown in Fig. 13.2) processes the input sequence in both forward and backward directions, capturing long-range dependencies more effectively than a standard LSTM.
  - Parameters: It uses 128 units and incorporates a dropout rate of 0.3 for both the input and recurrent connections to prevent overfitting.

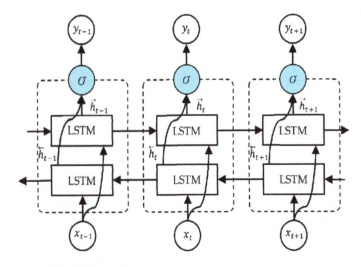

Figure 13.2: BiLSTM architecture.

Equation (13.1) explains the operations performed in BiLSTM units:

$$h_t = \sigma(w_1 x_t + w_2 h_{t-1}) \times \tanh(C_{t-1}),$$
$$h_t = \sigma(w_3 x_t + w_4 h'_{t+1}) \times \tanh(C'_{t+1}),$$
$$o_t = w_t h_t + w_t h'_t. \tag{13.1}$$

- Conv1D layer:
  - The Conv1D layer applies convolutional filters to the sequence of hidden states from the BiLSTM layer, capturing local temporal patterns in the data.
  - Parameters: It uses 128 filters, each with a kernel size of 3, and employs the ReLU activation function.
- Dropout layer:
  - Dropout is a regularization technique that helps prevent overfitting by randomly setting a number of input units to zero during each update cycle.
  - Parameter: This layer uses a dropout rate of 0.2.
- Batch normalization:
  - Batch normalization normalizes the input of each layer to improve the stability and performance of the training process.
- Second Conv1D and activation layers:
  - The model includes an additional Conv1D layer with 64 filters and a kernel size of 3, followed by a ReLU activation layer in order to further process the output of the previous convolutional layer.
- MaxPooling1D:
  - The max-pooling layer uses the largest value within a user-specified window to downsample the input representation, hence reducing the dimensionality of the feature maps.
  - Parameter: This layer uses a pooling size of 4.
- Flatten layer:
  - The flatten layer converts the 2D output of the Conv1D layers into a 1D feature vector and prepares it for the dense layers.
- Second dropout layer:
  - A second dropout layer with a dropout rate of 0.2 is used to further prevent overfitting.
- Dense layer:
  - A fixed-size vector is produced by the fully connected dense layer, and nonlinearity is added by passing the vector through a ReLU activation function.
  - Parameters: This layer contains 128 units.
- Output layer:
  - The final binary classification is obtained by passing the single unit that is produced by the final dense layer through a sigmoid activation function.
  - Parameter: This layer has 1 unit.
    The architecture of CNN-BiLSTM model used in our proposed work is shown in Fig. 13.3.

13 Performance comparison of different deep learning ensemble models — 233

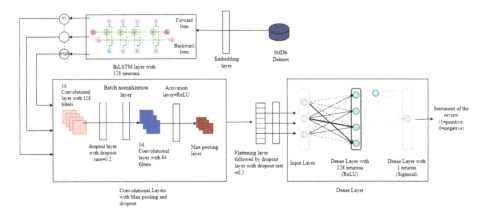

Figure 13.3: CNN-BiLSTM model architecture.

13.3.3.2 2D-CNN model

The custom 2D-CNN model (as shown in Fig. 13.4) is designed to capture spatial features from the input text data and make binary classifications for IMDb sentiment analysis. The following is a detailed description of the model architecture:

- Embedding layer:
  - Input: Sequences of integers representing words from a vocabulary size of 5,000.
  - Output: Dense vectors of dimension 200 to capture the semantic meaning of the words.
- Reshape layer:
  - The reshape layer transforms the 3D tensor output from the embedding layer into a 4D tensor, adding an extra dimension required for the 2D convolutional layers.
- Custom convolutional layer: The custom convolutional model performs convolutions and poolings with different filter sizes to capture different spatial features from the input sequences.
  - Input shape: (sequence_length, embedding_dimension, 1)
  - Number of filters: 200 filters for each convolution operation
  - Filter sizes: 2, 3, 4, and 5
  - Convolution and pooling operations:
    * The model applies four different convolution filters of varying sizes (2, 3, 4, and 5).
    * Each filter size captures different n-gram features from the input sequences.
    * Max-pooling is applied after each convolution to extract the most relevant features.

234 — A. Das et al.

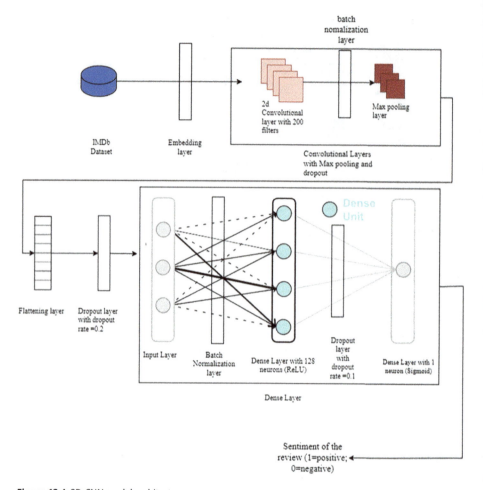

Figure 13.4: 2D-CNN model architecture.

- Concatenation:
  * The output feature maps from all convolutional operations are concatenated into a single feature vector.
- Dropout layer:
  - Dropout is used with a dropout rate of 0.2 and includes randomly changing some of the input units to zero during training in order to prevent overfitting.
- Flatten layer:
  - The flatten layer converts the 2D output of the convolutional layers into a 1D feature vector, setting it up for the fully connected dense layers.
- Fully connected dense layers:
  - Two dense layers of 8 and 1 units respectively are added after flattening the feature vector.

- ReLU activation functions are applied to introduce nonlinearity.
- In order to speed up and stabilize the training process, batch normalization is used.
- Output layer:
  - The final binary classification is obtained by passing the single unit that is produced by the final dense layer through a sigmoid activation function.

13.3.3.3 GRU-CNN model

The CNN-GRU model (as illustrated in Fig. 13.5) is designed to capture both spatial and temporal features from the input text data and make binary classifications for IMDb sentiment analysis. The following is a detailed explanation of the model architecture:
- Embedding layer:
  - Input: Sequences of integers representing words from a vocabulary size of 10,000.
  - Output: Dense vectors of dimension 200, which capture the semantic meaning of the words.
- Convolutional layers:
  - First Conv1D layer:
    * Filters: 128 filters
    * Kernel Size: 3
    * Activation: ReLU
    * Padding: Valid

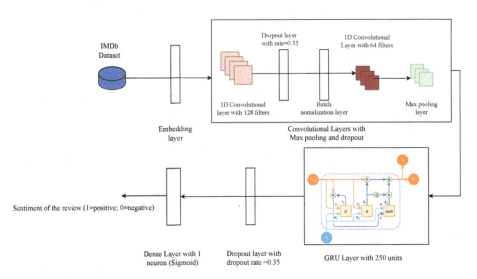

Figure 13.5: CNN-GRU model architecture.

* Purpose: to captures local spatial patterns in the input sequences.
 - Dropout layer:
   * Dropout is applied with a dropout rate of 0.35 to prevent overfitting by randomly setting a fraction of input units to zero during training.
 - Batch normalization layer:
   * Batch normalization normalizes the input of each layer to improve the stability and performance of the training process.
 - Second Conv1D Layer:
   * Filters: 64 filters
   * Kernel Size: 3
   * Activation: ReLU
   * Padding: Valid
 - MaxPooling Layer:
   * Pooling Size: 4
   * Purpose: Further captures spatial features and downsamples the input representation.
- GRU layer:
 - Description: The GRU layer processes the input sequences, effectively capturing sequential dependencies and long-range temporal patterns.
 - Units: 250 units
 - Dropout layer:
   * Description: Dropout is applied with a dropout rate of 0.35 to prevent overfitting.
- Dense classification layer:
 - Description: The final dense layer outputs a single unit, which is passed through a sigmoid activation function to produce the final binary classification.

13.3.4 Model training

Each model was trained using the Adam optimizer, which adapts the learning rate during training and is well suited for handling large datasets and models. The binary cross-entropy loss function was used for binary classification tasks. The dataset was divided into training and validation sets, with an 80-20 split. Early stopping was used to avoid overfitting, and training was stopped after a predetermined number of epochs when the validation performance did not improve.

13.3.5 Ensemble learning

Ensemble learning [22] is a powerful machine learning paradigm that has exhibited obvious advantages in many applications. An ensemble in the context of machine learning can be broadly defined as a machine learning system that is constructed from a set of individual models working in parallel, whose outputs are combined using a decision fusion technique to provide a single solution to a particular problem. The performance of an ensemble method depends on a number of factors, including the training and combination of the initial models.

Some of the methods we have employed are:

1. Majority voting: Majority voting (Fig. 13.6) trains a variety of machine learning models are trained on the same dataset, each using a unique set of techniques or approaches. When it comes time to predict, the final prediction is determined by the majority vote of each model [14].

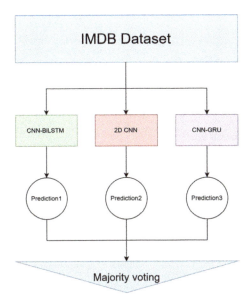

Final Prediction P=mode(Prediction1,Prediction2,Prediction3)

Figure 13.6: Majority voting algorithm.

2. Weighted averaging: In weighted averaging (Fig. 13.7), the base model with higher predictive power is more important. The sum of the weights would equal one [15].
3. Stacking: Combining different estimators to reduce their biases is known as stacking. The aggregated predictions from each estimator are input into the final estimator, which computes the final forecast and is also referred to as a meta-model. The final estimator is trained by cross-validation [16]. The two meta-models used were:
   a. Logistic regression: Logistic regression (Fig. 13.8) is a statistical model that estimates the probability of a discrete outcome given an input variable. The most common logistic regression models yield a binary outcome [12].

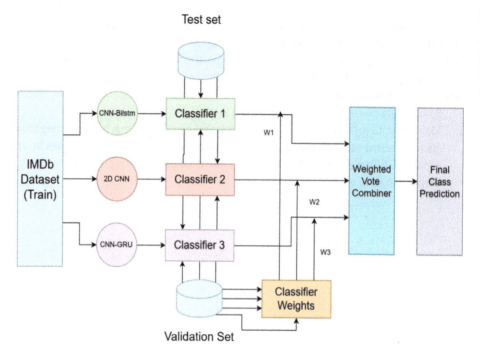

Figure 13.7: Weighted average algorithm.

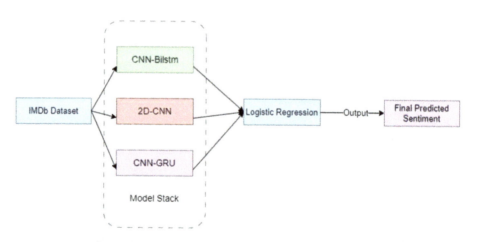

Figure 13.8: Stacking algorithm with logistic regression.

b. Support vector machine: Support vector machines (Fig. 13.9) are supervised maximum margin models with associated learning algorithms that analyze data for classification analysis [13].

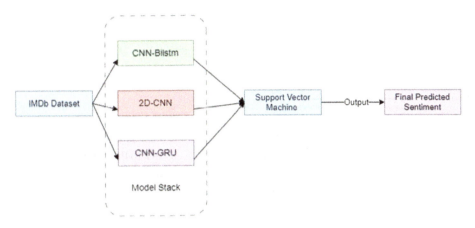

Figure 13.9: Stacking algorithm with support vector machine.

13.4 Results

13.4.1 Dataset used

The IMDB dataset (Fig. 13.10) was first introduced by Andrew Maas et al. in 2011 and used by a word vector learning model in the same paper. This dataset consists of 50,000 reviews scraped from the IMDB website, with at maximum of 30 reviews from each movie. The dataset is divided into equal halves for training and testing, and each half has an equal number of positive and negative reviews. Reviews with ratings below and equal to 4 stars are labeled as negative, and reviews with ratings equal to and above 7 stars are labeled as positive. Neutral reviews are excluded, making it suitable for binary sentiment classification [23]. The data used is legitimate and open to everyone. The IMDB

```
Positive Example:
    Although  this   was   obviously   a   low-budget
production, the performances and the songs in this
movie are worth seeing. One of Walken's few musical
roles to date. (he is a marvelous dancer and singer
and he demonstrates his acrobatic skills as well -
watch  for  the  cartwheel!)  Also  starring  Jason
Connery. A great children's story and very likable
characters.

Negative Example:
    Not only is it a disgustingly made low-budget
bad-acted   movie,  but   the   plot   itself  is  just
STUPID!!!
    A mystic man that eats women? (And by the looks,
not virgin ones)
    Ridiculous!!! If you've got nothing better to do
(like sleeping) you should watch this. Yeah right.
```

Figure 13.10: Example of positive and negative sentiments.

Table 13.1: Distribution of sentiments across training and validation sets.

Dataset Split	Positive	Negative
Training	12,500	12,500
Validation	12,500	12,500

dataset also ignores personally identifiable information, such as a person's name, age, or identity, i. e., a review from this dataset can't be traced back to the person who posted the review. Table 13.1 shows the distribution of the sentiments, taken from IMDB dataset, used for both the training and validation purposes.

13.4.2 Performance metrics

The evaluation metric used in this research work is accuracy. The parameters of accuracy are defined as follows:

- True positives (α) are the total number of reviews that are classified as positive but are actually positive.
- False positives (β) are all the reviews that are classified as negative but are actually positive.
- True negative (γ) refers to the total number of reviews that are classified as negative but aren't actually negative.
- False negative (δ) reviews are all the reviews that are marked as positive but are actually negative.

The ratio of accurately predicted reviews to the total number of reviews is used to determine accuracy:

$$\text{Accuracy} = \frac{\alpha + \gamma}{\alpha + \beta + \gamma + \delta}. \tag{13.2}$$

The ratio of reviews successfully predicted as positive to all reviews correctly predicted as positive is used to determine precision:

$$\text{Precision} = \frac{\alpha}{\alpha + \beta}. \tag{13.3}$$

The ratio of reviews that are accurately predicted to be positive reviews to all of the reviews in this class is used to compute recall:

$$\text{Recall} = \frac{\alpha}{\alpha + \gamma}. \tag{13.4}$$

The harmonic mean of recall and precision is used to determine the F1-score:

$$\text{F1-score} = \frac{2 \times \text{Precision} \times \text{Recall}}{\text{Precision} + \text{Recall}}. \tag{13.5}$$

When combined, these metrics provide a comprehensive evaluation of the effectiveness of the model, weighing the trade-off between recall and accuracy to produce the F1-score, which serves as a measure of overall effectiveness.

These metrics collectively provide a comprehensive evaluation of the model's performance, balancing the trade-off between precision and recall to give an overall measure of effectiveness through the F1-score.

13.4.3 Experiment results

In these experiments, we assessed the performance of three deep learning networks developed for the IMDb dataset: CNN-BiLSTM, 2D-CNN, and CNN-GRU.

We further enhanced our analysis by employing ensemble techniques. Specifically, we combined the predictions of these models using ensemble methods such as majority voting, weighted average, and stacking. For stacking, we used both Logistic Regression and Support Vector Machine (SVM) as meta-classifiers. These ensemble techniques allowed us to leverage the different strengths of each model, ultimately improving the overall predictive performance and robustness of our ensemble model.

We have used Google Colab's TPU v2 engine for training.

We will now present various metrics for our models, including accuracy vs. epoch, loss vs. epoch, precision, recall, F1-score, and testing accuracy. These metrics (given in Table 13.2) will provide insights into the effectiveness and performance of our models across different training epochs and evaluation criteria.

Table 13.2: Compilation of the different evaluation metrics of the basic deep learning models after individual training.

	Accuracy	Precision	F1-Score	Recall
BiLSTM-CNN	0.88164	0.87525	0.88264	0.89016
2D-CNN	0.88424	0.84415	0.89061	0.94248
CNN-GRU	0.89080	0.86537	0.89447	0.92560

13.4.3.1 Results of the BiLSTM-CNN model

The BiLSTM-CNN model was trained over 5 epochs, using 100-dimensional embeddings and a dropout rate of 0.2. This training configuration resulted in a validation loss of 0.2774 and a validation accuracy of 89.30 %. From Table 13.2 we can infer that this model has the highest precision among the three models, which is 0.87525, while the test accuracy, F1-score, and recall are 0.88164, 0.88264, and 0.89016 respectively. As shown in Fig. 13.11, both the training loss and the validation loss converge after 5 epochs. At the same time, in Fig. 13.12, both accuracies stop growing significantly. And the confusion

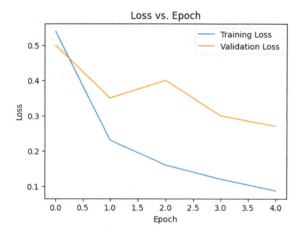

Figure 13.11: Loss vs. Epochs plot for the BiLSTM-CNN model with the number of embeddings set to 100 and the dropout rate set to 0.2.

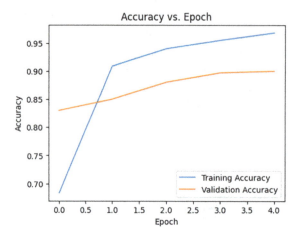

Figure 13.12: Accuracy vs. Epochs plot for the BiLSTM-CNN model.

matrix in Fig. 13.13 shows the number of true positives, true negatives, false positives and false negatives, where the positive class corresponds to a positive sentiment (1) and the negative class corresponds to a negative sentiment (0). In Fig. 13.13 we can see that 11127 out of 12500 positive test cases and 10914 out of 12500 negative test cases were correctly predicted.

13.4.3.2 Results of the 2D CNN model

The 2D CNN model was trained with an embedding dimension of 200 and a dropout rate of 0.2 across 10 epochs. With this arrangement, the validation accuracy was 88.46 % and

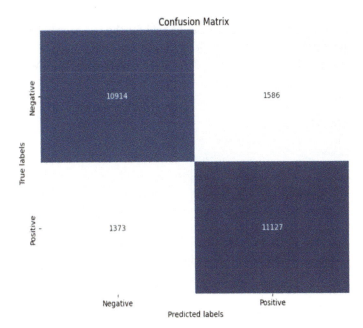

Figure 13.13: Confusion matrix for the BiLSTM-CNN model.

the validation loss was 0.3153. The model produced an F1-score of 0.89061, a recall of 0.94258, a precision of 0.84415 and a test accuracy of 0.88424. Table 13.2 shows that this model has the highest recall among the three models. In addition the test accuracy was reported to be 88.24 %. As depicted in Fig. 13.14, both the training loss and the valida-

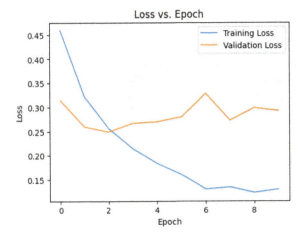

Figure 13.14: Loss vs. Epoch plot for the 2D CNN model with the number of embeddings set to 200 and the dropout rate set to 0.2.

tion loss converge after 10 epochs. And the same can be said for the two accuracies in Fig. 13.15. The confusion matrix for this model is shown in Fig. 13.16. In Fig. 13.16, a total of 11781 out of 12500 positive test cases 10325 out of the 12500 negative test cases were predicted correctly.

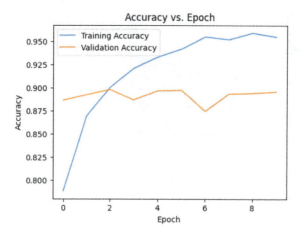

Figure 13.15: Accuracy vs. Epoch plot for the 2D CNN model.

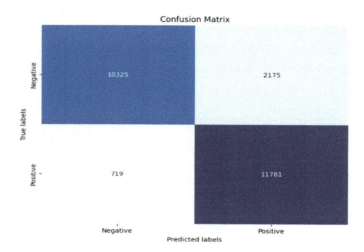

Figure 13.16: Confusion matrix plot for the 2D CNN model.

13.4.3.3 Results of the CNN-GRU model

The CNN-GRU model was trained over 5 epochs with 200-dimensional embeddings and a dropout rate of 0.35. With this training setup, a validation accuracy of 89.10 % and a validation loss of 0.2754 were obtained. The model obtained a recall of 0.92560, and a precision of 0.86537 in terms of performance measures. Compared to the other models in Table 13.2, the F1-score and the test accuracy were the highest at 0.89447 and 0.89080 respectively. As depicted in Fig. 13.17 and Fig. 13.18, both the losses and both the accuracies converge after 5 epochs. The confusion matrix is shown in Fig. 13.19. In Fig. 13.19,

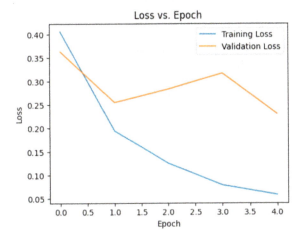

Figure 13.17: Loss vs. Epoch plot for the CNN-GRU model with the number of embeddings set to 200 and the dropout rate set to 0.35.

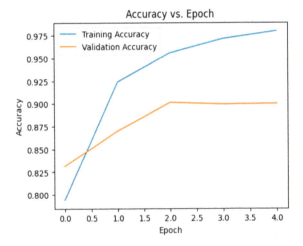

Figure 13.18: Accuracy vs. Epoch plot for the CNN-GRU model.

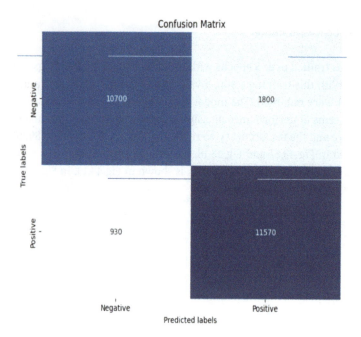

Figure 13.19: Confusion Matrix for the CNN-GRU model.

a total of 11570 out of 12500 positive test cases 10700 out of the 12500 negative test cases were predicted correctly.

13.4.3.4 Results of ensemble methods

Our previous model, using a bagging ensemble of 5 basic learners with 2 BiLSTM layers, 1 CNN layer, and 0.5 dropout rate, yielded a test accuracy of 87 %. We have mentioned the test accuracies achieved for each of the ensembles we have worked on in Table 13.2. Our current weighted average ensemble of 3 base learners has improved upon this, achieving an accuracy of 90.6 %, showing a 3.6 % improvement over the bagging ensemble and an improvement of at least 1.5 % over the base models (Table 13.3). The test accuracies of the researched ensemble techniques have been recorded in Table 13.3. The ensemble models are on par with the several prominent current research efforts, as observed in Table 13.4.

13.4.4 Comparison with previous works

In the following table (Table 13.4), we have compiled the previously noted works done on the IMDB dataset, each with different methodologies in various fields, such as machine learning, deep neural networks, transformers, etc. The current benchmark is achieved

Table 13.3: Ensemble techniques and their test accuracies.

Ensemble techniques	Test Accuracy
Weighted Average	**90.6 %**
Majority Voting	90.4 %
Stacking with Logistic Regression	89.9 %
Stacking with SVM	87.6 %
Bagging Ensemble	87 %

Table 13.4: Comparison with previous works on the IMDB dataset.

References	Year	Method	Task	Accuracy (%)
Ding et al. [24]	2021	ALBERT	Sentence level Sentiment Classification	89.05
Tan et al. [25]	2022	RoBERTa-LSTM Transformer and Recurrent Neural Network	Sentiment Classification	92.96
Uysal and Murphey [26]	2017	CNN, LSTM, CNN+LSTM	Document-level Sentiment Classification	89.1
Zulqarnain et al. [27]	2021	Enhanced Gated Recurrent Unit with Auto-Encoder	Solving Text Classification Problems	90.8
Wankhade et al. [28]	2022	CBVoSD: context-based vectors over sentiment domain	Ensemble model for review classification	89.4
Ahmad et al. [29]	2019	To measure the performance of SVM using the grid-search technique	Pre-processing (TF-IDF, Stop words, Stemming, words to keep, n-gram tokenizing)	87.2
Cen et al. [30]	2020	CNN	Sentiment Analysis	88.22
Das et al.	**2024**	**Weighted Average of three deep learning models**	**Sentiment Analysis**	**90.6**

by Tan et al. in 2022 with their transformer and recurrent neural network based model 'ROBERTA-LSTM' which reaches an accuracy of 92.96 % and thereby outperforming our model by some margin, with a much larger training time period.

13.5 Conclusion & future works

13.5.1 Conclusion

In conclusion, our study evaluated the performance of three deep learning models—CNN-BiLSTM, 2D CNN, and CNN-GRU—on the IMDb dataset. Leveraging ensemble techniques including weighted average, majority voting, and stacking with logistic regression and SVM meta-classifiers, we combined the strengths of individual models, resulting in enhanced predictive performance and robustness.

Notably, majority voting came in second at 90.4 %, with the weighted average ensemble achieving the best test accuracy at 90.6 %. The accuracy of stacking with SVM was significantly lower at 87.6 % than that of stacking using logistic regression, which achieved an accuracy of 89.9 %. These results highlight the effectiveness of ensemble techniques are in improving model performance.

Our investigation, carried out on the Colab TPU v2 engine, indicates potential ways to optimize of sentiment analysis tasks, as shown by the various metrics—accuracy, precision, recall, and F1 score—between various models and ensemble approaches. Our work not only sheds light on model performance, but also emphasizes the trade-offs between training efficiency and accuracy.

Although our ensemble approach does not reach the state-of-the-art performance levels of transformer-based models, it has notable advantages. Although our ensemble method may not match the peak performance achieved by transformers, it significantly reduces training time while still achieving respectable levels of accuracy.

13.5.2 Future works

13.5.2.1 Architecture exploration

The next step is to test future neural network architectures (e. g., attention-based ones). Attention mechanisms could improve performance and sentiment prediction by focusing the model on the most relevant sections of the input data.

13.5.2.2 Data augmentation

We intend to use data augmentation techniques to artificially expand our dataset, which will help improve generalization. That is, these can involve techniques such as synonym replacement, back translation, and noise injection, all of which can contribute to a more diversified training set, leading to reduced overfitting.

13.5.2.3 Model interpretability

Planning to add interpretability to our sentiment analysis model to increase the interpretability of our sentiment analysis models, we would like to apply some interpretability approaches such as SHAP (SHapley Additive exPlanations) and LIME (Local Interpretable Model-agnostic Explanations). Using these strategies, we will be able to gain insight into the model's decision-making process by determining which characteristics have the most influence on the sentiment forecasts.

13.5.2.4 Novel neural network architectures

We will explore new, custom neural network architectures (or hybrid models) that we have not worked with on before that could perform better. This means either trying out new combinations of existing models, or developing a model based on an entirely new architecture that is closer to the characteristics of sentiment analysis.

13.5.2.5 Cross-lingual sentiment analysis

Another interesting direction is to combine of our work with cross-lingual sentiment analysis. By fine-tuning our models on multilingual datasets, we will make our models language-independent, enabling sentiment analysis across multiple languages, thus extending the application of our models in the diversity of linguistic environments.

Bibliography

[1] Zulqarnain, M., Ghazali, R., Aamir, M., et al. (2024). An efficient two-state GRU based on feature attention mechanism for sentiment analysis. Multimed. Tools Appl., 83, 3085–3110. https://doi.org/10.1007/s11042-022-13339-4.
[2] Tan, K. L., Lee, C. P. & Lim, K. M. (2023). A survey of sentiment analysis: approaches, datasets, and future research. Appl. Sci., 13, 4550. https://doi.org/10.3390/app13074550.
[3] Hung, L. & Alias, S. (2023). Beyond sentiment analysis: a review of recent trends in text-based sentiment analysis and emotion detection. J. Adv. Comput. Intell. Intell. Inform., 27, 84–95. https://doi.org/10.20965/jaciii.2023.p0084.
[4] Harikrishnan, H. & Varadarajan, V. (2022). Sentiment analysis on movie reviews dataset using support vector machines and ensemble learning. Int. J. Inf. Technol. Web Eng., 17, 1–23. https://doi.org/10.4018/IJITWE.311428.
[5] Pang, B., Lee, L. & Vaithyanathan, S. (2002). Thumbs up? Sentiment classification using machine learning techniques. In Proceedings of the 2002 Conference on Empirical Methods in Natural Language Processing (EMNLP 2002) (pp. 79–86). Association for Computational Linguistics.
[6] Bordoloi, M. & Biswas, S. K. (2023). Sentiment analysis: a survey on design framework, applications and future scopes. Artif. Intell. Rev., 56, 12505–12560. https://doi.org/10.1007/s10462-023-10442-2.
[7] Hota, H. S., Sharma, D. K. & Verma, N. Lexicon-based sentiment analysis using Twitter data: a case of COVID-19 outbreak in India and abroad. Data Sci. COVID-19, 2021, 275–295. https://doi.org/10.1016/B978-0-12-824536-1.00015-0. Epub 2021 May 21. PMCID: PMC8989068.
[8] Ahmad, M., Aftab, S., Shah Muhammad, S. & Ahmad, S. (2017). Machine learning techniques for sentiment analysis: a review. Int. J. Multidiscip. Sci. Eng., 8(3), 27.
[9] Zhu, L., Xu, M., Bao, Y., Xu, Y. & Kong, X. (2022). Deep learning for aspect-based sentiment analysis: a review. PeerJ Comput. Sci., 8, e1044. https://doi.org/10.7717/peerj-cs.1044. PMID: 36092006; PMCID: PMC9454971.
[10] Karak, G., Mishra, S., Bandyopadhyay, A., Rohith, P. R. S. & Rathore, H. (2022). Sentiment analysis of IMDb movie reviews: a comparative analysis of feature selection and feature extraction techniques. In A. Abraham et al. (Eds.), Hybrid Intelligent Systems. HIS 2021. Lecture Notes in Networks and Systems (Vol. 420). Cham: Springer. https://doi.org/10.1007/978-3-030-96305-7_27.

[11] Nasukawa, T. & Yi, J. (2003). Sentiment analysis: capturing favorability using natural language processing. In Proceedings of the 2nd international conference on Knowledge capture (K-CAP '03) (pp. 70–77). New York, NY, USA: Association for Computing Machinery. https://doi.org/10.1145/945645.945658.
[12] Reddy, R. & Kumar, U. M. (2023). Classification of user's review using modified logistic regression technique. Int. J. Syst. Assur. Eng. Manag., https://doi.org/10.1007/s13198-022-01711-4.
[13] Harikrishnan, H. & Varadarajan, V. (2022). Sentiment analysis on movie reviews dataset using support vector machines and ensemble learning. Int. J. Inf. Technol. Web Eng., 17, 1–23 https://doi.org/10.4018/IJITWE.311428.
[14] Parveen, R., Shrivastava, N. & Tripathi, P. (2020). Sentiment classification of movie reviews by supervised machine learning approaches using ensemble learning & voted algorithm. In 2nd International Conference on Data, Engineering and Applications (IDEA), Bhopal, India (pp. 1–6). https://doi.org/10.1109/IDEA49133.2020.9170684.
[15] Sultana, N. & Islam, M. (2020). Meta classifier-based ensemble learning for sentiment classification. https://doi.org/10.1007/978-981-13-7564-4_7.
[16] Mohammed, A. & Kora, R. (2023). A comprehensive review on ensemble deep learning: opportunities and challenges. J. King Saud Univ, Comput. Inf. Sci., 35(2), 757–774. 2023, ISSN 1319-1578. https://doi.org/10.1016/j.jksuci.2023.01.014.
[17] Yenter, A. & Verma, A. (2017). Deep CNN-LSTM with combined kernels from multiple branches for IMDb review sentiment analysis. In 2017 IEEE 8th Annual Ubiquitous Computing, Electronics and Mobile Communication Conference (UEMCON) (pp. 540–546).
[18] Gupta, C., Chawla, G., Rawlley, K., Bisht, K. & Sharma, M. (2021). Senti_ALSTM: sentiment analysis of movie reviews using attention-based-LSTM. In A. Abraham, O. Castillo and D. Virmani (Eds.), Proceedings of 3rd International Conference on Computing Informatics and Networks. Lecture Notes in Networks and Systems (Vol. 167). Singapore: Springer. https://doi.org/10.1007/978-981-15-9712-1_18.
[19] Dang, C. N., Moreno-García, M. N. & De la Prieta, F. (2021). Hybrid deep learning models for sentiment analysis. Complexity, 2021, Article ID 9986920, 16 pages, 2021. https://doi.org/10.1155/2021/9986920.
[20] Shiri, F. M., et al. (2023). A comprehensive overview and comparative analysis on deep learning models: CNN, RNN, LSTM, GRU. arXiv preprint arXiv:2305.17473.
[21] Singh, S. K. & Singla, N. (2023). Sentiment analysis on IMDB review dataset. Journal of Computers, Mechanical and Management.
[22] Huang, F., Xie, G. & Xiao, R. (2009). Research on ensemble learning. In 2009 International Conference on Artificial Intelligence and Computational Intelligence, Shanghai, China (pp. 249–252). https://doi.org/10.1109/AICI.2009.235.
[23] Maas, A. L., Daly, R. E., Pham, P. T., Huang, D., Ng, A. Y. & Potts, C. (2011). Learning word vectors for sentiment analysis. In Proceedings of the 49th Annual Meeting of the Association for Computational Linguistics: Human Language Technologies (pp. 142–150). Portland, Oregon, USA: Association for Computational Linguistics.
[24] Ding, Z., Qi, Y. & Lin, D. (2021). Albert-based sentiment analysis of movie review. In 2021 4th International Conference on Advanced Electronic Materials, Computers and Software Engineering (AEMCSE), Changsha, China (pp. 1243–1246).
[25] Tan, K. L., Lee, C. P., Anbananthen, K. S. M. & Lim, K. M. (2022). RoBERTa-LSTM: a hybrid model for sentiment analysis with transformer and recurrent neural network. IEEE Access, 10, 21517–21525. 2022. https://doi.org/10.1109/ACCESS.2022.3152828.
[26] Uysal, A. K. & Murphey, Y. L. (2017). Sentiment classification: feature selection based approaches versus deep learning. In 2017 IEEE International Conference on Computer and Information Technology (CIT) (pp. 23–30). IEEE.
[27] Zulqarnain, M., Alsaedi, A. K. Z., Sheikh, R., et al. (2024). An improved gated recurrent unit based on auto encoder for sentiment analysis. Int. J. Inf. Technol., 16, 587–599. https://doi.org/10.1007/s41870-023-01600-4.

[28] Wankhade, M., Rao, A. C. S. & Kulkarni, C. (2022). A survey on sentiment analysis methods, applications, and challenges. Artif. Intell. Rev., 55, 5731–5780.
[29] Badr, E. M., Salam, M. A., Ali, M. & Ahmed, H. (2019). Social media sentiment analysis using machine learning and optimization techniques. Int. J. Comput. Appl., 975, 8887.
[30] Cen, P., Zhang, K. & Zheng, D. (2020). Sentiment analysis using deep learning approach. J. Artif. Intell., 2, 17–27. https://doi.org/10.32604/jai.2020.010132.

Aarya Vilas Karanjawane, Suresh Jagtap, Anupam Mukherjee, and Varsha Umesh Ghate

14 Elevating standards in homoeopathic medicine: chemometric standardization of medicinal plant for quality assurance

Abstract: In the field of homeopathy, maintaining the quality and consistency of medicinal plants is fundamental to ensuring effective treatment outcomes. However, the inherent variability among these plants poses a significant challenge to quality assurance efforts. Chemometric standardization offers a promising solution, using statistical and mathematical methods to enhance data accuracy and refine analytical processes. This comprehensive approach includes preprocessing techniques, calibration methods, and validation procedures, all directed towards improving product quality and safety. By adopting chemometric standardization, homeopathic practitioners can effectively address issues such as ensuring batch-to-batch consistency, authenticating botanicals, and detecting potential adulterants. Consequently, this strategy strengthens the reliability of medicinal products and gives patients greater confidence regarding the efficacy of homeopathic treatments. Moreover, the use of chemometric standardization facilitates compliance with regulatory requirements, further enhancing patient safety and trust. The establishment of standardized protocols and guidelines requires collaborative effort between academia, industry, and regulatory bodies. By working together,

---

Acknowledgement: The authors are grateful to the authorities of Bharati Vidyapeeth (Deemed to be University) Pune, India. Authors are thankful to Prof. Dr. Avinash R. Mhetre, I/C Principal, BV (DTU) HMC, Pune and Prof. Dr. Anita S. Patil, Dean, (FoH). The authors also extend sincere thanks to the Directorate of Homoeopathy, Department of Health and Family Welfare, Government of West Bengal.

Author contributions: AK: Conceptualization; Writing original draft; Visualization. SJ: Conceptualization; Methodology; Validation; Formal analysis; Writing review & editing. AM: Conceptualization; Methodology; Validation; Formal analysis; Writing review & editing. VUG: Conceptualization; Methodology; Validation; Writing original draft; Visualization.

Conflict of interest: Nil.

Financial support: Nil.

Aarya Vilas Karanjawane, Varsha Umesh Ghate, Department of Homoeopathic Pharmacy, Bharati Vidyapeeth (Deemed to be University), Homoeopathic Medical College & Post Graduate Research Centre, Hospital, Pune 411043, India, e-mails: aarya.karanjawane@bharatividyapeeth.edu, varshaghate29@gmail.com
Suresh Jagtap, Department of Herbal Medicine, Interactive Research School for Health Affairs (IRSHA), Bharati Vidyapeeth (Deemed to be University), Pune 411043, India, e-mail: suresh.jagtap@bharatividyapeeth.edu
Anupam Mukherjee, Department of Health and Family Welfare, West Bengal Homoeopathic Health Service Government of West Bengal, Kolkata 700091, India, e-mail: anupam.dr.98@gmail.com

https://doi.org/10.1515/9783111504667-014

stakeholders can ensure consistent implementation of chemometric standardization practices, ultimately enhancing the credibility and efficacy of homeopathic medicinal products. In essence, the adoption of chemometric standardization represents a pivotal step toward improving product quality, regulatory compliance, and overall patient well-being within the field of homeopathy.

Keywords: Homeopathy, chemometric standardization, analytical techniques, quality assurance, medicinal plants

14.1 Introduction

Homeopathy, founded by Dr. C. F. Samuel Hahnemann in 1796, uses remedies derived from various sources including plants, animals, and minerals [1]. While medicinal plants are crucial in both traditional and homeopathic medicine due to their abundant phytoconstituents [2], ensuring the quality and consistency of these remedies remains a challenge due to their inherent variability [3]. Chemometric standardization, using mathematical and statistical methods, has emerged as a solution for quality assurance in medicinal plants [4]. Using analytical techniques such as chromatography and spectroscopy, chemometrics helps to characterize chemical profiles, identify bioactive compounds, and detect contaminants [5]. Despite its growing application in herbal medicine [6], there is a gap in the use of chemometric standardization for quality assurance of homeopathic medicinal plants [7], which requires further research to establish standardized protocols and guidelines. The authors sought to elucidate the concept of chemometric standardization and its potential significance in ensuring the quality assurance of medicinal plants used in homeopathy.

14.2 Origin and development of chemometrics

Chemical science is known by the term 'Chemometrics,' which was first used by the Swedish scientist Svante Wold in 1971 [8]. Combining mathematics, statistics, and formal logic, chemometrics offers theories and techniques for measuring chemicals as well as new methods for analyzing various types of spectroscopic and chemical measurement data. Additionally, chemometrics can be used in chemistry to maximize relevant chemical information and optimize experimental protocols [9, 10]. Since the early 20th century, chemometrics has developed rapidly. Chemometrics has been driven by two factors: (1) the abundance of data generated by today's multi-element and multi-component equipment, from which chemometric techniques must be applied to extract critical information; and (2) the widespread use of computers, which enable the processing of complex data [11, 12]. In the twenty-first century, chemometrics represents a significant advancement in the software development of analytical instruments [13, 14, 15]. In addition to providing new concepts and techniques for building innovative, multidimensional, and hyphenated equipment, it promotes the intellectualization of equipment. Expert systems, artificial neural networks, high-dimensional data analysis, artificial intelligence in chemistry, and research on microcomputers have all advanced significantly along with the rapid growth of microcomputers, which have enabled the creation and retrieval of chemical spectrum libraries. Chemical chemometrics is developing rapidly along with analytical chemistry [16, 17].

14.3 Chemometric standardization

Chemometric standardization in analytical chemistry plays a crucial role in improving data accuracy by addressing instrument discrepancies, experimental variables, and sample matrix effects. This approach employs sophisticated statistical techniques to enhance precision and comprehensibility, making it invaluable to researchers in a variety of disciplines. In the context of homeopathy, where remedies are frequently derived from highly diluted plant extracts, chemometric standardization becomes even more critical. By applying chemometric techniques to analyze the chemical composition of medicinal plants, homeopaths can ensure the consistency and potency of their remedies, thereby enhancing their quality and efficacy. (See Figure 14.1 for the key components of chemometric standardization.)

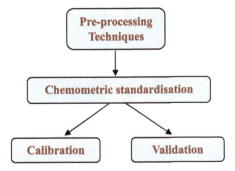

Figure 14.1: Key components of chemometric standardization.

14.4 Details of the key components of chemometric standardization

1. *Preprocessing Techniques*: Preprocessing techniques refine data quality and improve statistical model performance by removing undesired variation, enhancing relevant information, and rectifying systematic errors, tailored to data characteristics and analysis objectives.

2. *Calibration Methods*: Calibration methods train instruments for accurate results by creating mathematical models from known samples, establishing relationships between measured signals and analyte concentrations, and enabling precise quantification.
3. *Validation*: Validation verifies model reliability, accuracy, and robustness by assessing performance with new or unseen data, ensuring trustworthy results.

14.5 Steps involved in chemometric standardization

By following the steps mentioned below (Fig. 14.2), chemometric standardization aims to minimize variation in data and ensure consistent and accurate results across different instruments and laboratories. This is particularly important in fields such as spectroscopy, chromatography, and other analytical techniques where standardization increases the reliability and comparability of measurements.

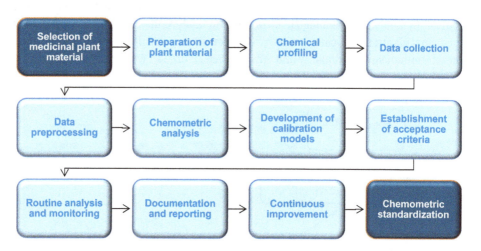

Figure 14.2: Steps involved in chemometric standardization.

14.6 Uses of chemometric standardization

Chemometric standardization is valuable in homeopathy, because it ensures the quality and consistency of herbal remedies. It precisely identifies and quantifies active ingredients, aiding in the selection of extraction methods and dilution ratios. It also detects contaminants, ensuring high quality ingredients. Chemometric analysis accounts for natural plant variability, helping to develop standardized protocols for sourcing and processing. This approach helps meet regulatory requirements and enhances the credibility of homeopathy. In conclusion, chemometric standardization is essential to raising the standards of homeopathic medicine by ensuring quality, safety, and efficacy.

14.7 Application of chemometrics in medicinal plants (Mps)

1. *Authenticity*: An important first step in assessing the efficacy of a drug prepared from a plant source is authenticity verification. There are a few unique components to every medicinal plant. As a result, by examining the components, particularly the respective chemical ratios, it is possible to identify medicinal plants and distinguish them from imitations.
2. *Efficacy and consistency*: The chemical components and concentrations of herbal remedies have a direct bearing on their efficacy. The degree of consistency might fluctuate depending on factors such as climate, harvesting season, cultivation methods, and storage techniques. Small variations in fingerprint concentrations may have an impact on the quality of the medicinal plant, but smaller variations between species can be used to distinguish between them when analyzing the recorded fingerprints. Fingerprints from medicinal plants can be used to effectively classify and discriminate using Principal Component Analysis (PCA), Successive Signal Correction (SSC), and Linear Discriminant Analysis (LDA) [18].

14.8 Prospects

The impact of chemometrics in the field of medicinal plants is widely acknowledged. It plays a crucial role in refining experimental techniques, extracting valuable insights from chromatographic data, and separating mixtures into linear components. While chemometrics is recognized as a valuable tool for assessing the quality of herbal drugs (HDs), [19, 20] it's important to note that standardization of the chromatographic fingerprint of HDs may not always provide a comprehensive representation of all compounds. Despite the existence of numerous monographs for herbal quality evaluation in certain countries, there is still a need for a universally valid standard to ensure accurate scientific quality assessment [21].

14.9 Closing Statement

In conclusion, chemometric standardization offers a scientifically based method to ensure the quality and consistency of medicinal plants in homeopathy. By integrating this approach from raw material analysis to final product quality control, manufacturers can meet regulatory standards, enhance efficacy, and ensure patient safety. Further research and collaboration between academia, industry, and regulatory bodies are essential to establish universal protocols. Embracing chemometric standardization enhances the credibility of homeopathic medicinal products and ensures reliable therapeutic outcomes for patients worldwide.

Bibliography

[1] Ghosh, A. K. (2018). History of development of homoeopathy in India. Indian J. Hist. Sci., 53(1), 76–83.
[2] Shankar, P. R., Kumar, K., Shankar, S. R. & Rao, R. K. S. (2011). Quality control methods for herbal materials. In Herbal Technologies.
[3] Kumar, S., Yadav, A., Yadav, M., et al. (2017). Effect of climate change on phytochemical diversity, total phenolic content and in vitro antioxidant activity of Aloe vera (L.) Burm.f. BMC Res. Notes, 10, 60.
[4] Dwivedi, V. & Chauhan, A. (2021). Chemometric tools for quality control of herbal medicines: a review. J. Pharm. Anal., 11(2), 111–124.
[5] Wang, J., van der Heijden, R., Verpoorte, R. & van der Greef, J. (2007). Quality control of herbal material and phytopharmaceuticals with MS and NMR based metabolic fingerprinting. Planta Med., 73(7), 681–694.
[6] Mishra, P., Kumar, A. & Nagireddy, A. (2014). Application of chemometrics in quality control and standardization of traditional medicine and dietary supplements. Phytochem. Rev., 13(2), 321–331.
[7] Marzotto, M., Bonafini, C., Olioso, D., Baruzzi, A., Bettinetti, L. & Di Leva, F. (2020). Protocol for the quality control of homeopathic medicines: the Italian model. Homeopathy, 109(4), 213–220.
[8] Wold, S. & Sjöström, M. (1998). Chemometrics present and future success. Chemom. Intell. Lab. Syst., 44, 3–14.
[9] Jurgen, W. E. (2004). Chemometrics in analytical chemistry. Anal. Bioanal. Chem., 380, 368–369.
[10] Kateman, G. (1983). Meeting reports: International conference on Chemometrics in Analytical Chemistry. Trends Anal. Chem., 2(3), 11–12.
[11] Yu, R. Q. (1991). Introduction of Chemometrics. Hunan Educ Press.
[12] Daniel, K. W. & Mok, C. F. T. (2006). Chemical information of Chinese medicines: a challenge to chemist. Chemom. Intell. Lab. Syst., 26, 210–217.
[13] Li, Y. J. & Zhu, L. (2005). Initial study on the way of chemometrics into our country. J. Xinchang Agric. Coll., 19, 87–89.
[14] Wu, H. L., Liang, Y. Z. & Yu, R. Q. (1991) Analytical chemometrics. Anal. Lab., 18, 94–100.
[15] Liang, Y. Z. & Yu, R. Q. (1991). The development of chemometrics in China. Chemistry, 10, 14–18.
[16] Yu, R. Q. (1992). Chemometrics in China. Chemom. Intell. Lab. Syst., 14, 23–39.
[17] Wold, S. (1991). Chemometrics, why, what and where to next? J. Pharm. Biomed. Anal., 9, 589–596.
[18] Liang, K. X., Wu, H. & Su, W. (2014). A Rapid UPLC-PAD fingerprint analysis of Chrysanthemum morifolium ramat combined with chemometrics methods. Food Anal. Method., 7, 197–204.
[19] Gad, L. H. A., El-Ahmady, S. H., Abou-Shoer, M. I., et al. (2013). Application of chemometrics in authentication of herbal medicines: a review. Phytochem. Anal., 24(1), 1–24.
[20] Tistaert, M. C., Dejaegher, B. & Heyden, Y. V. (2011). Chromatographic separation techniques and data handling methods for herbal fingerprints: a review. Anal. Chim. Acta, 690, 148–161.
[21] Springfield, N. E., Eagles, P. & Scott, G. (2005). Quality assessment of South African herbal medicines by means of HPLC fingerprinting. J. Ethnopharmacol., 101, 75–83.

Varsha Umesh Ghate, Ajay G. Namdeo, Abhay Harsulkar,
Anupam Mukherjee, Yashwant Chavan, Suresh Jagtap, Devasis Pradhan,
and Mehdi Gheisari

15 Evaluation of genetic diversity in *Rauvolfia* species using Random Amplification of Polymorphic DNA (RAPD) technique

Abstract: Background: *Rauvolfia serpentina* (L.) Benth. ex Kurz is one of the threatened medicinal plants. Owing to demand and scarcity, *R. serpentina* roots are adulterated or substituted with other Rauvolfia species, but in homoeopathy only *Rauvolfia serpentina* species are used to prepare mother tincture or dilutions.
Methods: For identification and discrimination based on genetic information among *R. serpentina*, *R. densiflora*, *R. tetraphylla*, *R. vomitoria*, and *R. micrantha*, DNA fingerprints were developed with RAPD analysis using 12 random primers by standard protocol. Genetic polymorphism was quantified by generating a similarity matrix based on the presence or absence of polymorphic bands.
Results: The obtained dendrogram represents the genetic relationships among the samples. As per the analysis, *R. serpentina* and *R. densiflora* are most closely related species; whereas *R. tetraphyla* and *R. vomitoria* have maximum genetic distance indicating their distant phylogenetic relation.
Conclusion: These findings emphasize importance of RAPD analysis in identifying genetic differences among various *Rauvolfia* species. Furthermore, DNA fingerprinting

---

Varsha Umesh Ghate, Department of Homoeopathic Pharmacy, Bharati Vidyapeeth (Deemed to be University), Homoeopathic Medical College & Post Graduate Research Centre, Hospital, Pune 411043, India, e-mail: varshaghate29@gmail.com
Ajay G. Namdeo, Department of Pharmaceutical Sciences, HNB Garhwal Central University, Srinagar 246174, Uttarakhand, India, e-mail: ajay.namdeo@bharatividyapeeth.edu
Abhay Harsulkar, Department of Pharmaceutical Biotechnology, Bharati Vidyapeeth (Deemed to be University), Poona College of Pharmacy, Pune 411038, India, e-mail: abhay.harsulkar@bharatividyapeeth.edu
Anupam Mukherjee, Department of Health and Family Welfare, West Bengal Homoeopathic Health Service, Government of West Bengal, Kolkatta 711104, India, e-mail: anupam.dr.98@gmail.com
Yashwant Chavan, R & D Department, geneOmbio Technologies Pvt Ltd, Vedant, Sr. No. 39/3, Yogi Park, Baner, Pune 411045, India, e-mail: yashvant.chavan@geneombiotechnologies.com
Suresh Jagtap, Department of Medicinal Plant Medicine, Bharati Vidyapeeth (Deemed to be University), Interactive Research School for Health Affairs (IRSHA), Pune 411043, India, e-mail: suresh.jagtap@bharatividyapeeth.edu
Devasis Pradhan, Department of Electronics & Communication Engineering, Acharya Institute of Technology, Bangalore 560107, Karnataka, India, e-mail: devasispradhan@acharya.ac.in
Mehdi Gheisari, Department of Cognitive Computing, Institute of Computer Science and Engineering, Saveetha School of Engineering, Saveetha Institute of Medical and Technical Sciences, Chennai 602105, India, e-mail: mehdi.ghesari61@gmail.com

https://doi.org/10.1515/9783111504667-015

can holds the potential in supporting the pharmaceutical and nutraceutical industries by facilitating standardization and quality evaluation of medicinal plants.

Keywords: *Rauvolfia* species, DNA fingerprinting, genetic diversity, RAPD PCR, quality control

15.1 Introduction

Homeopathic medicines are prepared from various natural sources. Most of these are prepared from one or more parts of the plant, even some that are poisonous and carnivorous. Therefore, medicinal plants represent a significant reservoir of bioactive natural compounds that hold great importance for the pharmaceutical sector. The secondary metabolites present in medicinal plants serve as essential components of complementary and alternative therapies. Ensuring the quality of these medicines is crucial not only for their clinical outcomes but also for the medicinal plant industry and traditional medicinal systems that rely on these industries. The evaluation of medicinal plant quality should commence from the moment raw materials are acquired, rather than solely at the end of the production process [1]. This proactive approach to quality assessment is vital to guarantee the safety and efficacy of medicinal plants. Rigorous quality control measures are applied to medicinal plants and their preparations to ensure adherence to predefined standards. The quality control procedures involve regular assessments of the identity, purity, and content of characteristic compounds within medicinal plants. In homeopathic prescriptions, the dilution is dependent on the quantity of compounds

---

Acknowledgement: The authors are grateful to authorities of Bharati Vidyapeeth (Deemed to be University), Pune, India for providing financial assistance for this research work. The authors are also grateful to Prof. Dr. Avinash R. Mhetre, I/C Principal; Prof. Dr. Anita S. Patil, Dean – Faculty of Homeopathy and PG-Coordinator, Bharati Vidyapeeth (Deemed to be University) Homeopathic Medical College, Pune and Prof. Dr. Pramod Kumar Singh, Principal, Dr. M. P. K. Homeopathic Medical College, Hospital & Research Centre for this unmatched support and guidance to improve this article. The authors also extend sincere thanks to the Directorate of Homeopathy, Department of Health and Family Welfare, Government of West Bengal for the constant support.

Author contribution: VUG: Conceptualization; Methodology; Design; Writing original draft; Visualization; Resources; Project administration. AN: Methodology; Design; Validation; Software; Formal analysis; Writing an original draft. AH: Methodology; Validation; Software; Formal analysis; Writing review & editing. AM: Conceptualization; Methodology; Validation; Formal analysis; Writing review & editing. YC: Methodology; Writing review & editing; Visualization; Resources. SJ: Conceptualization; Methodology; Validation; Formal analysis; Writing review & editing.

Funding: Financial Support for this research work has been received from the Bharati Vidyapeeth (Deemed to be University), Pune, India.

Conflict of interest (if any): "None to declare".

Ethics approval: "None to declare".

present in medicinal plants. Furthermore, a specific botanical name of the plant is mentioned in the Homeopathic Pharmacopeia. These evaluations are performed to verify that the medicinal plant meets established quality criteria. By conducting thorough quality control checks, the medicinal plant industry can maintain the integrity and reliability of its products, thereby ensuring the safety and effectiveness of medicinal plants for consumers [2, 3].

Fingerprinting is the most precise and reliable approach for determining the quality of medicinal plants because it is independent of plant stage or season. DNA fingerprinting has developed into an incredibly significant tool for genotype identification in both wild and cultivated plant species [4]. The World Health Organization has authorized DNA fingerprint analysis as a preferred technique for ensuring the quality of medicinal plant samples [5]. DNA fingerprinting, a gold standard technique, is especially helpful for the authenticity of medicinal plants, particularly to identify botanical species that are closely similar to one another. This technique is also useful in monitoring adulteration, regulating the extraction process, or assessing the quality of a finished product [6]. RAPD, RFLP, and AFLP, as well as SSR sequencing of the rDNA-ITS region, are all important methods for DNA bar-coding and DNA fingerprinting [7]. *Rauvolfia serpentina* is one of the essential threatened medicinal plants native to South Asia, known as Indian Snake-root or Sarpagandha. This is a woody shrub belonging to the Apocynaceae family [8]. More than 250 alkaloids, notably *Reserpine* and *Rescinnamine* are the important active components in the roots of *R. serpentina*. Due to its therapeutic uses, it is a well-known plant in both AYUSH and Western medical systems [9]. But, the critically endangered species list includes *Rauvolfia serpentina* [10].

Owing to high demand and scarcity, *Rauvolfia serpentina* roots are commonly adulterated or substituted with other *Rauvolfia* species [11]. However in homeopathy only *Rauvolfia serpentina* species is used to prepare mother tinctures or dilutions. Thus, using the Random Amplification of Polymorphic DNA (RAPD) technique, the current study was carried out to assess genetic diversity in a selected group of five *Rauvolfia* species, including *R. serpentina, R. densiflora, R. tetraphylla, R. vomitoria,* and *R. micrantha*.

15.2 Experiment

15.2.1 Material and methods

15.2.1.1 Plant material

Rauvolfia species including *R. serpentina, R. densiflora, R. tetraphylla, R. vomitoria,* and *R. micrantha* were used in the present investigation. Dried root powder samples of exploitable size from a minimum of three-year-old plants were collected from Natural Remedies Pvt. Ltd., Bengaluru, Karnataka.

15.2.1.2 Genomic DNA isolation

Genomic DNA was extracted from harvested root samples of these *Rauvolfia* species by adopting the procedure outlined by Dellaporta et al. (1983) with minor modifications [12]. Approximately 20 mg dry plant material was homogenized using a mortar pestle and liquid nitrogen. The resulting powdered samples were immediately transferred to a new microcentrifuge tube, and 400 µL Plant Lysis Buffer was added. The buffer was composed of 100 mM Tris-HCl (pH 8.0), 25 mM EDTA (pH 8.0), 1.5 M NaCl, 2 % CTAB, 0.2 % β-mercapto ethanol (v/v) and 1 % PVP (w/v) and mixed well to form a slurry and incubated at 65 °C for 60 minutes.

Before centrifugation at 12,000 rpm for 12 minutes at room temperature, an equal volume of chloroform: isoamyl alcohol (24: 1 v/v) was added to the extract. After 30 minutes of incubation at room temperature, an equal volume of isopropanol and half an equal volume of 5 M NaCl were added to the supernatant, followed by centrifugation (Effendorf Centrifuge 5804R) at 12,000 rpm for 12 minutes. The resulting pellet was centrifuged at 12,000 rpm for 12 minutes while being cleaned with 70 % ethanol.

The dried DNA pellet was dissolved in Tris-EDTA (TE) buffer. Three microliters of *RNase* A (10 mg/ml) were added, and the mixture was incubated for 1 hour at 37 °C. Thereafter, chloroform: isoamyl alcohol (24:1) was used twice to extract the DNA pellet, and the mixture was centrifuged at 12,000 rpm for 10 minutes at room temperature. Cold absolute ethanol was added to the aqueous phase, and DNA was separated as a pellet by centrifuging at 12,000 rpm for 10 minutes, followed by two washes in 70 % ethanol. The DNA was then air-dried and dissolved in 100 µL of TE buffer. Using a UV-2600 spectrophotometer (LT-291 Labtronics), five aliquots of genomic DNA from five plants were quantified by measuring absorbance at 260 nm. Stock DNA was diluted to make a working solution of 10 ng/µl for RAPD-PCR analysis.

15.2.1.3 RAPD PCR

Unlike normal PCR which uses two primers, RAPD only uses one primer with an arbitrary sequence. Therefore, amplification in the RAPD process occurs anywhere along a genome that contains two complementary sequences to the primer which are within the length limits of PCR (~3 kb). These protocols work well for random 10-mers. Each RAPD PCR reaction contained 5 µL of diluted genomic DNA (~50 ng), 1X PCR buffer, 2.5 mM $MgCl_2$, 0.1 mM of each dNTP 0.2 mM of RAPD primer, and 1 Unit of *Taq DNA Polymerase* (Thermo Fisher Scientific). The final volume of each reaction was 25.0 µL adjusted using nuclease-free water. The reaction mix was prepared for all samples and added into 200 µL PCR tubes. Genomic DNA was added later to each tube. Agarose gel electrophoresis of the RAPD products was performed using 1.5 % (w/v) agarose gel using standard 0.5X TBE gel electrophoresis buffer. The DNA molecules were resolved at 5 V/cm until the tracking dye migrated two-thirds of the distance through the gel. Bands were detected under a UV transilluminator. Gel images were recorded using the BIO-RAD GelDoc-XR gel documentation system.

15.2.1.4 Data analysis

For RAPD analysis, amplified products were graded according to whether each primer's band was present (assigned a value of 1) or not (assigned a value of 0). Only distinct and unambiguous bands were scored when evaluating the banding patterns of each primer. Based on the amplified bands' migration in relation to a molecular size marker (a DNA ladder ranging from 100 bp to 3 Kb, ExcelBand, SMOBIO), the size of the amplified bands was calculated in nucleotide base pairs (bp). Discrete variables were used to enter the data into a binary data matrix. The Unweighted Pair Group Method with Arithmetic Mean (UPGMA) was used to calculate Jaccard's coefficient of similarity and create a dendrogram based on the similarity coefficients. Cluster analysis was performed using the software NTSYSpc version 2.2 (Exeter Software, Setauket, NY, USA).

15.2.1.5 RAPD primers used in this study

Table 15.1: RAPD primers.

S. No.	Primer name	Nucleotide sequence (5'-3')
1	OPA08	GTGACGTAGG
2	OPA10	GTGATCGCAG
3	OPB12	CCTTGACGCA
4	OPB10	CTGCTGGGAC
5	OPM05	GGGAACGTGT
6	OPA04	AATCGGGCTG
7	OPA11	CAATCGCCGT
8	OPA07	GAAACGGGTG
9	OPM06	CTGGGCAACT
10	OPX07	GAGCGAGGCT

15.3 Results and discussion

15.3.1 RAPD

The RAPD analysis was performed for five samples using ten different random primers (refer Table 15.1). The agarose gel electrophoresis image shows considerable polymorphism among all five samples (Figure 15.1). In all ten primers, the profiles of DNA frag-

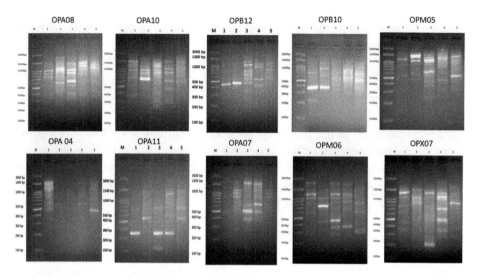

Figure 15.1: Agarose Gel electrophoresis of RAPD PCR for *R. serpentina*, *R. densiflora*, *R. tetraphylla*, *R. vomitoria*, *R. micrantha*. Lane M: 100 bp + 3 k DNA Ladder; Lane 1: *R. serpentina*; Lane 2: *R. densiflora*; Lane 3: *R. tetraphylla*; Lane 4: *R. vomitoria*; Lane 5: *R. micrantha*.

ments found for all the samples were not identical. With these primers, DNA fragment length polymorphisms were observed with few similar-sized fragments. The higher-intensity bands may be due to the amplification of repetitive DNA sequences, the influence of neighboring sequences on hybridization to the target sequence, or fewer mismatches to the target sequence. In contrast, the lower-intensity bands may have been generated inefficiently because of a higher degree of mismatch between the primer and the target sequence [13]. 5 µL of 100 bp + 3 k DNA Ladder (Excel Band, SMOBIO) was loaded in one lane for confirmation of the size of the amplicon using a reference ladder.

15.3.2 Similarity matrix

RAPD data were converted to binary data in the form of '0' wherever no bands were seen and '1' wherever a band was observed for scoring of RAPD bands. This data was further converted to sequence format for the construction of the dendrogram. The number of base substitutions per site in the samples was studied. Analyses were conducted using the Maximum Composite Likelihood model [14]. This analysis involved five nucleotide sequences. All ambiguous positions were removed for each sequence pair (pairwise deletion option). There were a total of 710 positions in the final dataset. Evolutionary analyses were conducted in MEGA11 [15]. Primer OPB12 showed higher polymorphism (65 %) whereas primer OPA07 showed the lowest polymorphism (51.52 %) among all the primers (refer Table 15.2). All the primers showed high degree of polymorphism which provides crucial information about genetic variability among the five samples studied.

Table 15.2: Percentage of polymorphism based on RAPD fragments.

Sr. No.	Primer	Total bands	Polymorphic bands	% polymorphism
1	OPA08	46	29	63.04
2	OPA10	48	25	52.08
3	OPB12	47	25	53.19
4	OPB10	20	13	65.00
5	OPM05	44	24	54.55
6	OPA04	27	16	59.26
7	OPA11	34	20	58.82
8	OPA07	33	17	51.52
9	OPM06	44	24	54.55
10	OPX07	52	27	51.92

15.3.3 Distance matrix analysis

It shows that the *R. serpentina* and *R. densiflora* are the most closely related, whereas *R. serpentina* and *R. micrantha* exhibit the highest genetic distance based on RAPD polymorphism (Table 15.3).

Table 15.3: Distance matrix analysis.

Sr. No.	Rauvolfia species	R. serpentina	R. densiflora	R. tetraphylla	R. vomitoria	R. micrantha
1	R. serpentina	0.000	0.141	0.165	0.241	0.208
2	R. densiflora	0.141	0.000	0.194	0.226	0.221
3	R. tetraphylla	0.165	0.194	0.000	0.272	0.225
4	R. vomitoria	0.241	0.226	0.272	0.000	0.142
5	R. micrantha	0.208	0.221	0.225	0.142	0.000

15.3.4 Dendrogram

The following dendrogram was drawn using MEGA11 software. Briefly, all the RAPD bands were scored in binary format. Data from all primers was used for the construction of the UPGMA tree [16]. The UPGMA tree also shows clear differentiation among all the species as different branches with variable bootstrap values are formed for each species. A Neighbor-Joining phylogenetic tree constructed using RAPD data obtained from all five *Rauvolfia* species (Figure 15.2).

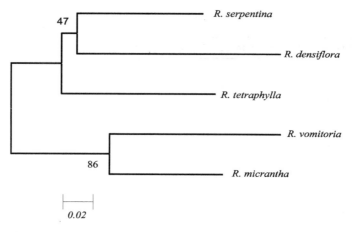

Figure 15.2: Dendrogram analysis.

15.3.5 RAPD data

The evolutionary history was inferred using the Neighbor-Joining method [17]. The percentage of replicate trees in which the associated taxa clustered together in the bootstrap test (500 replicates) is shown next to the branches [18]. The tree is drawn to scale, with branch lengths in the same units as those of the evolutionary distances used to infer the phylogenetic tree. The evolutionary distances were computed using the Maximum Composite Likelihood method [19] and are expressed in units of the number of base substitutions per site. This analysis involved 10 nucleotide sequences. All ambiguous positions were removed for each sequence pair (pairwise deletion option). There were a total of 710 positions in the final dataset. Evolutionary analyses were conducted using MEGA11 [20].

To establish effective plant conservation strategies, it is crucial to recognize and characterize variations within and among plant species. In the case of several medicinally significant plants, a combination of morphological and molecular indicators has proven to be valuable markers for evaluating genetic diversity [21]. In the present study, the possibility of adulteration with respect to genetic diversity in *Rauvolfia* species was assessed using Random Amplified Polymorphic DNA (RAPD) analysis [22]. Previous research and pharmaceutical applications have mainly focused on *R. serpentina*, while other *Rauvolfia* species are used or supplied as adulterants or substitutes in preparations involving *Rauvolfia serpentina* [22]. Therefore, the current study aimed to investigate the genetic diversity in various *Rauvolfia* species, including *R. serpentina, R. densiflora, R. tetraphylla, R. vomitoria,* and *R. micrantha*. DNA fingerprints were developed for these species to facilitate genetic analysis and aid in the establishment of conservation strategies. The results of the genetic analysis revealed significant genetic diversity among the analyzed samples based on RAPD patterns using different primers.

Out of the ten primers used in the study, all generated polymorphic bands, with no two primers producing identical band profiles. In total, the primers produced 60 intervals of different-sized fragments and a total of 404 DNA fragments. Each sample exhibited two bands consistently across all primers. The dendrogram analysis indicated genetic polymorphism among all the samples, providing evidence for differentiation among the plant species. According to the analysis it is evident that *R. serpentina* and *R. densiflora* are the most closely related species; whereas *R. tetraphyla* and *R. vomitoria* have the maximum genetic distance indicating their distant phylogenetic relationship. Therefore, the major polymorphic bands obtained through RAPD analysis hold utility for distinguishing between these *Rauvolfia* species. The findings of this study contribute to the understanding of genetic diversity in *Rauvolfia* species from Maharashtra and can aid in the formulation of conservation strategies for these plants.

15.4 Conclusions

The research findings emphasize the importance of utilizing RAPD analysis in identifying the genetic differences among various *Rauvolfia* species. According to the analysis, *R. serpentina* and *R. densiflora* are most closely related species; whereas *R. tetraphyla* and *R. vomitoria* have maximum genetic distance indicating their distant phylogenetic relationship. The RAPD primers used in this study can also be used for the discrimination of other species, as these show excellent polymorphism in the studied samples. Furthermore, DNA fingerprinting holds the potential in supporting the pharmaceutical and nutraceutical industries by facilitating standardization and quality evaluation of medicinal plants.

Bibliography

[1] Murugesan, L., Shanmugaramasamy, K. & Kaliappan, I. (2023). A Systematic review of analytical methods for quantification of natural indole alkaloids from *Catharanthus* and *Rauvolfia* species. Res. J. Pharmacogn., 10(1), 57–66. https://doi.org/10.22127/rjp.2022.359342.1970.
[2] Choi, D. W., Kim, J. H., Cho, S. Y., Kim, D. H. & Chang, S. Y. (2002). Regulation ad quality control of medicinal plant drugs in Korea. Toxicology, 181–182: 581–586.
[3] Minocha, S. (2017). Short review on DNA-fingerprinting and standardization of medicinal plant drugs. Int. J. Med. Biomed. Stud., 1(2), 1–9.
[4] Nybom, H., Weising, K. & Rotter, B. (2014). DNA fingerprinting in botany: past, present, future. Invest. Genet., 5(1), 1–35.
[5] Kumar, S. & Mishra, S. (2020). Recent Advances in Molecular Biology and Plant Physiology. New Delhi: AkiNik publication.
[6] Rohela, G. K., Bylla, P., Pendli, S., Rajender, K., Dharavath, B. & Thammidala, C. R. (2018). ISSR marker-based DNA profiling studies in *Rauwolfia* species. Ann. Plant Sci., 7(5), 2289–2295.

[7] Ahmad, W., Muhammad, K., Hussain, A., et al. (2017). DNA fingerprinting of essential commercialized medicinal plants from Pakistan. Am. J. Plant Sci., 08(09), 2119–2132.
[8] Kumar, S., Kumari, D. & Genus, S. B. (2022). *Rauvolfia*: a review of its ethnopharmacology, phytochemistry, quality control/quality assurance, pharmacological activities and clinical evidence. J. Ethnopharmacol., 295, 115357.
[9] Sulaiman, C. T., Jyothi, C. K., Unnithan, J. K., Prabhukumar, K. M. & Balachandran, I. (2020). Identification of suitable substitute for Sarpagandha (*Rauvolfia serpentina* (L.) Benth. ex Kurz) by phytochemical and pharmacological evaluation. Beni-Suef Univ. J. Basic Appl. Sci., 9, 1–11.
[10] Varnika, V., Sharma, R., Singh, A., Shalini, S. & Sharma, N. (2020). Micropropagation and screening of phytocompounds present among in vitro raised and wild plants of *Rauvolfia serpentine*. Walailak J. Sci. Technol., 17(11), 1177–1193.
[11] Bindu, S., Rameshkumar, K. B., Kumar, B., Singh, A. & Anilkumar, C. (2014). Distribution of reserpine in *Rauvolfia* species from India – HPTLC and LC–MS studies. Ind. Crop. Prod., 62, 430–436.
[12] Dellaporta, S. L., Wood, J. & Hicks, J. B. (1983). A plant DNA minipreparation version II. Plant Mol. Biol. Report., 1, 19–22.
[13] Semagn, K., Bjornstad, Å., Skinnes, H., Marøy, A. G., Tarkegne, Y. & William, M. (2006). Distribution of DArT, AFLP, and SSR markers in a genetic linkage map of a doubled-haploid hexaploid wheat population. Genome, 49(5), 545–555.
[14] Kumar, S. & Gadagkar, S. R. (2000). Efficiency of the neighbor-joining method in reconstructing deep and shallow evolutionary relationships in large phylogenies. J. Mol. Evol., 51(6), 544–553.
[15] Tamura, K., Stecher, G. & Kumar, S. (2021). MEGA11: Molecular evolutionary genetics analysis version 11. Mol. Biol. Evol., 38(7), 3022–3027.
[16] Iruela, M., Rubio, J., Cubero, J. I., Gil, J. & Millán, T. (2002). Phylogenetic analysis in the genus *Cicer* and cultivated chickpea using RAPD and ISSR markers. Theor. Appl. Genet., 104(4), 643–651.
[17] Saitou, N. & Nei, M. (1987). The neighbor-joining method: a new method for reconstructing phylogenetic trees. Mol. Biol. Eval., 4(4), 406–425.
[18] Felsenstein, J. (1985). Confidence limits on Phylogenies: an approach using the bootstrap. Evolution, 39(4), 783–791.
[19] Tamura, K., Nei, M. & Kumar, S. (2004). Prospects for inferring very large phylogenies by using the neighbor-joining method. Proc. Nat. Acad. Sci., 101(30), 11030–11035.
[20] Tamura, K., Stecher, G. & Kumar, S. (2021). MEGA11: Molecular evolutionary genetics analysis version 11. Mol. Biol. Evol., 38(7), 3022–3027.
[21] Mahesh, R., Kumar, N. & Sujin, R. (2008). Molecular analysis in *Rauvolfia tetraphylla* L. using RAPD markers. Ethnobot. Leafl., 12, 1129–1136.
[22] Nair, V. D., Raj, R. P. D., Panneerselvam, R. & Gopi, R. (2014). Assessment of diversity among populations of *Rauvolfia serpentina* Benth. Ex. Kurtz. from Southern Western Ghats of India, based on chemical profiling, horticultural traits, and RAPD analysis. Fitoterapia, 92, 46–60.

Index

ablation study 174
accuracy 154–156, 167, 169, 171–173, 176–179
activity recognition 153
Adam optimizer 167, 168
ADASYN 159
Advanced Life Support 185, 188
advances in molecular biology 12
analytical techniques 254
ant colony optimization (ACO) 81
artificial intelligence (AI) 45, 47, 48, 71, 77, 184, 185, 187, 188
artificial intelligence in chemistry 255
aspect-based analysis 227
Atomwise's Ebola drug discovery 11, 14, 23
attention-based 153
AUC scores 169
automatic sleep staging 153

Basic Life Support 185, 188
batch normalization 232, 236
batch size 168
Bidirectional Long Short-Term Memory 231
Bidirectional LSTM 229, 231
bioinformatics 124
bioinformatics in drug discovery 12
biomedical data mining 127
biomedical image classification 153
blockchain technology 71, 80, 86, 88
breast cancer 110
breast cancer classification 109
Brood parasitism 134
Brownian Motion Search Algorithm 109

cancer analysis 153
cancer classification 128
Cardiovascular Risk Prediction 79
Caregiver Scheduling 81
challenges in machine learning implementation 21
chemometric standardization 253–258
chemotherapy optimization 79
chromatography 254, 256
class imbalance 154, 159, 172
classification 239
classification accuracy 121, 142, 228
clinical trials 11, 12, 24
clustering Techniques 78
CNN 59, 64

https://doi.org/10.1515/9783111504667-016

collaboration in ML-driven drug discovery 21
compound screening and prioritization 20
comprehensive evaluation 117
computational chemistry 14, 19, 25
Concatenation 234
confusion matrix 119, 143, 168–171, 173, 174, 243–245
Constraint Programming (CP) 81
convolutional neural networks 229
Cuckoo Search algorithm 128
curse of dimensionality 128

data accuracy 253, 255
data analysis in drug development 19
data analytics 61, 63
data augmentation 21
data availability and quality in drug discovery 21
data integration 83
data integration and standards 21
de novo drug design 11, 13, 18, 19, 22, 23, 25
Decision Tree 27, 28, 36, 77, 100
Decision Tree algorithm 100
deep learning (DL) 59, 61, 64, 66, 78, 88, 153
deep learning algorithms 225, 227
DeepMind's AlphaFold for protein folding 11
DeepSleepNet 155
dense layer 232, 234–236
detection 249
diabetes management 71, 79, 84
diagnosis of complex diseases 146
dimensionality reduction 128
disease management 71, 72, 74, 77, 78, 88
DNA fingerprinting 259–261, 267
dropout 231, 232, 234, 236, 241, 245, 246
dropout layers 167
Drug Adherence Monitoring 78
drug discovery 72, 77, 78
drug discovery and development 11, 13, 15

ECG 156
EEG 152–156
electronic health records 60
embedding 230, 231, 233, 235, 241–243, 245
embedding_dimension 233
Emerging AI Technologies 88
EMG 152, 156
emotion detection 227

ensemble 155, 179, 227–229, 233
ensemble learning techniques 147
ensemble models 225
entropy 210, 211
entropy concept 210
EOG 152, 156
epoch 152, 167–169, 236, 241, 242, 244, 245
ethical concerns in ML 21
European Data Format (EDF) 157
evaluation metric 167
Expanded Sleep-EDF 176, 177
explainable AI 11, 21, 22, 24
extremely randomized tree 128

F1-score 155, 156, 167, 176, 240, 241, 243, 245, 248
false negative 167
false positive 167
FDA Adverse Event Reporting System (FAERS) 41, 43
feature engineering 230
feature selection (FS) techniques 110
feature selection 128, 153
fine-grained sentiment 227
flatten 232, 234
FNN 154
Food and Drug Administration (FDA) 41, 48
future of ML in drug development 24

gene expression data 127
gene selection 109
General Data Protection Regulation (GDPR) 48
genetic diversity 260, 261, 266, 267
genomics 71, 78, 87, 88
global adoption 74
Gramian Angular Field (GAF) images 179
green logistics 71
gated recurrent unit (GRU) 153, 155, 162, 164, 167, 174, 176, 178, 179, 229

Health Insurance Portability and Accountability Act (HIPAA) 48
healthcare 59–68
healthcare systems 68
high-dimensional data 110
high-throughput screening technologies 17
home healthcare (HHC) 71, 83, 85, 88
homeopathy 253, 254, 256–258
homoeopathy 259
hybrid algorithms 83
hybrid approach to gene selection 128

hyperparameter 228–230
hypnograms 157
HySleep_Net 153, 156, 164, 167–169, 174, 176–179
HySleep_Net model 153

IITNet 154
Intensive Care Unit 185, 188
interpretable AI 124
interval analysis 210, 212
Inventory Management 81
ISRUC 153, 156, 159, 162, 168, 173, 174, 176, 178

kappa statistics 154
k-means clustering 78
K-Nearest Neighbor (KNN) 98, 127
K-Nearest Neighbor algorithm 98

language 250

lead compound discovery 12
Learning-Rate 168
Leave-One-Out Cross-Validation 117
Lévy flight 134
lexicon 226, 228, 249
ligand-based virtual screening 17
linear regression 127
logistic regression (LR) 27, 28, 35, 36, 101, 227–230, 237, 238, 241, 247
long short-term memory 229
LSTM networks 153, 162, 163

machine learning (ML) 27, 29–32, 34, 38, 41–43, 45–47, 49–54, 184, 185, 187, 188, 199, 204
machine learning in drug discovery 19, 21, 22
manual feature extraction 154, 156
max-pooling 232, 233
MaxPooling 232, 236
medicinal plants 253–255, 257, 259–261, 267
MedWheels 183–185, 199, 202, 203
metaheuristics 81
microarray datasets 116
Mixed-Integer Linear Programming (MILP) 80
model complexity 116
models 231
multi-omics integration 124
MVF-SleepNet 155

Naïve Bayes 102
National Heart-Lung-Blood Institute 159
natural 225, 249

natural catastrophes 209
natural language processing (NLP) 88, 225, 228
network 247
neural networks 78, 88
normalization 235
NREM 1 152, 171–174
NREM 2 152, 171–174
NREM 3 152, 171, 173

operations research 71, 80, 83
optimization 71–73, 80–82, 88
optimization algorithm 110, 149
Optimizing Drug Dosages 78
overfitting 229, 231, 232, 234, 236, 248
oversampling 157–159

Particle Swarm Optimization (PSO) 81
performance 154, 155, 162, 167–169, 173, 176–179
personalized medicine 125, 147
pharmacophore model 16
pharmacophore modeling 15
phylogenetic analysis 259, 266, 267
PhysioNet 157
PNN 154
polymorphism 259, 263–265, 267
precision-recall curve 144, 120
precision 176, 229, 240, 241, 243, 245, 248
predictive analytics 61–63, 65–68, 71, 72, 77–80, 83–85, 87, 88
predictive modeling 147
Principal Component Analysis (PCA) 257
prognostic and predictive modeling 147
proposed hybrid BMSA-SVM 117
PSG 154–157, 159, 160, 166, 178, 179

quality assurance 253, 254
quality control 260, 261
quantitative structure-activity relationship (QSAR) 14, 15, 20, 25

Radial Basis Function 116
Random Forest 27–29, 36, 77, 99
random forest classifier 139, 156
RAPD PCR 260, 262
Rauvolfia species 259–262, 265–267
real time tracking 198, 199, 202
recall 167, 176, 228, 229, 240, 241, 243, 245, 248
Receiver Operating Characteristic (ROC) 145, 169, 171, 173, 174

Receiver Operating Characteristic (ROC) curve 120
recommendation systems 66
recurrent neural network 247
recurrent neural networks (RNNs) 78, 93, 229
redundancy and irrelevant genes 109
regression 248, 250
regression models 77
regulatory compliance in drug discovery 21
ReLU 166, 168
REM 152, 173, 174
remote monitoring 71, 72, 85
rescue management 207, 208
rescue model 210, 215
reshape 233
RNN 59, 66
robustness of feature selection 129
ROC curves 145

scikit-learn 162
screening and prioritization 20
semantic similarities 230
sensitivity analysis 216, 217
sentiment 229
sentiment classification 225, 228, 230, 247, 249, 250
SHHS 153, 154, 156, 159, 160, 162, 168, 172, 176, 178
sigmoid kernels 116
Simulation Models 81
sleep disorders 152, 153, 156, 159
Sleep-EDF 153, 154, 156, 157, 160, 162, 168, 169, 171, 172, 176, 177
Sleep-EDF 78 153, 156, 160, 162, 168, 171, 176
Sleep-EDF Exp 153
SMOTE 157, 159
Softmax 167, 168
spatial and temporal dependencies 153
spectrogram 179
spectroscopy 254, 256
stacking 227, 229, 237–239, 241, 247, 248
Stacking Logistics Regression Random Forest Decision Tree model (SLRD) 27, 28, 36
stochastic optimization 113
stochastic programming 81
strong discriminatory capability 121
structure-based virtual screening 17
support vector machine (SVM) 33, 36, 102, 109, 142, 227–229, 238, 239, 241

target identification 11, 16, 17, 19
telemedicine 71–77, 83, 84, 86–88

Time-Series Analysis 78
training 227, 229–232, 234–237, 239, 240, 248
true negative 167
true positive 167

validation 156, 217, 227, 236, 237, 240–243, 245
validation sets 167
vanishing gradients 163
variance filter 128
variational autoencoders (VAEs) 18

VGG-16 155
virtual screening 11, 13, 16, 17, 20, 22–25
virtual screening workflow 16
voting 227–229, 237, 241, 247, 248

weighted 248
weighted average 238, 241, 246, 247
weighted averaging 237

XGBoost 27, 28, 35, 36

www.ingramcontent.com/pod-product-compliance
Lightning Source LLC
Jackson TN
JSHW060922090825
88997JS00008B/22